Praise for *This Mortal Coil*

A *Guardian, Economist* and *Prospect* Book of the Year

'Surprisingly upbeat ... The chapters on plague are the most interesting in the book, perhaps because they are so resonant and show how lucky we are to live in the age of the vaccine ... Full of curious facts' *The Times*

'Told in five acts like a Shakespearean tragedy, Andrew Doig's book considers our vulnerabilities and vices, from typhoid to tobacco ... A compelling story that is made admirably accessible' *Financial Times*

'You might expect a book on this morbid theme to be forbidding or sombre. This one is neither. Instead Mr Doig, a biochemist at the University of Manchester, tells an empowering story of human ingenuity' *Economist*

'The way we humans have died has changed profoundly over history: from famine and pestilence, to modern lifestyle diseases like obesity, heart disease and diabetes. In this gripping book, Andrew Doig explores the fascinating biology of our own mortality and, crucially, what death can teach us about life' Prof. Lewis Dartnell, author of *Origins: How the Earth Shaped Human History*

'An absorbing read ... A gripping and fascinating book; informative and seasoned with dry humour' *Mail on Sunday*

'Wry, insightful and optimistic, *This Mortal Coil* brings a compassionate yet amused eye to one of the last great taboos. Essential reading for us all' Matthew Cobb, Baillie Gifford Prize-shortlisted author of *The Idea of the Brain*

'An utterly fascinating history of death, this masterful volume traces changes in the causes of mortality over the centuries' Waterstones

'The most fascinating book I've read in a long time. As much about how we live as it is about h   zola, author of *The Clockwork Girl*

'Rather than being a depressing read, the book actually gives a wonderful long-term perspective on our current situation … This intriguing and detailed discussion of death and its causes provides a bedrock of context to look at how we might tackle mortality going forward … Oddly life-affirming stuff' *Big Issue*

'The story of how we die is deeply entwined with all of science, technology, economics, global health, sociology and human behaviour – in other words, pretty much everything. Which amounts to a book that is profound and original' Daniel M. Davis, author of *The Beautiful Cure* and *The Secret Body*

'A fascinating, clear-eyed study of the major causes of death humanity has faced through the ages … Doig's attention to detail, personable style and clear explanations make the book easily accessible, even for those with little knowledge of biology or medicine … The obvious beauty of *This Mortal Coil* is that in being a history of death, it is also a history of life, and a brilliant, fascinating one at that' *Scotsman*

'Andrew Doig tackles the complex and unsettling history of mortality with matter of fact and clarity but also with tenderness and humanity. This is a remarkable debut interspersing history with science to create a mille feuille of what it means to be human' Helen Carr, author of *The Red Prince*

ANDREW DOIG is Professor of Biochemistry at the University of Manchester. He studied natural science and chemistry at the University of Cambridge, and biochemistry at Stanford University Medical School. He became a lecturer in Manchester in 1994, where he has been ever since. His research is on computational biology, neuroscience, dementia, developmental biology and proteins. *This Mortal Coil* is his first book.

THIS MORTAL COIL

A History of Death

Andrew Doig

BLOOMSBURY PUBLISHING

LONDON · OXFORD · NEW YORK · NEW DELHI · SYDNEY

BLOOMSBURY PUBLISHING
Bloomsbury Publishing Plc
50 Bedford Square, London, WC1B 3DP, UK
29 Earlsfort Terrace, Dublin 2, Ireland

BLOOMSBURY, BLOOMSBURY PUBLISHING and the Diana logo are trademarks of
Bloomsbury Publishing Plc

First published in Great Britain 2022
This edition published 2023

A catalogue record for this book is available from the British Library

ISBN: HB: 978-1-5266-2441-3; TPB: 978-1-5266-2442-0; PB: 978-1-5266-2439-0;
EBOOK: 978-1-5266-2440-6; EPDF: 978-1-5266-4641-5

2 4 6 8 10 9 7 5 3 1

Typeset by Newgen KnowledgeWorks Pvt. Ltd., Chennai, India
Printed and bound in Great Britain by CPI Group (UK) Ltd, Croydon CR0 4YY

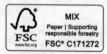

To find out more about our authors and books visit www.bloomsbury.com
and sign up for our newsletters

To Penny, Lucy and Sarah

For in that sleep of death what dreams may come,
when we have shuffled off this mortal coil,
must give us pause.

William Shakespeare, *Hamlet*, 1599/1601

Contents

Introduction:
The Four Horsemen of Siena

And so many died that all believed that it was the end of the world.

Agnolo di Tura del Grasso, *The Plague in Siena: An Italian Chronicle*, 1348

Six hundred years after the Franks, Goths, Saxons and other invaders brought down the Western Roman Empire, their lands had developed into nations that we still recognise today: France, England, Spain and Germany. Here, from 1000 to 1300, the climate grew warmer, forests were cleared and cultivated, towns were founded and farming methods improved. New inventions of paper, the compass, windmills, gunpowder and reading glasses, with better ships and mechanical clocks, drove economic growth and trade. Greater wealth funded new universities, magnificent Gothic cathedrals, literature and music. Famine was still present, but the structure of medieval society, with its threefold division into those who pray, those who fight and those who work, remained strong. All this was to be stretched to breaking point by the catastrophic Black Death, which struck Europe in the 1340s.

In 1347, Siena was one of the richest and most beautiful cities in Central Italy, with its prosperity based on moneylending, the wool trade and military strength. Visitors would have seen the impressive seat of government, the Palazzo Pubblico, and a spectacular cathedral undergoing construction work that was intended to more than double its size. By the thirteenth century Siena was able to match Florence, its great rival thirty miles to the north, and was steadily expanding the size of its republic.

Shoemaker and tax collector Agnolo di Tura del Grasso produced a chronicle of events in Siena from 1300 to 1351, based on his own observations, consultation of public records and personal experience. He provides one of the best contemporary accounts that we have for the deadliest disease that has ever afflicted humanity – plague.

Plague entered Tuscany through the port of Pisa in January 1348. It took two months to travel upstream to Florence, then made its way south to Siena. Di Tura tells us that: 'The mortality began in Siena in May [1348]. It was a cruel and horrible thing ... the victims died almost immediately. They would swell beneath their armpits and in their groins, and fall over dead while talking. Father abandoned child, wife husband, one brother another.'[1]

The enormous death rate made normal Christian funerals impossible. No one could be found to bury the dead. Families had to leave their corpses in ditches or take them to great pits, where they were often buried without a priest to officiate. Poor Di Tura lost all his children: 'And I ... buried my five children with my own hands. And there were also those who were so sparsely covered with earth that the dogs dragged them forth and devoured many bodies throughout the city. There was no one who wept for any death, for all awaited death ... And no medicine or any other defence availed.'

Di Tura estimated that three-quarters of the population of the city and suburbs of Siena died – about 80,000 people in just five months. Society collapsed:

And those that survived were like persons distraught and almost without feeling. And many walls and other things were abandoned, and all the mines of silver and gold and copper that existed in Sienese territory were abandoned as is seen; for in the countryside many more people died, many lands and villages were abandoned, and no one remained there. I will not write of the cruelty that there was in the countryside, of the wolves and wild beasts that ate the poorly buried corpses. The city of Siena seemed almost uninhabited, for almost no one was found in the city. And then, when the pestilence abated, all who survived gave themselves over to pleasures: monks, priests, nuns, and lay men and women all enjoyed themselves, and none worried about spending and gambling. And everyone thought himself rich because he had escaped and regained the world.[1]

The story of plague in Siena and the testimony of Agnolo di Tura graphically show the devastation that plague could cause. While the Black Death is an extreme example, sudden death at the hands of various infectious diseases was common for thousands of years, certainly from when we started farming and living in cities. Thankfully, it is now rare. Even though we rightly worry about infections like influenza, pneumonia or Covid-19, their power does not come close to that of cholera, smallpox or plague. Yet the details of the events in Siena reveal two other leading causes of death that we have also largely overcome, namely famine and war.

The harvest failed in Tuscany in 1346 and hailstorms destroyed crops the year after.[2] Hungry, malnourished people moved from the countryside to the city, in search of food, work and charity. Their living conditions would magnify the effects of the Black Death, as the disease was swiftly transmitted in overcrowded and dirty neighbourhoods. Famine kills mainly by promoting infectious disease and magnifying its dangers, so the plague struck Siena at its most vulnerable, following two years of famine.

The city states of Italy, and their powerful neighbours, like France, Spain and the Ottoman Empire, were routinely engaged in conflict with each other. Wars were endemic throughout Italy and the rest of Europe. Rather than using their own citizens as soldiers, Italian wars were typically fought by mercenaries who engaged in sieges, fed themselves by looting, and deliberately destroyed crops, livestock and buildings in enemy territory, reducing peasants to destitution and famine. Armies made use of plague, waiting for the disease to ravage a city before sending in an occupying force.

Siena had been largely successful in warfare for hundreds of years, right up to the fateful 1340s, expanding their state to the coast. All this came to a sudden halt with the plague. Industry, construction, agriculture and government simply stopped. When politics did resume, the city council was reduced in size by one-third, as so many of the city elite had died. Tuscany was full of abandoned buildings, ghost towns, overgrown fields and returning forest.[2] The oligarchy that had ruled Siena for sixty-eight years was overthrown in 1355, leading to a century of unstable governments and revolutions.[1] Unpaid mercenary companies took control of the countryside, terrorising and looting. Taking advantage of the new situation, rival states began to eat into

Sienese territory. The end finally came in 1555, when the republic surrendered to King Philip of Spain, who promptly handed Siena over to their bitter rivals, Florence. It was not until the twentieth century that Siena's population returned to pre-plague levels, which is one reason why it has preserved its beautiful medieval city centre. The cathedral remains unfinished.

Plague, Famine and War, together with Death itself, were thus the Four Horsemen of the Medieval Apocalypse. Today, our main causes of death are utterly different: namely heart failure, cancer, stroke and dementia. We have gone from a world in which death from disease or violence were likely to strike down anyone at any age, and where famine was just one or two harvest failures away, to one where in many countries an excess of food is more of a problem than a lack of it, and death before sixty is seen as shockingly young. How we live has changed in innumerable ways, reflected in how we die. The aim of this book is to show how this happened.

What are the main causes of death in the modern world? In total, 56,873,804 people died in 2016. Some died in a hospital bed, suffering from cancerous tumours, soothed by morphine and in the company of loved ones. Many had infectious diseases, with their immune systems unable to fight off deadly microbes. Some had only had a few hours of life after birth, due to birth defects, genetic abnormalities or a traumatic delivery. Others had fatal accidents – on the road, by drowning or in a fire. Some took their own lives, using weapons or drugs to end it all. Currently, the most frequent cause of death worldwide is coronary heart disease, more simply known as a heart attack. Stroke is the second biggest killer. Next, we have lung diseases, including asthma, emphysema and pneumonia. Fatal cancers are split into various categories, but if these are all grouped together, then cancer kills almost as many people as heart disease.

This current situation, where people now die mainly from non-communicable diseases like cancer, is entirely new. Why have the reasons we die changed so much? Our species evolved when we lived in small bands in a dangerous, violent world, where many died from accidents or at the hands of other people. Farming and the establishment of the first states brought security, but at the dreadful cost of chronic malnutrition, alongside a life devoted to backbreaking and tedious work for the overwhelming majority. In addition, close contact with animals over thousands of years meant that many pathogenic organisms jumped the species barrier, bringing new diseases to literally plague us. Higher population densities and lack of sanitation kept the diseases circulating, so that infectious disease became the leading cause of death.

Success in tackling infectious diseases came from understanding how and why they occurred. It was only in the late nineteenth century that it was finally accepted that disease could be spread by infectious microorganisms, driving the provision of clean water, homes and clothing, free from deadly microbes, vermin and parasites. Combining our understanding of the true causes of infectious disease with a scientific approach gave us vaccines and drug-discovery programmes. The result was a huge decline in infectious disease and a rising life expectancy from the mid-nineteenth century onwards.

While heart disease, stroke, lung disease, diabetes and cancer were bound to become more significant as life expectancy increased, our changing lifestyles also played a major part in promoting them. We now eat too much, particularly junk food, use drugs, smoke cigarettes, overindulge in alcohol and avoid exercise. Still, we continue to live longer, leading to the growing prevalence of neurodegenerative diseases that are common in the elderly, like Parkinson's, Alzheimer's and other forms of dementia.

On top of examining the ways we live and die today, we shall also look to the future and see how we are entering the next healthcare revolution, where many more of the current causes of death will be defeated, using new technologies like stem cells, organ transplants and genetic modification. The story of the causes of human death and how we have overcome so many of them is, therefore, also a story of growing medical knowledge and better social organisation, of achievement and, looking to the future, of promise.

PART I

CAUSES OF DEATH

... finding some Truths and not-commonly-believed opinions to arise from my meditations upon these neglected Papers, I proceeded further to consider what benefit the knowledge of the same would bring to the world ... with some real fruit from those ayrie blossoms.

John Graunt, *Natural and Political OBSERVATIONS Mentioned in a following Index and made upon the Bills of Mortality,* 1662[1]

1

What is Death?

On 15 April 1989 Liverpool were due to play Nottingham Forest in an FA Cup semi-final football match at Sheffield Wednesday's Hillsborough ground. Slow traffic meant that many Liverpool fans arrived late, so just before kick-off several thousand were still outside, eager to get in. Police therefore opened a set of gates leading to the already overcrowded central section of a concrete terrace, where spectators would stand to watch the game. Between the terrace and the pitch was high steel fencing, installed to stop anyone getting onto the field. The barriers worked far too well. As the late arrivals rushed into the back of the terraces, those at the front were pushed and crushed against the fencing. Ninety-six people died and 766 were injured.

Tony Bland was an eighteen-year-old Liverpool supporter who had travelled to the game with two friends. His ribs were crushed and his lungs were punctured, which interrupted the supply of oxygen to his brain. This caused catastrophic and irreversible damage to his higher brain centres, leaving him in a persistent vegetative state, unable to see, hear or feel anything. His brainstem, however, was still functioning, keeping his heart, breathing and digestion working. In the eyes of the law at the time, this meant that he was alive, even though he had no chance of recovery. As long as he was fed through a tube and provided with medical treatment, his body was expected to live for many more years. Tony's doctors and parents came to the view that no useful purpose was served by continuing his medical care, so the artificial feeding and other measures keeping his body alive should end. They were concerned, however, that this might constitute a criminal offence, particularly after a coroner said that in his view, removing the feeding tube would count as murder. The case went to the High Court of Justice for advice.

After considering the moral and ethical issues raised by the case, the judges agreed that:

> It is perfectly reasonable for the responsible doctors to conclude that there is no affirmative benefit to Anthony Bland in continuing the invasive medical procedures necessary to sustain his life. Having so concluded, they are neither entitled nor under a duty to continue such medical care. Therefore, they will not be guilty of murder if they discontinue such care.[1]

Treatment was withdrawn on 3 March 1993, twenty-two years after Tony was born.

The lethal immovable barriers in football stadiums were later removed and grounds were converted to all-seater stadiums, removing the dangerous terraces. Prosecutions related to the Hillsborough disaster are still ongoing. The questions are: how old was Tony Bland when he died? Eighteen or twenty-two? Did he die from the injuries on the day or from the withdrawal of treatment?

Death was once defined as when breathing and the heart stopped. In order to tell whether someone is alive, a mirror could be held over someone's nose – to see if it misted up – to detect very shallow breathing. Alternatively, if someone is alive, then a light shone in their eyes would make the pupils contract. Pressing the nail bed would cause pain and a response. An uncooked onion held under the nose might make someone wake up. Emptying of the bowels and bladder is also a bad sign. More exotic methods to tell whether someone was dead included: 'pour vinegar and salt or warm urine in the mouth', 'put insects in the ear' and 'cut the soles of the feet with razor blades'.[2] Nipple pinching was also popular.

None of these methods are foolproof, leading to many people's ultimate horror of being buried alive. This was not a completely irrational worry. In 1896 the London Association for the Prevention of Premature Burial was founded. This campaigned for reforms to ensure that those buried were definitely dead, after finding more than a hundred reports of people apparently being buried alive. A popular way to avoid this was to use a safety coffin, where a rope could be pulled from inside the coffin to ring a bell.

While many safety coffins of various designs were sold, there is no record of anyone ever coming back from the grave as a result of using one. Cremation instead of burial was a possible alternative, as revival after incineration is impossible. Cremation was strongly opposed by the church and tradition, however, and hence illegal in the UK until 1884.

Blunders can also occur simply from mistaken identity. In 2012, a forty-one-year-old car washer from Brazil, called Gilberto Araújo, showed up at his own wake. A co-worker at the car wash, who looked similar to Araújo, had been murdered. The police got Araújo's brother to identify the body at the morgue and he got it wrong. After a friend told Araújo about his own funeral, he had to show up to it to convince everyone that it wasn't him in the coffin.[3]

First-aid courses teach how to perform resuscitation when someone's heart or breathing has stopped; after a drowning, for example. In this situation, you should never stop trying to revive your patient and must continue until a medical professional arrives to take over. There have been many cases of people incorrectly deciding that someone has died, so mouth-to-mouth resuscitation or chest compressions were stopped too soon. If you are not medically trained, you can never conclude that someone has died, even if you are sure that they are not breathing and have had no heartbeat for a long time. Mouth-to-mouth resuscitation or pumping on the heart by hand could still be keeping the brain alive.

Modern definitions of death centre upon the idea of brain death, rather than cessation of breathing, heartbeat, response to pain or pupil dilation. Loss of blood flow or breathing can cause death only when lack of oxygen is prolonged enough to cause irreversible destruction of the brain. This normally takes about six minutes. The brain is the seat of our consciousness and thinking – hence it is the only organ that cannot be transplanted without a change of identity. Brain death can be defined as the total and irreversible ending of neuronal activity, recognised by irreversible coma, absent brainstem reflexes and no breathing.[4] A first-aider is obviously unable to diagnose brain death, which is why they should never give up resuscitation.

A rare exception to this rule would be if the head is detached from the body, when even a rank amateur in medicine can confidently conclude that the patient has gone to meet their maker. During the French Revolution, however, it was noted that a head chopped off by a guillotine could apparently live for about ten seconds.[5]

Why is the brainstem singled out to determine death, rather than any other part of the brain? The brainstem is located at the bottom centre of the brain. Motor and sensory neurons travel through the brainstem to connect the upper brain to the spinal cord. It coordinates motor-control signals sent from the brain to the body, is required for alertness and arousal, and controls fundamental life-supporting functions, such as breathing, blood pressure, digestion and heart rate. Without a functioning brainstem, we have no chance of consciousness or maintaining basic bodily functions. Ten important cranial nerves are connected directly to the brainstem. Brainstem activity can therefore be assessed by seeing whether reflexes mediated by these cranial nerves are functioning. For example, the pupil in the eye should contract or expand in response to light or darkness; touching the cornea in the eye should make someone blink; moving the head swiftly from side to side should make the eyes move; and poking the throat should cause gagging and coughing. All these reflexes require only a functioning brainstem and are not under conscious control, so it isn't possible to dilate or contract your pupils just by thinking about it. Diagnosis of brain death can be confirmed by checking that there is no blood flow in the brain using MRI or that electrical activity is absent using an electroencephalogram.

Using brain death and brainstem activity to determine whether someone is alive (or dead) is not without its problems, as the brain has distinct parts. What if some parts are working, but some are not? If someone is in an intermediate state between being conscious and having no brain activity at all, then defining death is not straightforward.

A coma is a state of consciousness from which a person cannot be woken. The sleep/wake cycle is not working, and the body does not respond to stimuli such as speech or pain. Consciousness requires a functioning cerebral cortex, as well as a brainstem. The cerebral cortex is responsible for higher thought: language, understanding, memory, attention, perception and so on. Coma can be caused by intoxication, poisoning, stroke, head injury, heart attack, blood loss, low glucose levels and many other conditions. After these traumas, the body enters a comatose state to give it an opportunity to recover. Coma might also be induced deliberately, using drugs to help recovery from brain injury. Comas usually last a few days to a few weeks, though recovery after many years is possible.

In a vegetative state, someone is awake, but not aware. This means that they can perform basic functions like sleeping, coughing, swallowing and opening their eyes, but not more complex thought processes. They won't follow moving objects with their eyes, respond to speech or show emotions. This might be caused by brain damage from injury, or possibly a neurodegenerative condition like Alzheimer's disease.[6] Recovery from a long-term vegetative state is highly unlikely.

Locked-in syndrome is a horrible condition, where the patient is unable to move anything except the eyes, yet is still conscious. It usually incurable, though the insomnia drug Zolpidem has shown some potential in promoting recovery.[7] In the worst cases, even the eyes cannot be moved. Here, the brainstem is damaged, but not the upper brain, including the cerebral cortex. It is easy to mistake for coma, but the patient's experience is entirely different, as they are awake but helpless. Complete locked-in syndrome can be identified using modern brain-imaging methods. For example, if we ask someone with locked-in syndrome to imagine playing tennis, then a specific part of the brain will light up.

The status of people with these kinds of conditions is an ongoing and difficult area of debate, involving law, ethics and medicine. The case of Tony Bland is just one example of the challenging issues involved.

2

Observations Made Upon the Bills of Mortality

In December 1592 the plague returned to London. Seventeen thousand people would shuffle off this mortal coil as a result, including three of William Shakespeare's sisters, one of his brothers and his son Hamnet. Plague had been the most terrifying and lethal disease in Europe for the previous thousand years. Little could be done to prevent it, as it was so infectious, other than frequently ineffective quarantine measures. There was no cure.

Following an example set by several north Italian cities, in 1592 civil authorities in London started to keep track of exactly how many people the disease was killing each week, published as Bills of Mortality.[1] These data were the foundation of recording statistics on causes of death, a vital measure for understanding public health. Their introduction marked the birth of public health records in modern Europe.

In 1592 the following orders, with the authority of the Lord Mayor of London, were passed 'to be used in the tyme of the Infeccon of the Plague within the Cittie and Liberties of London':

> That in or for every parishe there shal be appointed twoe sober Ancient Woemen, to be sworne to be viewers of the boddies of such as shall dye in tyme of Infeccon, which woemen shall imediatly, uppon suche there Viewes by vertewe of there Oath, make true reporte to the Constable of that precincte where such personn shall dye or be infected.[2]

These 'sober Ancient Woemen' were known as the 'searchers of the dead'. They were appointed by London parishes to view every fresh corpse and record its cause of death, and were summoned by the ringing of a bell. They performed this central task in the recording of public health in England for more than 250 years. Their data was used to compile Bills of Mortality that recorded the locations of deaths and listed a cause. Attributing a death to plague, as opposed to any other disease such as smallpox or spotted fever, was not easy, since the symptoms and signs of the plague varied greatly and were not easy to read. This meant the searchers had to examine every bloated and rotting corpse for the presence of telltale buboes.

Identifying a plague victim could have dire consequences, since parish officials then had to board up a plague house, trapping all its inhabitants inside until none had contracted the disease for twenty-eight days. A plague house was marked with a red cross and the words 'Lord have mercy upon us' on the door, with a watchman standing guard outside to stop anyone entering or leaving. Unfortunately, infected rats couldn't read, so didn't know that they were also supposed to stay in the sealed house. Quarantine was often a death sentence for all the members of a household, so searchers were under great pressure not to brand a house as infected. Similarly, relatives could also try to press or bribe searchers not to record causes of death with high stigma, such as suicide or syphilis.

As searchers were repeatedly exposed to corpses, they were at high risk of spreading disease themselves. They were therefore made to carry a red wand as they went about their business, to warn people to stay away. They had to keep away from crowds and walk down streets near the channels carrying refuse. Not only were they shunned, but they were also at risk of being accused of witchcraft, since they were mostly old widows who spied on their neighbours and made life-or-death decisions in mysterious ways. Being a searcher of the dead has to be one of the most unpleasant jobs of all time. However, as they were paid per corpse, a new outbreak of plague provided a healthy cash bonus.

Searchers' results were given to clerks in each parish, who compiled the data. Searchers had little or no medical training and their inconsistencies and ignorance were much criticised by those who tried to use their data (such as by John Graunt – more on him later – who said that searchers 'after the mist off a cup of ale, and the bribe of a two groat fee, instead of one' were unable to decipher correctly the cause of death).

The Diseases and Casualties this Week.

Abortive — 2	Imposthume — 1
Aged — 32	Infants — 7
Bleeding — 1	Kingsevill — 1
Childbed — 5	Mouldfallen — 1
Chrisoms — 9	Kild accidentally with a Carbine, at St. Michael Wood-street — 1
Collick — 1	Overlaid — 1
Consumption — 65	Rickets — 9
Convulsion — 41	Rising of the Lights — 2
Cough — 5	Rupture — 2
Dropsie — 43	Scalded in a Brewers Mash, at St. Giles Cripplegate — 1
Drowned at S Kathar. Tower — 1	Scurvy — 4
Feaver — 47	Spotted Feaver — 2
Flox and Small-pox — 15	Stilborn — 13
Flux — 3	Stopping of the Stomach — 11
Found dead in the Street at Stepney — 1	Suddenly — 1
Griping in the Guts — 15	Surfeit — 7
	Teeth — 27
	Tissick — 12
	Ulcer — 1
	Vomiting — 1
	Winde — 1
	Wormes — 1

Christned { Males — 121 Females — 111 In all — 232	Buried { Males — 195 Females — 198 In all — 393	} Plague — 0		

Decreased in the Burials this Week — 69

Parishes clear of the Plague — 130   Parishes Infected — 0

The Assize of Bread set forth by Order of the Lord Maier and Court of Aldermen, A penny Wheaten Loaf to contain Eleven Ounces, and three half-penny White Loaves the like weight.

Bill of Mortality for 21–28 February 1664.

The authorities of the City of London used the bills to track plague epidemics and to respond accordingly. For example, theatres were obliged to close when plague deaths were more than thirty per week, as people in the close-packed audiences could easily infect each other.[3] Before 1592, bills seem to have been produced only in times of high mortality, so that rulers could track the progression of plague. Weekly bills began to be printed every Thursday in 1593 and sold well. Readers could use the data to decide whether it was safe to visit public places in London, for instance, rather as we might consult a weather forecast to see whether climbing a mountain is a good idea tomorrow. In 1665, John Bell wrote in his *London Remembrancer*, which also analysed the bills, 'the Bill of Mortality is of very great use … it giveth a general notice of the Plague, and a particular Accompt of the places which are therewith infected, to the end such places may be shunned and avoided.'[1] At first the bills listed only the total numbers christened and buried, divided into dying either from plague or from something else. From 1629, however, the causes of death were quantified under about sixty headings, and the total christenings and deaths separated by sex. You could also check the current bread situation (see figure on page 17). Present-day World Health Organization (WHO) data quantifying causes of death can be traced back to these bills.

TABLE 1 *Examples of causes of death recorded in Bills of Mortality.*

Cause of death	Likely meaning and comments
Aged	Dying of 'old age' is not usually an acceptable term on a death certificate any more. More than sixty or seventy years counted as 'aged'.
Affrighted	Frightened to death. Perhaps a stress-induced heart attack or stroke?
Apoplex	Bleeding in internal organs (haemorrhage).
Childbed	Childbed fever. Infection caught after giving birth.
Chrysome	A child in the first month of life.
Consumption	Tuberculosis.
Cut of the stone	Gallstones.

Distracted	Perhaps they wandered in front of a galloping horse and cart.
Dropsie	Abnormal swelling of the body caused by the build-up of clear watery fluid. Often caused by kidney or heart disease.
Evil	Maybe King's Evil (scrofula).
Faintnesse	Epilepsy?
Falling sickness	Epilepsy.
Feaver	Any infection that causes high temperature.
Flux	Dysentery. Infectious diarrheal disease. Sometimes called 'bloody flux'.
Griping in the guts	Sudden, sharp pain in your stomach or bowels. Appendicitis?
Infants	A young child. Likely to have died from infectious disease.
Kings evill	Scrofula. Tuberculosis of neck and lymph glands. Thought to be curable by a king laying hands on sufferers. Many monarchs spent long periods of time trying to cure King's Evil in this way.
Melancholia	Depression.
Miasma	Poisonous vapours thought (incorrectly) to pollute the air and cause disease. Some kind of infectious disease.
Overlaid	Suffocation of a baby by its mother. Presumably accidental, though quite possibly killing an unwanted child.
Paines in the head	Meningitis? Brain haemorrhage?
Palsie	Paralysis.
Planet-struck	A sudden severe malady or paralysis, perhaps caused by an especially bad horoscope that day. Astrology was a serious business then.

Purples	A rash due to spontaneous bleeding in the skin. Possibly a symptom of various severe illnesses, such as bacterial endocarditis or cerebrospinal meningitis.
Rising of the lights	A rather poetic name for coughing your lungs up. Probably croup, an infection of the windpipe or larynx, characterised by a hoarse, barking cough and breathing difficulties. 'Lights' is an old word for lungs, still available under this name at a traditional butcher's.
Scalded in a brewer's mash at St Giles Cripplegate	Speaks for itself.
Sighing	Maybe asthma?
Sinking of the spirits	Depression?
Stopping of the stomach	Appendicitis?
Suddenly	Hopelessly vague. Heart attack? Stroke? Haemorrhage?
Sweating sickness	Infectious and often fatal epidemic disease affecting England in the fifteenth century. Exactly what it was is a mystery.
Teeth	Infant that died when teething.
Trouble and oppression	Surprisingly lethal.
Spanish disease	Syphilis. Diseases with stigma were often attributed to other nations.

The Bill of Mortality (page 17) shows a very good week, with not a single person dying of plague across 130 parishes. Only Anglican christenings were recorded, rather than all births, so the figures do not, for example, include Quakers, Dissenters, Jews or Roman Catholics. Around one-third of the London population was thus left out. In addition, many new parents failed to notify authorities of a birth, to avoid paying a fee. The 393 people who did die were afflicted by a sometimes puzzling set of conditions. Table 1 lists some of the reasons for dying found in the bills. There is substantial uncertainty on what many of these reasons might actually mean. This isn't just due to the poor medical knowledge of the searchers. The identification of diseases from the past based on contemporary descriptions is always fraught with difficulties. Symptoms were not well described, texts can be hard to interpret, and pathogens can mutate very rapidly, changing symptoms.

Apparently, not a single person died of dementia, cancer or heart disease this week, though these could have been recorded under other terms, such as 'aged' or 'suddenly'. In any event, infectious disease was undoubtedly the leading cause of death. The Bill of Mortality for 15–22 August 1665 (overleaf), just eighteen months after the data for 21–28 February 1664, shows that the total weekly death toll has leapt from 393 to 5,319, with plague going from zero to 3,880, affecting 96 of the 130 parishes reporting. Cancer is recorded now, but there were only two cases.

Comparing the two bills also shows evidence of deliberate falsification by the searchers and parish clerks. The number of deaths attributed to the usefully vague 'Feaver' has increased from 47 to 353 – these were mostly likely to be plague as well. Searchers and parish officers were often under pressure to change a record from plague to anything else to avoid the otherwise compulsory shutting up of the house. Just comparing these two bills shows the highly intermittent nature of plague. Normally it is dormant with no deaths, but occasionally it spreads ferociously, killing thousands per week. This pattern of most years showing very few deaths from plague with occasional epidemic years is clear from the existing data available from 1560 to 1665.[4]

The last year in which London suffered a major plague outbreak was 1665, as described by Samuel Pepys in his famous diaries. Around 100,000 died – a quarter of the population of the city in eighteen months. People fled the city if they could; King Charles II, for example, moved to Salisbury. Cart drivers did indeed travel the streets calling, 'Bring out your dead!', removing piles of bodies. The next year most of the city was destroyed by the Great Fire of London. Rebuilding the city as an environment less suitable for rats may have inadvertently helped ensure that plague was much less of a problem for London after 1665.

The Diseases and Casualties this Week.

Abortive	6	Kingsevil	10
Aged	54	Lethargy	1
Apoplexie	1	Murthered at Stepney	1
Bedridden	1	Palsie	2
Cancer	2	Plague	3880
Childbed	23	Plurisie	1
Chrisomes	15	Quinsie	6
Collick	1	Rickets	23
Consumption	174	Rising of the Lights	19
Convulsion	88	Rupture	2
Dropsie	40	Sciatica	1
Drowned 2, one at St. Kath- Tower, and one at Lambeth	2	Scowring	13
Feaver	353	Scurvy	1
Fistula	1	Sore legge	1
Flox and Small-pox	10	Spotted Feaver and Purples	190
Flux	2	Starved at Nurse	1
Found dead in the Street at St. Bartholomew the Less	1	Stilborn	8
Frighted	1	Stone	2
Gangrene	1	Stopping of the stomach	16
Gowt	1	Strangury	1
Grief	1	Suddenly	1
Griping in the Guts	74	Surfeit	87
Jaundies	3	Teeth	113
Imposthume	18	Thrush	3
Infants	21	Tissick	6
Kild by a fall down stairs at St. Thomas Apostle	1	Ulcer	2
		Vomiting	7
		Winde	8
		Wormes	18

Christned { Males — 83, Females — 83, In all — 166 } Buried { Males — 2656, Females — 2663, In all — 5319 } Plague — 3880.

Increased in the Burials this Week — 1289

Parishes clear of the Plague — 34. Parishes Infected — 96

The Assize of Bread set forth by Order of the Lord Maior and Court of Aldermen. A penny Wheaten Loaf to contain Nine Ounces and a half, and three half-penny White Loaves the like weight.

Bill of Mortality for 15–22 August 1665.

Little use was made of the information tabulated in the Bills of Mortality for nearly a hundred years, other than tracking plague outbreaks. All this was to change in 1662.

Actuaries deal with risk management related to the financial sector, such as working out the cost of life insurance. In order to do this, it is essential to be able to estimate the life expectancy of the person seeking to take out the insurance. John Graunt was the first person to make such calculations, using the Bills of Mortality data, and published in his great and still perfectly readable work, *Natural and Political OBSERVATIONS Mentioned in a following Index and made upon the Bills of Mortality: With reference to the Government, Religion, Trade, Growth, Ayre, Diseases, and the Several Changes of the said CITY*, which first appeared in 1662.[5]

Graunt's day job was as a haberdasher, selling cloth from a shop that he inherited from his father (now within the London financial district). He was also a part-time captain of a band of soldiers. We don't really know what inspired Graunt to start his analysis of the Bills of Mortality. He said of his original interest: 'I know not by what accident engaged my thoughts,' and later spoke of his 'long and serious perusal of all the bills'.[5]

Cities and countries operated in the seventeenth century without any idea of how many people actually lived there. Clearly, it was possible for a major city like London to be governed by the Lord Mayor and king without this most basic information. Graunt had spoken with several 'men of great experience' who believed that the population of London was 6 or 7 million. Graunt realised that this could not be right, since only 15,000 were buried each year. If the population was 6 million, then this meant that only one in 400 would die each year. Graunt was quite sure that life expectancy was less than 400 years. He sought to find more accurate estimates.

First, he considered that each woman of childbearing age would give birth once every two years. From 12,000 births per year, this gives 24,000 so-called 'Teeming women'. If half of adult women are teeming and each woman lives in a family of eight ('the Man, and his Wife, three Children, and three Servants, or Lodgers'), we have a population of 24,000 x 2 x 8 = 384,000.

Secondly, from a personal survey, he found that three out of eleven families had suffered a death in the previous year. So 13,000 deaths in total x 11/3 again gives 48,000 families. Eight people per family means 48,000 x 8 = 384,000 total population again.

Finally, Graunt used a map of London to calculate the population from the number of houses, getting about the same result. Graunt therefore knew that London had about 400,000 people, far fewer than previously thought. This meant that the king could now work out how many potential 'fighting men' were available for his armies.

While crude, these calculations were an enormous improvement on the previous wild guesses in the absence of any census. It is also excellent practice to use a variety of methods for the same job, and reassuring to get the same answer.

Graunt was nervous about including his population estimates in his *Observations*, since taking a census was the 'sin of David'. According to Chronicles I, chapter 21, Satan tempted King David to count his population using a census. David found that 1.57 million soldiers lived in Israel and Judah. God was so angry that David had done this that he gave David a choice of three punishments for his sin (for mysterious reasons): either three years of famine, three months of fleeing before his enemies, or three days of plague. David couldn't decide, so God chose plague for him and 70,000 men died. Graunt had therefore been 'frighted with that misunderstood example of David, from attempting any computation of the people of this populous place'. He overcame his fear, however, and included his census in his *Observations*.

Graunt invented the life table, a key tool in population and actuarial work. Life tables show how many people die at each age. Table 2 (below) shows Graunt's data as we might present it today. We start with 100

TABLE 2 *John Graunt's first life table.*

Age	Probability of dying in range	Number alive at start of range	Number dying in range	Life expectancy at start of range (years)
0–6	0.36	100	36	15
6–16	0.38	64	24	16
16–26	0.38	40	15	15
26–36	0.36	25	9	14
36–46	0.38	16	6	13
46–56	0.40	10	4	10
56–66	0.50	6	3	7
66–76	0.67	3	2	3
>76	1.0	1	1	5

babies born in 1661. Only 64 of them will live to the age of 6 and only 10 to the age of 46. Life expectancy at birth was only 15; life expectancy at the age of 36 was 13 more years. From the ages of 6 to 56, the probability of dying each year is about 4 per cent; younger or older than this range, it is even higher. We see why people had so many children, as only one in four could be expected to live to their mid-twenties.

London was without doubt an unhealthy place to live. Graunt pointed out that in the forty years from 1603, the Bills recorded 363,935 burials and 330,747 christenings. While more burials than christenings suggests that the population of London must be declining, this was contradicted by a 'daily increase of Buildings upon new Foundations, and by the turning of great Palacious Houses into small Tenements'.[5] Graunt had an explanation, though: 'It is therefore certain, that London is supplied with People from out of the Countrey.'[5] In the seventeenth century, cities were much less healthy ('most Smoaky, and Stinking'[5]) than rural areas; nevertheless, thousands continued to move to them.

Graunt found an excess of births of boys to girls, by a ratio of 14:13, and suggested that this is because more young men die violent deaths (slain in wars, killed by mischance, drowned at sea), are executed, emigrate, or do not have children as they become unmarried fellows of colleges. These factors would alter the numbers to equality when it came to the populations of marriageable age. Table 3 (page 26) gives Graunt's subdivisions of 229,250 deaths over a twenty-year period in London, using his terms and groupings. It has little in common with the present-day statistics (shown in Table 4, page 31). By far the largest category in Table 3 is 'diseases of children under five'.

Graunt also noted that rickets was not reported at all before 1634 and had been increasing since then. He therefore concluded that rickets was a new disease. We now know that rickets can be caused by a lack of vitamin D, often due to children not getting enough sunlight. As such, it was highly unlikely to have first appeared in 1634. Instead, the growth of rickets suggests either that searchers were more aware of the disease and so were reporting it more often, or that more children were suffering from it as London grew smokier. Consumption of oily fish, rich in vitamin D, may also have declined as the Thames became more polluted. What was important was that Graunt was reporting that new diseases can appear, and that their numbers can fluctuate.

TABLE 3 *Causes of death over a twenty-year period for Church of England burials in London in the early seventeenth century, according to John Graunt.*

Cause	Number of deaths
Diseases of Children under five (Thrush, Convulsion, Rickets, Teeth, and Worms; and as Abortives, Chrysomes, Infants, Liver-grown, and Over-laid)	71,124
Small-Pox, Swine-Pox, and Measles and Worms	12,210
Outward Griefs (Cancers, Fistulaes, Sores, Ulcers, broken and bruised Limbs, Impostumes, Itch, King's-evil, Leprosie, Scald-head, Swine-Pox, Wens)	4,000
Notorious diseases	
Apoplex	1,306
Cut of the Stone	38
Falling Sickness	74
Dead in the Streets	243
Gout	134
Head-ach	51
Jaundice	998
Lethargy	67
Leprosie	6
Lunatick	158
Overlaid and Starved	529
Palsie	423
Rupture	201
Stone and Strangury	863
Sciatica	5
Suddenly	454

Casualties	
Bleeding	69
Burnt and Scalded	125
Drowned	829
Excessive drinking	2
Frighted	22
Grief	279
Hanged themselves	222
Kill'd by several accidents	1,021
Murdered	86
Poysoned	14
Smothered	26
Shot	7
Starved	51
Vomiting	136

By subdividing the total population by sex, location, profession and so on, it was now possible to measure the effects of these factors on human health, so founding the science of epidemiology: the study of the distribution and causes of disease and health-related states. Graunt is thus regarded as one of the founders of statistics, demographics, actuarial science and epidemiology, all from one slim volume. He showed that valid conclusions could be deduced for the likely experience of a group of people, even though what will happen to a single individual was impossible to predict. This was a contentious issue, as making predictions about the behaviour of people could be interpreted as denying free will.

Contemporaries were highly impressed with Graunt's *Observations*.[6] Within a month he was proposed and accepted for membership into the Royal Society, then, as now, the most prestigious scientific society in Britain. Five editions of the *Observations* were published in England and elsewhere in Europe over the next fourteen years. Survival rates were used to cost life insurance by the Dutch prime minister, Johan De Witt, inspired by Graunt's methods. Life-table data, as used by John Graunt, remains the basis for many kinds of future projections.

Classifying death is needed to determine public health needs and to understand how the causes of death have changed across time. Standardisation of classification of diseases arose from efforts of public health officials in the nineteenth century, such as William Farr, the first medical statistician for the General Register Office of England and Wales. He pointed out the inadequacies of the Bills of Mortality, writing in 1842:

> The advantages of a uniform statistical nomenclature, however imperfect, are so obvious, that it is surprising no attention has been paid to its enforcement in Bills of Mortality. Each disease has, in many instances, been denoted by three or four terms, and each term has been applied to as many different diseases: vague, inconvenient names have been employed, or complications have been registered instead of primary diseases. The nomenclature is of as much importance in this department of inquiry as weights and measures in the physical sciences, and should be settled without delay.[7]

Because of arguments along these lines, the first International Statistical Congress, held in Brussels in 1853, asked William Farr and Dr Marc d'Espine of Geneva to create an internationally applicable, uniform classification of causes of death. Two years later Farr and d'Espine submitted separate lists, based on different principles. Farr's classification used five main groups: epidemic diseases, constitutional (general) diseases, local diseases, organised by location in the body, developmental diseases, and diseases caused by violence. D'Espine classified diseases according to their nature (for example, affecting blood). Since both these two proposals were sensible, they were combined to give a list of 139 definitions of causes of death.

While a definite step forward from the Bills of Mortality, where a cause of death was assigned at the whims of a searcher, the Congress's list remained contentious and hence was still not used everywhere. Therefore, the International Statistical Institute, at its meeting in Vienna in 1891, charged a committee, chaired by Jacques Bertillon, chief of statistical services of the City of Paris, to prepare a new classification of causes of death. In 1893, Bertillon presented his report in Chicago. His proposal was based on a classification used by the City of Paris, which used Farr's principles, and best practice in France, Germany and Switzerland. The Bertillon Classification of Causes of Death, later known as the International Classification of Diseases (ICD) was approved and was adopted by many countries and cities, such as Canada, Mexico and the United States in 1898.[8] We therefore have had reliable data on causes of death for more than 120 years. Before this time, diagnosis and records of why people died were decidedly suspect.

The ICD has been revised about every ten years since, to take into account new medical knowledge, and is now run by the WHO. We are currently using ICD-11, released in 2019.[9] The twenty most common causes of death today are shown in Table 4 (page 31). We know these numbers because the WHO keeps records of deaths, collating information from every country.[10] The 55 million deaths are divided into thousands of categories. The dominance of non-communicable diseases, like heart disease, stroke, cancer, dementia and diabetes is plain, though infectious diseases have by no means gone away.

ICD codes are defined so that a doctor anywhere in the world should be able to make the same assignment. For example, category 2 means malignant cancer and 2E65 is breast cancer; category 8 is diseases of the nervous system, and 8A40 is multiple sclerosis.[9]

In the UK, most people die, not unexpectedly, in a hospital, hospice or at home. When this happens, the doctor attending during their last illness issues a medical certificate of the cause of death (MCCD). Many of us are familiar with a death certificate, which also has a cause of death, but the MCCD is a bit more complicated. It includes the following sections:

CAUSE OF DEATH

I (a) Disease or condition directly leading to death

_____

  (b) Other disease or condition, if any, leading to I (a)

_____

  (c) Other disease or condition, if any, leading to I (b)

_____

II Other significant conditions CONTRIBUTING TO THE
   DEATH but not related to the disease or condition causing it

_____

Suppose a doctor has an HIV-positive patient who develops
AIDS, drastically weakening their immune system. They then
catch a nasty fungal infection in their blood from a bug called
Cryptococcus, which in this case is fatal. The patient is a smoker,
which has led to emphysema, making them more likely to be
infected by *Cryptococcus*.[12] The doctor records this information on
the MCCD as shown here:

INTERNATIONAL FORM OF MEDICAL CERTIFICATE OF CAUSE OF DEATH

	Cause of death		Approximate interval between onset and death
I Disease or condition directly leading to death*	(a)	Cryptococcus septicaemia	3 months
		due to (or as a consequence of)	
Antecedent causes Morbid conditions, if any, giving rise to the above cause, stating the underlying condition last	(b)	AIDS	2 years
		due to (or as a consequence of)	
	(c)	HIV Infection	8 years
		due to (or as a consequence of)	
	(d)		
II Other significant conditions contributing to the death, but not related to the disease or condition causing it		Smoking	25 years

*This does not mean the mode of dying, e.g. heart failure, respiratory failure.
It means the disease, injury, or complication that caused death.

Example of an MCCD form for someone who died from AIDS.

TABLE 4 *Top 20 causes of death in the world, 2019.[11]*

Cause	Number of deaths (thousands)
Ischaemic heart disease	8,885
Stroke	6,194
Chronic obstructive pulmonary disease	3,228
Lower respiratory infections	2,593
Neonatal conditions	2,038
Trachea, bronchus, lung cancers	1,784
Alzheimer's disease and other dementias	1,639
Diarrhoeal diseases	1,519
Diabetes mellitus	1,496
Kidney diseases	1,334
Cirrhosis of the liver	1,315
Road injury	1,282
Tuberculosis	1,208
Hypertensive heart disease	1,149
Colon and rectum cancers	916
Stomach cancer	831
Self-harm	703
Falls	684
HIV/AIDS	675
Breast cancer	640

While this procedure might seem straightforward enough, many issues can complicate matters. Firstly, not all deaths occur from natural causes where the reasons for death are obvious to a doctor. When the death is classed as unnatural, the legal world needs to get involved in the form of a coroner. Unnatural deaths are those caused by violence, poisoning, self-harm, neglect, a medical procedure or an injury in a job. Coroners also investigate if the cause of death is unknown or suspicious, if the deceased was in prison, or cannot be identified. A coroner can order a post-mortem examination (autopsy) to be carried out by a pathologist. Permission to carry out a post-mortem examination can also occasionally be sought by a doctor with relatives' consent. The doctor might want to investigate why a death from an illness was sudden, for example, and perhaps uncover another condition that they were not aware of.

The law can get more involved if an inquest is required by a coroner. Here the aim is to determine the cause of a person's death, rather than put an individual on trial. The procedure works like a trial, though, with a coroner in place of a judge, witnesses and occasionally a jury. The conclusion can be natural death, accidental death, misadventure, suicide or murder. If it is murder, or death through negligence, then criminal prosecution can follow.

Suspected suicides are always dealt with by a coroner. Here they will only conclude that suicide was the cause of death if this is beyond reasonable doubt, as in a criminal trial. The requirement for greater evidence and the social stigma of suicide means that many deaths recorded as accidents were probably suicides in reality – poisonings or car crashes, for instance. The number of reported suicides is therefore an underestimate. Doctors will also report deaths in different ways. Most contentious is part II on the MCCD, the existing conditions contributing to a death. If an overweight smoker dies from heart failure, some doctors will put obesity or smoking as a contributing factor; others will not, perhaps in the interests of sensitivity to the family. Relatives might be upset if they think that the deceased brought their premature death on themselves.

In the UK, once an MCCD has been issued, a relative needs to register the death at a register office to obtain a death certificate. In the UK, this death registry data is passed to the National Office of Statistics, where the information is collated and passed on to the WHO. Thanks to this work, thousands of modern-day John Graunts can now compare causes of death in different places, confident of using public health data based on a common understanding of the causes of death to discover ways to prevent and treat disease.

3

Live Long and Prosper

Life expectancy is the single most important indicator of general well-being. Life expectancy has varied greatly throughout history, from about thirty in ancient and medieval times to more than eighty in the healthiest and wealthiest countries today. It takes a major change in how people live to cause a significant alteration in life expectancy, such as industrialisation, a large-scale war, famine, an epidemic or curing an important disease like smallpox. Historical events can thus cause both short- or long-term changes to life expectancy. Here we will look at how life expectancy has varied over thousands of years and across the world, reflecting the broadest changes in human health.

Life expectancy at birth is defined as how long, on average, a newborn can expect to live, if current death rates do not change. In the UK in 2015, life expectancies at birth were 79.2 for men and 82.9 for women. These are typical values for a Western European country and place the UK at 20 in the world league table.[1] Top of the list is Japan, with 80.5 for men and 86.8 for women, followed by Switzerland, Singapore, Australia and Spain. Affluent countries in East Asia and Europe, plus Canada, Australia and New Zealand, make up all the top 25. Averaging men and women, the USA is placed 31 at 79.3, between Costa Rica and Cuba. China is at 53 with a life expectancy of 76.1 years, Russia is at 110 with 70.5 and India is at 125 with 68.3. All but one of the bottom 37 are sub-Saharan African – the only non-African country is Afghanistan. Last is Sierra Leone, with 49.3 for men and 50.8 for women.

Life expectancy is, of course, a single number. Much more informative is to consider the likelihood of dying at any age. The graph below shows the number of deaths at different ages for men and women. It neatly demonstrates how men are more likely to die at a younger age than women and that newborns have the same risk of dying as someone aged sixty. The complete data is in Appendix 1 (page 302), which also shows how these numbers can be used to calculate life expectancy at any age, not just birth.

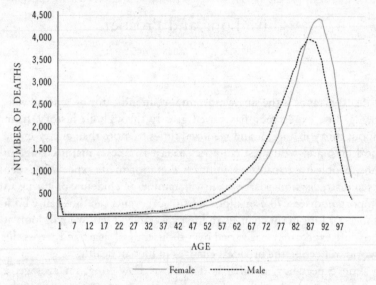

Number of deaths for each age within a total population of 100,000 males and 100,000 females, UK 2014–16.[2]

How long people used to live is hard to know, however, as accurate information was rarely kept. Often no records were kept at all. Tombstones are an obvious source of dates of birth and death, but they will be biased towards those that could afford them, and even in rich families, infant deaths might not be recorded in this way. The weather can also erode tombstone inscriptions. In the absence of any written (or carved) records, we can be left with skeletons as our main source of information. Potentially, a graveyard can be used to reconstruct the population picture of an entire city, giving the number of people who died at each age, their sex, birth rates, death rates, family size, population size, and effects of nutrition, disease and physical exertion.

Some conditions related to health are easily detectable in skeletons (for example, height, arthritis and fractures). It is possible to test whether a woman ever had children from pelvic bone changes resulting from childbirth. If we assume that we have the skeletons of every person who lived near the site, then we can get an accurate picture of the entire community.[3]

We shall look at four examples of life expectancies in the past, chosen partly because their data is accurate compared to other places at the time. These are: ancient Greece, the Roman Empire, English nobility in the Middle Ages, and France since 1816.

Two of the largest cities of classical Greece were Athens and Corinth. Twentieth-century excavations of graves from these cities dated 650–350 BCE show the following:

Male mean age at death	44
Female mean age at death	36
Births per adult female	4.5
Sex ratio, male to female, children	145:100
Sex ratio, male to female, adults	129:100

The excess of males is puzzling.[4] Perhaps the data is biased, as female adult bones tend to decay a little faster than males. Another possibility when high male-to-female ratios are seen is that infanticide is practised, with baby girls more likely to be killed than boys. More likely is that the ashes of males tended to be buried in those particular cemeteries in urns, while women's ashes were buried urn-less, unless they were of high status. About one-third of the burials were of children younger than fifteen, so a high birth rate and marrying young was essential to maintain the population.

Estimating the population structure of the Roman Empire is tricky, as quality data is lacking. Nevertheless, we can try. The figure overleaf shows survival curves for Roman males and females in the first and second centuries CE, using University of Michigan Professor of Classics Bruce Frier's model life table,[5] compiled from a variety of data sources, such as written records and tombstones. Some of the best surviving data for ordinary subjects of the Roman Empire can be found in 300 census returns, containing entries for more than 1,100 persons, filed in Roman Egypt during the first to third centuries CE. Egyptian life expectancy at birth was then somewhere between twenty-two and twenty-five.[6] The UK in 2016 is included for comparison below. We start with 100,000 people, then plot the number who survive to each age. Thus 50 per cent of Roman females lived to the age of twelve, while 50 per cent of Roman males only lived to the age of seven. In the modern world, most will live more than eighty years; in Roman times only a tiny proportion lived that long.

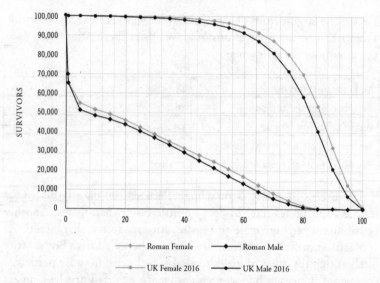

Survival curves for the Roman Empire compared to the present day.

The data plotted in this graph translates to an appallingly low life expectancy at birth of twenty-five years for females and twenty-three years for males, substantially worse than ancient Athens and Corinth. Infant mortality rates were extremely high. If a child reached the age of five, then their life expectancies jumped up to forty for females and thirty-nine for males. These curves can only be rough estimates, and there must have been substantial variations across the empire and in different times. We do have a single surviving life table

TABLE 5 *Ulpian's life table.*

Age x	Life expectancy at age x
0–20	30
20–25	28
25–30	25
30–35	22
35–40	20
40–50	59-x
50–55	9
55–60	7
60+	5

from the ancient world, called Ulpian's table.[7, 8] Table 5 (above) shows Ulpian's data, which was used to help make the survival curves in the figure opposite. While the numbers are intriguing, it is not clear what exactly they mean. The life expectancies might be the average (mean) number of years left to live or they could be the median number of years (the age to which half the people will live). It is also unclear what the table was used for. It may have been used to calculate taxes on an inherited property.[9] Slaves counted as property, and the value of a slave depended on how many years' work you could expect to get out of them. The data therefore probably gives life expectancies for slaves. Hence, the tax payable on a twenty-seven-year-old slave would be five times greater than a sixty-five-year-old slave, as the twenty-seven-year-old has a life expectancy of twenty-five more years, while that of the sixty-five-year-old is just five more years. Free, common people in the Roman Empire are likely to have lived longer than slaves, but perhaps not. A rich slave owner would want to keep their property alive, for instance, but a sick or starving free man might well be on his own. The quality of life of a slave could vary enormously. An educated scribe in a rich household could be well treated and hence have a good chance of reaching old age; a worker in the Spanish silver mines would not.

Roman death rates were so high for several reasons:

- Roman medicine was ineffective in the face of infectious diseases, which killed most people.
- The great majority of the population suffered from poor nutrition, making them less able to fight off infections.
- Even though Roman engineers were excellent at building aqueducts, sewers and so on, these were still inadequate to stop the spread of waterborne disease. The shared water in the highly popular public baths was not at all clean.
- The famed Roman roads linking large cities and trading ships across the Mediterranean helped rapidly to spread any new diseases.
- Roman government did very little to implement measures to limit disease outbreaks, such as imposing quarantines and eradicating vermin.[5]

Making a serious attempt to tackle these issues did not take place in Europe for another thousand years.

We have written records for some families in the Middle Ages, primarily nobility. Here is one example: Edward Plantagenet married Eleanor of Castile in 1254; he was fifteen and she thirteen. Eleanor had a stillborn daughter the next year. Even though their marriage was arranged for political reasons and the couple were very young, they had a deeply loving relationship, as the twelve Eleanor crosses that mark the route of her funeral procession from Lincoln to Charing Cross in London suggest.[10] Eleanor and Edward had at least sixteen children in total. Noble women like Eleanor would have had wet nurses to breastfeed their children. As breastfeeding acts as a contraceptive, this meant that Eleanor was able to have children more closely spaced in ages than most women of the time. After Eleanor died in 1290 at the age of forty-nine, Edward married Margaret of France, with whom he had a further three children. Edward's children are listed in Table 6. There is some uncertainty about the children who were stillborn or died as babies. Eleanor is also likely to have had miscarriages that were not recorded.

Edward Plantagenet was king of England from 1272 to 1307, reigning as Edward I. As well as giving the Scots and the French

TABLE 6 *Offspring of King Edward I of England.*

With Eleanor of Castile	Years lived	Age at death
Daughter of unknown name	1255	Stillborn
Katherine	1261–64	3
Joan	1265–65	<1
John	1266–71	5
Henry	1268–74	6
Eleanor	1269–98	29
Juliana	1271	<1
Joan	1272–1307	35
Alphonso	1273–84	11
Margaret	1275–1333	58
Berengaria	1276–78	2
Daughter of unknown name	1278	<1
Mary	1279–1332	53
Son of unknown name	1281	<1
Elizabeth	1282–1316	34
Edward	1284–1327	43
With Margaret of France		
Thomas	1300–38	38
Edmund	1301–30	29
Eleanor	1306–10	4

a sound thrashing on the field of battle, a vital duty of a king was to provide a son and heir to inherit the kingdom, thus avoiding the potential disaster of anarchy, lack of leadership, or civil war from an unclear succession or a child monarch. Edward and Eleanor had five sons and eleven daughters. Only Edward, their fifth son and sixteenth child, lived to adulthood to become King Edward II. Eleanor therefore had to become pregnant and give birth at least sixteen times before she managed to produce a son fortunate enough to survive childhood. Ten or more of her children died before she did, including her first five. The average lifespan of Edward's nineteen children is just eighteen, and only half lived to be six. Edward and Eleanor had the best standard of living available at the time. Not having enough food was not an issue, for example, which it often was for most people. Yet with all their money and power, they could do nothing about the deaths, over and over again, of their children. Deep grief must have been a normal condition and parents lived in fear whenever a child picked up a new infection.

The consensus among historians, putting together all these data, is that life expectancy in the Middle Ages was between thirty and forty.[11] This was before the arrival of the Black Death, which, as we shall see, made things much, much worse.

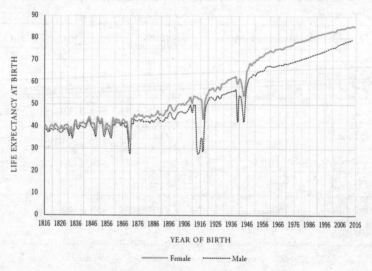

Life expectancy at birth in France, 1816–2016.[12]

Population data for every citizen of a country, including lifespan, only started to be rigorously collected in the nineteenth century. The figure above shows how life expectancy changed from 1816 to

2016 in France. France, which has kept quality data for 200 years, is a typical developed country. Over this time, life expectancy more than doubled, from 41.1 to 85.3 for women and 39.1 to 79.3 for men.

TABLE 7 *Historical events that have affected life expectancy in France since 1816.*

Year	Events and comments
1816–65	Little overall change. Brief dips are due to epidemics, such as cholera in 1832.
1870–71	Franco-Prussian War. A six-month war between the French Empire and an alliance of German states, led by Prussia. A major French defeat, including the Siege of Paris, that resulted in the unification of Germany under the Prussian Kaiser, the overthrow of French Emperor Napoleon III, and the transfer of the provinces of Alsace and Lorraine from France to Germany (storing up trouble for the future).
1871–1940	Increasing life expectancy mostly due to improvements for young people, such as childhood vaccinations and better nutrition.
1914–18	First World War. The French army suffered a horrific 1.4 million casualties. Only one village in the entire country suffered no deaths (Thierville in Normandy). Many more men died than women, leaving a generation of women without husbands.
1918–19	Spanish flu. One of the deadliest epidemics in history. The H1N1 strain of the influenza virus killed 50–100 million people worldwide. As a high proportion of these were young adults, Spanish flu had an especially severe effect on life expectancy. Years of malnutrition as a result of the war made people especially vulnerable to disease in many countries.

1929	Wall Street Crash and start of the Great Depression. Big increases in unemployment and homelessness.
1939–34	Second World War. France shows a double dip with minima at 1940 and 1944. 1940 saw the German invasion and defeat of the French army, so it was males that were mostly killed at this time. France was extensively bombed and became a battleground in 1944 after the Allied invasion on D-Day, affecting women more than in 1940. Male casualties were still higher than women, as many fought and died with Charles de Gaulle's Free French forces and others.
1946–55	End of food rationing, better nutrition. Introduction of antibiotics, led by penicillin. Rapid increase in life expectancy.
1955– present day	Increasing life expectancy mostly due to improvements for older people. Better treatments for heart disease, cancer and countless other diseases. Decrease in prevalence of smoking.

Another way of looking at this is that life expectancy in France increased on average by five hours per day since 1816. So, every day, the date of a French person's death gets closer by twenty-four hours due to the passing of time, but recedes by five hours, thanks to medicine, nutrition, sanitation, good government, trade, peace and so on. The early twenty-first century is the healthiest time ever to be alive. We shall look at how these gains were achieved in more detail later, but we can identify a number of historical events that affected life expectancy (Table 7, above). Bad things, like wars, show up as sudden dips, while good things, like antibiotics, cause permanent increases.

We can compare life expectancies in France in the past with present-day life expectancies in various countries. Life expectancy in France reached 50.1, the same as Sierra Leone now, in 1910. The country with the lowest life expectancy in the world now, therefore, has similar health to one of the richest just over a hundred years ago. In 1946 France reached the level of present-day Afghanistan (60.5 years). Afghanistan is now commonly seen as a failed state, with a dysfunctional government, civil wars, terrorism and severe damage by invasions by the USSR and USA. Yet it still has a higher life expectancy than France in the 1930s. France reached present-day Iraq in 1958 (68.9 years), North Korea in 1961 (70.6 years) and Iran in 1986 (75.5 years). Even the world's poorest countries have good life expectancies at present compared to rich countries in the recent past. All the poorest countries now are healthier than every country in the nineteenth century.

These huge recent changes in life expectancy are part of a phenomenon called the demographic transition. Women living in pre-industrial societies married young and had many children. Twenty pregnancies in a lifetime was not unusual, with a new baby every year or two. Despite these high birth rates, human populations only grew slowly, held back by chronic disease and malnutrition, with occasional devastating famines and epidemics. Life expectancy was about thirty, with high infant mortality, many children and few old people. In Korea, for example, so many children did not survive the first weeks of life that a celebration for a new baby was only held once it had survived a hundred days after birth in good health. The child could then be taken outdoors for the first time. High birth and death rates gave a roughly stable population.

A few hundred years ago in North America and Europe, we finally began to overcome our biggest killers. Trade, wealth, new foods and better farming practices allowed us to increase population without triggering famine. Improved housing, better nutrition and sanitation cut the incidence and death rates from infectious disease. The result was soaring population in Europe and the emigration of millions of Europeans.

People will have lots of children if they expect them to die young. Once people have confidence that their children will survive, and they will be looked after in old age, most choose to have just two. Fertility decline is also linked to female educational attainment and access to contraception. We therefore see a transition from a high birth rate/ high death rate society to one with low birth and death rates. The decrease in death rate takes place well before the decrease in birth rate, however. Typically, there is a generation where women have many children, as their mothers did, but nearly all survive to adulthood. The next generation then chooses to have far fewer children. This lag between a drop in the death rate and a decrease in the birth rate generates a huge increase in population while the shift is taking place.[13]

This switch in the way we reproduce is the demographic transition.[14] It is not especially dependent on where you live – all countries show a similar change. What varies is when the transition starts and how long it takes.

Most countries now have made it through the demographic transition. They have life expectancies above seventy-four, very low infant mortality (the death of a child before their first birthday), an increasing number of elderly people and a fertility rate of less than two children per woman. Thus, somewhat paradoxically, high life expectancy eventually causes a population decline. Data from three countries – Japan, Brazil and Ethiopia – are examples of the different stages of the demographic transition in Table 8 (below).

Japan underwent its demographic transition more than fifty years ago. Its excellent healthcare gives one of the highest life expectancies in the world and a very low infant mortality rate. Leading causes of death are coronary heart disease, cancer, stroke, lung disease and

TABLE 8 *Population data for Japan, Brazil and Ethiopia in 1960 and 2017.*[15,16]

Country	Japan		Brazil		Ethiopia	
Year	1960	2017	1960	2017	1960	2017
Infant mortality (per 1,000 births)	30.4	1.9	~170	14.8	~200	41.0
Life expectancy at birth	67.7	84.1	54.2	75.5	38.4	65.9
Population (millions)	92.5	126.8	72.2	207.8	22.1	106.4
Fertility rate (children per woman)	2.0	1.4	6.1	1.7	6.9	4.1
Rate of population change per year	+0.9%	-0.2%	+2.9%	+0.8%	+2.2%	+2.7%

suicide. Japan's fertility rate is only 1.4 and it has little immigration; hence its population is now falling by 0.2 per cent per year and the population is becoming more elderly. Most European countries are like Japan: they have fertility rates less than two and can only avoid a population decrease with substantial immigration.

Brazil underwent its demographic transition between 1960 and 2017, so shows huge changes in this time. Health has improved enormously: infant mortality plummeted from nearly one baby in five dying in its first year to only 1.5 per cent, and life expectancy increased by more than twenty years. Leading causes of death in Brazil are now coronary heart disease, cancer, stroke, lung disease and diabetes, as in most countries. Compared to Japan, Brazil has more deaths from violence and traffic accidents, but fewer from suicide. As usual, people's response to secure health is to have fewer children, so Brazil's fertility rate at 1.7 is now not much more than Japan's. While the Brazilian population has tripled since 1960, the decline in fertility means that the population is set to stabilise and then decrease from about 2030.[17] Most countries in Asia, North Africa and the Americas are now like Brazil, having made it through the demographic transition to reach a state with low birth and death rates, high life expectancy and a population set to peak soon.

Apart from failed states like Afghanistan and Yemen, life expectancy is lowest in sub-Saharan Africa. Even so, the demographic transition is under way in most African countries. Ethiopia provides an example. In 1960, it was in a high birth rate/high death rate condition with life expectancy less than forty. Now infant mortality is fourfold lower and life expectancy is up to 65.9. As a result, fertility is decreasing, down to 4.1 in 2017. The population is still growing fast, but the rate should drop substantially in the next few decades. Compared to Brazil and Japan, many more people in Ethiopia currently die from infectious diseases, notably influenza, pneumonia, diarrhoeal disease, tuberculosis, measles and HIV/AIDS, though coronary heart disease, cancer and stroke are also prevalent.[18] Ethiopia looks like Brazil did twenty years ago, also slowly turning into a population resembling that of Japan.

Table 9 (overleaf) shows some data for the whole world. We have seen great improvements since 1960, particularly in the last twenty years. The world is evening up, with the previous model of a country

TABLE 9 *World demographic data from 1960 to 2017.*[15,16]

Year	1960	1997	2017
Infant mortality (per 1,000 births)	126	58	29.4
Life expectancy at birth	52.7	66.9	72.2
Population (millions)	3,032	5,873	7,511
Fertility rate (children per woman)	5.0	2.8	2.4
Birth rate (per 1,000 people)	31.8	22.7	18.7
Death rate (per 1,000 people)	17.7	8.7	7.6

being either developed or developing and having enormous differences in health and wealth no longer valid.

These trends look set to spread and accelerate. Declining fertility rates, to well below 2.1 in most countries, means that the world population is set to peak just below 10 billion in 2064. The population structure is becoming top-heavy, with many elderly and retired people supported by a decreasing number of younger workers. The Middle East, North Africa and especially sub-Saharan Africa will take up a larger fraction of the world population, while Europe and East Asia plummet.[19] Exemplifying these changes, by 2100 the population of China is forecast to almost halve from its maximum to 700 million, while Nigeria nearly quadruples to 800 million, behind only India.

These data point to profound changes in causes of death during the transition and impressive advances in public health across the planet. How were these achieved? As we shall see, the world now has better governments, on the whole. An increasing number are democracies that act in the interests of their people, providing sanitation and healthcare, and avoiding war and famine, all based on increasing wealth. Infants benefit most from these changes.

Why do countries today have different life expectancies? A key observation was first made by American sociologist Samuel Preston in 1975, who plotted life expectancies against the wealth of a country, measured as Gross Domestic Product (GDP) per person. The graph opposite is a Preston curve, using 2015 data. The trendline shows a smoothed relationship between wealth and health. The curve always increases, so that richer countries tend to have better health. It is a logarithmic curve, however – far from a straight line. On the left, the curve is steep, where a small increase in wealth leads to a big jump in life expectancy. Reaching seventy years requires a GDP per person of $7,100; taking this up to 75 needs a big increase, more than doubling to $15,700.

Data for some individual countries are labelled. Those that are above the trendline are doing well, with good health for their wealth. Most impressive is Nepal, which has a life expectancy of eighty-one years, despite having a GDP per person of only $1,268. Many of the worst performers are in the Middle East, due to genetic disease, obesity and diabetes.

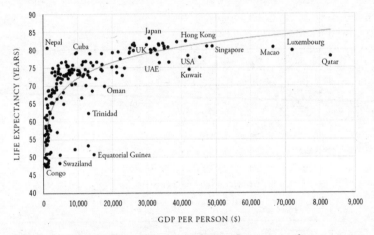

Correlation between life expectancy and gross domestic product per person, 2010. Data is from World Statistics: GDP and Life Expectancy.[20] The trendline equation is $y = 6.273\ ln(x) + 14.38$.

Does the Preston curve simply mean that richer countries provide better healthcare? It depends what the money is spent on and who benefits. A country might be wealthy but decide not to spend much on health. The money might also be spent inefficiently, advertising health-insurance companies and settling court cases rather than spending on patient care, for example. Being wealthy at least gives the option of providing extensive healthcare. A more informative measure is therefore to plot life expectancy against healthcare spending per person, rather than life expectancy versus GDP, which includes all economic activity. The figure below shows how health spending correlates with life expectancy for forty-four countries in 2013. The graph shows that spending more on health does indeed benefit health, but there are many outliers. Reaching a life expectancy of seventy-five requires a spend of about $1,000 per person per year, and eighty requires $3,200. Taking a country up to a life expectancy of seventy costs little and has great benefits. As with the previous figure, the curve flattens off, so spending more money provides smaller gains. Spain, Japan and South Korea are excellent-value health spenders, partly due to their healthy diets. Outliers below the curve include Russia and the USA. South Africa is exceptionally low due to HIV.

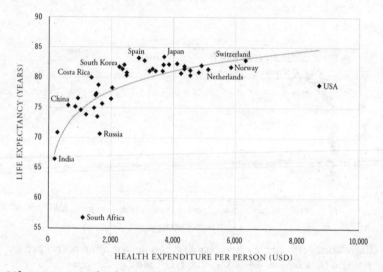

Life expectancy at birth versus health spend per person, 2013.[21] The trendline equation is $y = 4.73 \ln(x) + 41.84$.

Why does the USA have a poor life expectancy, despite spending far more on health than any other country?[22] Life expectancy in the USA is the same as Chile (78.8 years), yet USA spends $8,713 per person per year on health, while Chile spends just $1,623. Several things contribute to the dismal performance of the US health system. Administrative costs on the US health sector are excessive. Homicide and suicide rates are high in the US compared to other rich countries, as guns are easily available.

The USA also stands out for high levels of child mortality and death in childbirth; these lead to a higher death rate among young people, with a disproportionate effect on life expectancy. Health spending in the USA shows exceptional levels of inequality.[23] Nearly all affluent countries have healthcare protection coverage for all their citizens; in the USA, nearly 10 per cent still have no health insurance at all.

While the graphs opposite seem to suggest that greater wealth leads to better health, particularly if the money is spent sensibly, things may not be so simple. If spending is the only thing that matters, then the improvement in life expectancy over the past 150 years is simply due to growth in GDP. There clearly must be more to it than this: it doesn't matter how many doctors you employ to cure disease if cures don't exist. A life expectancy of just thirty before 1800 was not because there were no doctors. There were plenty of doctors but, unfortunately, pretty much everything they did was useless, if not downright harmful. Poor practices included: bleeding, inducing vomiting, spreading disease as they travelled from patient to patient without washing, and administering laxatives. A careful analysis suggests that at least 75 per cent of the improvements in health from 1930 to 1960 were due to factors other than growth in a country's income, like public health interventions and wide use of medical innovations such as the first antibiotics.[24, 25, 26]

Over time, the Preston curve is shifting upwards, meaning that health improves even if income does not. For example, in the 1930s an annual income per person of $400 (US 1963 dollars) would get you a life expectancy of fifty-four years; in the 1960s, the same income gave a life expectancy of sixty-six years.[24] Maybe this means that there is no need to increase overall wealth at all to improve health – it can happen anyway, thanks to medical advances. Vaccination is cheap.

The correlation between income and health is true for individuals, as well as countries. While rich people might be able to buy better healthcare, another possibility is that health is affected by how people see themselves in society. People at the bottom of the heap can feel psychological stress that worsens their immune systems and leads to behaviour that causes poor health, such as drug-taking.[27, 28] If this is true, then greater inequality in a society would lead to poorer health overall. If we want a general increase in health, we need to work towards a more equal society.[29]

PART II

INFECTIOUS DISEASE

All that would be required to prevent the disease would be such a close attention to cleanliness in cooking and eating, and to drainage and water supply, as is desirable at all times.

John Snow, *On the Mode of Communication of Cholera*, 1849[1]

4

The Black Death

For most of human history, life expectancy was about thirty. It only began to rise about 250 years ago, first in Europe and North America, and now in all countries. By 2016, worldwide life expectancy had tripled from Roman times, to seventy-two years.[1] This is by far the highest life expectancy that we have ever had. These simple statistics reflect profound changes in human health. Most importantly, the biggest killer in the past by far was infectious disease. Plague, smallpox, typhoid, cholera and malaria, to name but a few, each took the lives of hundreds of millions of people, often with little warning and after only a few days' illness.

Before we look at how infectious diseases were tackled and largely defeated, starting with plague, we need to set the scene by examining how we lived and how we died when we were hunter-gatherers. Hunting and gathering has been our species' way of life for most of our time on Earth, during which infectious disease was not such a large concern. Hunter-gatherers forage for plants and hunt animals for food and are usually nomadic. They live in temporary settlements in extended families, with an egalitarian social structure and shared possessions, and without any permanent leaders. Nowadays, the hunter-gatherer way of life persists only in a few places: the deserts of south-west Africa, the Amazon rainforest and the high Arctic. These communities offer insights into how we used to live, though we can question how representative present-day hunter-gatherers are of the Palaeolithic period, since they now tend to live in marginal land unsuitable for agriculture. The way of life of modern hunter-gatherers may also have significantly changed after contact with other societies – obtaining manufactured tools from trade, for instance. Nevertheless, looking at the lifestyles of contemporary hunter-gatherers should give some insight into how we used to live and die. In addition, studies of Palaeolithic skeletons and archaeological sites can indicate how healthy hunter-gatherers used to be and how they died.

Hunter-gatherers' diet was mostly vegetables, fruits, nuts and roots, with little or no dairy products, processed oils, salt, alcohol or caffeine. The only sugar would have been from fruit or honey. Our ancestors used an amazing range of plants for food and materials – 192 different types were found at the site of Abu Hureyra, a village in Syria inhabited by hunter-gatherers 12,000 years ago.[2] The varied diet and active lifestyles of hunter-gatherers meant that they were physically healthy, with heights not far short of modern people. Obesity was rare. Infant mortality was high, however; infanticide may have been practised when it was not possible to carry babies from site to site and in order to control populations. Prolonged breastfeeding in the absence of animal milk acted as a contraceptive, helping to space out births. Accidents were a common cause of death, including falls, broken bones, drowning, and injuries from animal bites, often during hunting. Hunter-gatherers would have known disease, such as bacterial infections caught from dirty water, wounds or animal bites. Many did live to an old age, so would have been affected by cancer, neurodegeneration and arthritis.

About 10,000 years ago, the greatest transformation ever in the way we live began with the onset of agriculture, bringing in the Neolithic period. Rather than gathering a variety of wild strains of plants, land was devoted to a limited number of crops – most importantly wheat, barley, maize, rice and millet. Crops were selected to have more useful characteristics: dense growth in tilled fields, long-term storage, many large seeds, a wide geographical range, being easy to harvest and so on. Farmers would tend to replant the best seed, so after thousands of years of this selection, farmed plants could end up looking very different from their wild cousins. Instead of being hunted, animals were captured, penned and protected. Sheep, goats, cattle and pigs were kept for food and clothing, while horses, camels, llamas and donkeys were used for transport. Domesticated animals were bred to produce more meat, milk or wool. They became more docile, tolerant of humans and had more offspring. People adapted too, with smaller teeth and mutations that allowed them to drink larger quantities of alcohol and milk.

Agriculture started independently in about ten areas, including the Middle East, the Indus Valley of Pakistan, the Yellow River of China, the Andes and Central America, before spreading across most of the planet. Sumeria, in what is now southern Iraq, was perhaps first: 10,000 years ago it was not arid as it is today; instead it was a rich, marshy country with trees and many wild animals. Settlements were on mounds above the wetlands.

With areas of land now devoted solely to food production, the amount of food produced per square mile increased hugely, allowing population densities to rise in parallel. New social classes and larger communities gave leaders wealth and power. Job specialisations appeared with merchants, craftsmen, soldiers, priests and others. Still, most people were farming and for them, the switch from hunting and gathering was a disaster for health.

Compared to fishing, hunting animals or gathering plants, farm work was a back-breaking chore, often taking far more hours in the day. Without constant defence, crops could be lost to weeds, rodents, fungi and insects. We can tell that people in Abu Hureyra had switched to farming by 9000 BCE because the skeletons of the women have deformed knees and bent toes, caused by long hours kneeling to grind grain for flour.[2] Rather than a varied diet, people were now consuming predominantly staple crops, often deficient in essential nutrients. Meat rich in protein, fat and iron might be missing altogether. People got smaller; their bones and teeth reveal nutritional problems – notably anaemia, as the cereals they were eating lacked fatty acids needed to take up iron.[3] A diet of mostly carbohydrate would be short of protein and vitamins. New diseases related to poor nutrition appeared, arising even if enough calories were consumed, like pellagra, beriberi and kwashiorkor. Malnutrition would have led to loss of fertility in both men and women.

Records of ancient epidemics are poor: many are not detectable in skeletons, and if all your scribes are killed, there is no one left to tell the tale. Nevertheless, it is striking that the world population of about 4 million in 10,000 BCE had increased to only 5 million in 5000 BCE,[4] despite the invention of agriculture which, for all its faults, should produce a lot more food than hunting and gathering. In addition, women could have many more children if they lived in the same place. Nomads had to space out their births, as they could not carry lots of babies. If farmers were generating substantially more food and women were having many more babies, then why wasn't there a population explosion?

On top of the nutritional problems came a vast array of new diseases. Most of the more than a thousand infectious diseases that currently affect humans are caused by microorganisms that once lived in animals but jumped the species barrier at some time in the last 10,000 years.[5] Measles, for example, comes from the rinderpest virus in cattle, and influenza comes from poultry. Living closely with animals, possibly even in the same buildings, meant a higher risk of catching their diseases and parasites. With thousands of people crowded together in cities, a single case of a new disease could easily spread. The first states in Mesopotamia – in modern Iraq – about 5,000 years ago were aware of the importance of contagion and made some efforts to stop the spread of disease by avoiding infected people, plus their cups, cutlery and bed linen.[6] Once sick, however, cures were not available.

The archaeological record and literature from the time show that the first states frequently collapsed, with massive population losses, destruction and abandonment of sites.[4, 7] While these catastrophes were undoubtedly sometimes caused by harvest failure from bad weather, invasions or floods, it is likely that many were a result of epidemics. The first people exposed to a new disease would have no natural resistance, so a whole city could be devastated. Tuberculosis, typhus and smallpox seem to have been some of the first diseases to have appeared as a result of agriculture.[8] A few fortunate people with the right genes might be able to tolerate the disease, so they and their children could survive it. Thus, natural selection would ensure that genes that enabled their owners to resist disease would spread. If the population was large enough, a disease might then become established as a highly infectious childhood disease. This could make the adapted group potentially deadly to another population that had never encountered that disease before.

In this way, over thousands of years, agricultural communities eventually acquired their own set of diseases that lived with them and their animals. Disaster could then strike when communities became linked through trade, expansion or migration. This happened about

2,000 years ago, when China, India, the Middle East and the Roman Empire first established regular trading links. As well as swapping silk and silver, they could also exchange their disease packages, triggering epidemics. In 165 CE, the Roman army had pushed east to attack its great rival the Parthian Empire and was besieging Seleucia on the Tigris in what is now Iraq. There the army caught a new deadly disease, called the Antonine Plague, which they brought back to Europe. The plague killed about a quarter of the people of Rome and devastated the army. Han China was hit by waves of epidemics at the same time, triggering rebellions and the eventual collapse of the dynasty. The nature of the Antonine Plague is not known, though smallpox is plausible.[9] In any event, this could well be an example of new trade links stretching across Asia allowing disease exchange and starting an epidemic.

Farm animals could also be wiped out by disease, with large herds allowing easy swapping of infections. The disappearance of one of the few species being farmed would cause famine, as the community's main source of meat, clothing or power vanished. Similarly, relying on just one crop for most of your calories would put your city at high risk of famine, if a new disease or pest destroyed your staple food.

Sanitation was not much of a problem for nomadic communities, who could leave their waste behind. However, spending your whole life at the same site created new problems of sewage disposal that would contaminate water sources and cause diarrheal disease. In Sumeria, for example, the only sources of drinking water were the rivers, but these had been polluted by all the cities upstream.

The onset of new diseases repeatedly obliterated settlements, which may be the primary cause of 5,000 years of population stagnation in the Neolithic. It took all this time for people to acquire resistance so that they could live at high densities with their animals.[10] The Neolithic was the most lethal period in history, largely thanks to infectious disease.[4]

The switch to states based on agriculture was the most profound change ever in the way we live, with enormous effects on human health. Unless you were one of the state's elite, life as a nomadic hunter-gatherer was a lot better in terms of health, diet and work.[11] American polymath Jared Diamond has argued that the advent of agriculture was the worst mistake in the history of the human race.[12]

The pay-off from farming is that turning over all the land to the crop of choice produces far more food, increasing populations and allowing a variety of job specialisations and socioeconomic groups to appear. High populations can only be maintained by farming. Moving from hunting and gathering to agriculture is therefore a one-way trip, unless the state has collapsed totally, with massive population losses (as did happen with the Maya in Central America, where their cities were abandoned by 900 CE, perhaps during a prolonged drought[13]).

Eventually, the advantages of having different social classes, technological advances and wealth creation within states paid off, when specialist scientists, scribes, doctors, engineers, politicians and others developed genuine improvements in our standard of living, with infectious diseases mostly prevented or cured. This has allowed us to return to, and even overtake, the good health we enjoyed in the Palaeolithic. Unfortunately, this took 10,000 years.

Plague is the worst infectious disease ever to beset humanity, being remarkably contagious, swift-acting and deadly. Two strains of plague, from separate transmission events from rodents to humans, caused the greatest epidemics recorded in history: the Plague of Justinian in the sixth century CE and the Black Death of the 1340s, which we have already encountered in Siena. While the DNA sequences of the plague microbe differed, their symptoms and lethality were much the same. Each killed around one-third of the population in the lands that they affected. We shall see how plague pandemics had profound effects on history, shaping the world to the present day. While plague could be largely controlled and prevented by the end of the seventeenth century by quarantine, fresh outbreaks were still capable of devastating cities up to the nineteenth century. Recent work on DNA from the plague-causing bacterium, *Yersinia pestis,* has shown that our relationship with plague goes back far before Justinian, devastating civilisations for many thousands of years.

In the year 527 CE, the most powerful man in the world was Justinian the Great, Emperor of the East Roman (Byzantine) Empire. He ruled over Europe, Turkey, Syria and Egypt from the great city of Constantinople, now Istanbul. Constantinople had been established 200 years earlier as a new capital on the site of the ancient Greek city of Byzantium by the Roman Emperor Constantine. Constantine poured wealth into the metropolis, setting it up as the richest and largest city in Europe for the next 800 years.

Justinian had inherited the throne at the age of forty-five after several years of effectively running the empire on behalf of his illiterate uncle, the Emperor Justin. He reformed the Roman legal system and undertook a new construction programme, culminating in the great church of Hagia Sophia. Hagia Sophia was the biggest building in the world at the time and still stands near the Sultan's Palace in Istanbul. Despite looting and vandalism by Crusaders and Turks, it remains a stunning building with an astonishing interior space, rising past walls, arches, sheets of marble, semi-domes, windows and mosaics to an enormous dome.

Even though the empire then contained 26 million people out of a world population of 200 million,[14] it was still only half the size that it had been. A hundred years earlier, the western half of the Roman Empire had collapsed after prolonged assault by barbarian tribes of Huns, Goths, Vandals and others. They had crossed the Rhine and Danube river borders and set up new kingdoms in France, Spain, Italy, North Africa and Britain. The richer, more populated eastern half withstood these attacks. Energetic, intelligent and ambitious, Justinian dreamed of fulfilling the re-conquest of the lost half of the Roman Empire, returning all the Mediterranean lands to the one true faith with himself at its head.

Justinian was not a general. Instead, from his palace in Constantinople, he despatched his fleets and armies like a chess master. His first success was in Tunisia, where the Vandal Kingdom was quickly destroyed by his top general Belisarius, helped by the local population, who loathed their new masters. By 541, his armies led by Belisarius and John the Eunuch had retaken most of Italy from the Goths. Justinian's dream was on track. It was not to last.

In 541, reports came to Constantinople of a deadly new disease in Egypt. The following year, ships transporting Egyptian grain brought the plague to the capital by also transporting infected rats. The disease tore through the city, with death rates of 5,000 per day. Death came so suddenly that people took to wearing name tags so that their bodies could be identified. Perhaps 40 per cent of the population of Constantinople died in just four months. Justinian himself caught the plague but survived. While plague affected people across Europe and

Asia, our best records of its effects are from writers in Constantinople, so the epidemic is named after Justinian. The total effect of the epidemic is hard to know for sure, though maybe 50 million people and nearly half the population of Europe died, with the disease spread by armies and trade.

Weakening of the empire due to population loss had terrible long-term effects. Loss of workers meant that many farms were abandoned, causing an eight-year famine. Decreased grain production caused prices to soar and tax revenues to decline. This did not stop the ruthless Justinian continuing to demand the same level of taxes from his much-reduced population so that he could continue with his military and construction projects. The wars in Italy dragged on, though with diminishing success. After such losses in population, the empire was only able to put out much smaller armies. The Italian campaign became a holding operation, a matter of clinging on to their earlier conquests. Italy was ruined after twenty years of fighting and the north fell to the Germanic Lombards shortly after Justinian died in 565.

Justinian's dream was defeated by an enemy that he could not see, did not understand and was helpless to stop. In the longer term, historians have often speculated that the conquest of Egypt, North Africa, Syria and Persia by the Arabs in the seventh and eighth centuries, inspired by the new religion of Islam, would not have been possible without the depopulation of the Byzantine and Persian empires by repeated plague epidemics,[15] though attributing the Arab conquests to just one cause stretches credibility to breaking point. Constantinople was unsuccessfully besieged by the Arabs from 674 to 678; if it had fallen, then it is likely that the whole empire would have collapsed and been taken over by the Arabs. Instead, the Byzantine Empire endured for nearly 1,000 years, only finally being conquered by the Turks in 1453. The Persian Sassanid Empire, which had also been decimated by the plague, was conquered by the Arabs in 651, leading to the slow replacement of Zoroastrianism by Islam, though Persian culture and language continued. Many places in Syria, Egypt and Libya have not recovered to this day from the Plague of Justinian, with previously tilled and irrigated fields abandoned to become pasture or even desert.[16]

After this first appearance of Justinian's plague, it returned intermittently over the next 200 years before its last outbreak and disappearance in 750, with the disease becoming more localised and less deadly, perhaps due to increased resistance in survivors. Plague was not to return to Europe for another 600 years, this time in the form of the Black Death.

What was plague? Many writers left gruesome descriptions of the deadly disease, giving us the following typical progression for the bubonic plague, the most common form of both Justinian's plague and the Black Death.

First came a severe headache, then a few hours later a fever and tiredness. The day after the fever started, the victim was so exhausted that they were unable to leave their beds. Their backs, arms and legs hurt, and nausea led to frequent vomiting. The next day hard, painful and burning swellings began to grow on the neck, inner thighs and armpits. This was new, indicating no ordinary disease. The swellings grew to the size of an orange and turned black. Sometimes the skin on the swellings would break, releasing foul-smelling pus and blood. The family could only watch helplessly, torn between comforting the victim in their agony and staying away to avoid infection themselves. Internal bleeding broke out throughout the body, with blood in vomit, urine, faeces and the lungs. Black boils and spots appeared as bleeding took place in the skin, causing immense pain everywhere. Fingers, toes, lips and the nose turned black, and their flesh died, causing frequent loss of these extremities and permanent disfigurement if the victim survived. All bodily fluids smelled revolting. The victim would lapse into delirium and coma before death came only a week after infection and a few days after the first symptoms. By this time, all the inhabitants of the house would probably have contracted the disease. Their survival was not likely. Even today, with modern medicine and antibiotics, the death rate is 10 per cent; untreated it is 80 per cent. The black swellings, known as buboes, are caused by bacteria congregating in the lymphatic system, which carries fluid around the body. Hence the name: bubonic plague.

Grim though bubonic plague undoubtedly is, it could be even worse. A less common, but even more deadly, form is pneumatic plague, where the bacteria infest the lungs, usually after inhaling droplets coughed into the air by an infected person or animal. Fever, headache, weakness and nausea rapidly progress to shortness of breath, chest pain and coughing up blood. This pneumonia-like stage lasts two to four days, before respiratory failure and inevitable death, if untreated with antibiotics. Septicaemic plague occurs when bacteria enter the bloodstream, causing blood clotting, bleeding into the skin and tissue death. It is almost always fatal, sometimes even on the same day that symptoms first appear.

The bacteria that cause plague, *Yersinia pestis*, live in small rodents (such as rats, squirrels, rabbits, marmots, prairie dogs and chipmunks) currently found in rural areas of Africa, Asia and the United States. *Y. pestis* can be transmitted to humans by bites from infected fleas, by humans handling infected animals via a cut in the skin or by inhaling infectious droplets coughed into the air by a sick animal or person.

In 1346 frightening rumours reached Europe that a plague epidemic was present to the east. Later known as the Black Death, it first spread from rodents (probably marmots) to humans living in grasslands in Central Asia. Plague is described on inscriptions on the graves of Nestorian Christians living in Kyrgyzstan in 1338. The Silk Roads passed through Central Asia, used by traders for thousands of years to link China to Europe. Mongols were also travelling vast distances across their huge new empire, which included Central Asia, China and the Middle East. While people had probably been infected by rodents in the region for thousands of years, the disease tended to remain localised, with a family group all killed but no others in the absence of long-distance travel. Now, however, frequent trade caravans and Mongol horsemen were transmitting new diseases between east and west. Chinese records of the time are sketchy and not well studied, but the Black Death strain of plague may well have been in China by 1331 or 1334 and could even have originated there. China certainly had big losses of population from 1330 to 1360, partly due to epidemics, as well as famines, natural disasters, political unrest and war, as the Mongol-led Yuan dynasty collapsed, to be replaced by the Ming. Surprisingly, plague does not seem to have reached India until a few hundred years later, even though northern India was ruled by sultans, who were trading with Persia and Central Asia.[17] Plague may have crossed the Sahara Desert, as cities in Ghana, Burkina Faso and Ethiopia show evidence of sudden population loss at the time of the Black Death.[18]

In 1347, ships brought infected rats and people into Mediterranean sea ports such as Messina, Pisa, Genoa and Venice, launching the deadliest epidemic ever to hit Europe. One of many entry points for the plague was a city called Caffa in the Crimea, on the shores of the Black Sea, held by the Italian trading city of Genoa. Caffa had been besieged by an army of Crimean Tartars, people related to Turks and Mongols, led by Khan Jani Beg. The Christian armies were trapped in the city for nearly three years, until the Tartars suddenly fell victim to disease.

Gabriele De' Mussi, from Piacenza near Genoa, described what happened, claiming that thousands died every day: 'All medical advice and attention was useless; the Tartars died as soon as the signs of disease appeared on their bodies: swellings in the armpit or groin caused by coagulating humours, followed by a putrid fever.'[19]

With his army rapidly dying, Khan Jani Beg was forced to give up his siege. He had a nasty parting shot for the Genoans, however: corpses were placed in catapults, then lobbed into the city. The number was overwhelming: even though the Genoans tried to dump them in the sea, the air and water were poisoned: '… the stench was so overwhelming that hardly one in several thousand was in a position to flee the remains of the Tartar army. Moreover, one infected man could carry the poison to others, and infect people and places with the disease by look alone. No one knew, or could discover, a means of defence.'

Ships fleeing Caffa to Genoa or Venice carried the plague with them.

When the sailors reached these places and mixed with the people there, it was as if they had brought evil spirits with them: every city, every settlement, every place was poisoned by the contagious pestilence, and their inhabitants, both men and women, died suddenly. And when one person had contracted the illness, he poisoned his whole family even as he fell and died, so that those preparing to bury his body were seized by death in the same way.[19, 20]

The overall mortality rate varied from city to city; in Florence, Venice and Paris half the population died, while Milan, Poland and the Basque Country got off relatively lightly. Death rates were so high that corpses were buried together in pits; rotting bodies lay in homes and streets. Doctors, monks and priests were particularly affected, as they were more likely to be in contact with the sick. From 1347 the plague moved across Europe from the Mediterranean ports. It headed north to France, Germany, Britain and Scandinavia, and then turned east, reaching Moscow in 1353. Ships from the Black Sea and Constantinople also took the plague to Alexandria in Egypt in 1347. Within two years it devastated cities across the Middle East, such as Antioch, Mecca, Baghdad and Jerusalem.

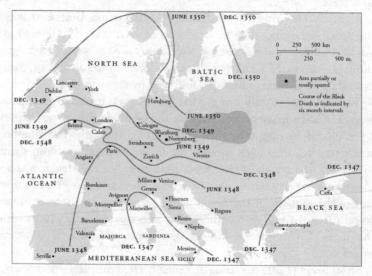

The Black Death in Europe.[21]

While the total death toll for the Black Death is quite uncertain, the numbers were clearly enormous; up to 60 per cent of the population of Europe died.[22] Often, six months after the first case in a city, more than half the population would have succumbed. It was the worst natural disaster ever in Europe. In densely populated parts of Italy, Spain and southern France, where plague might last a full four years, a staggering 80 per cent of the population could be lost.[23] By 1430, Europe's population was lower than it had been in 1290 and would not return to that level for hundreds of years. Now that plague was re-established by 1350, new epidemics took place every year somewhere in Europe for 400 years. For example, it broke out in

Venice twenty-two times between 1361 and 1528, then returned in 1576–7 to kill 50,000, almost a third of the population.

European society of the Middle Ages was shattered by the plague. Villages, industry and farmland were abandoned. Surviving peasants found that their labour was much more in demand so their wages, social mobility, legal rights and standard of living all improved. Many moved to towns. In a deeply religious society, turning to God was the main strategy to survive plague. God had to be very angry indeed to send the Black Death, so extreme measures were needed: people gave all their money to the Church, stopped their sinful behaviour, flogged themselves in public and murdered Jews. Nothing worked. Christianity's credibility thus took a beating.

Plague is the definitive example of a deadly epidemic disease. From the first appearance of the Plague of Justinian in the sixth century, it took 800 years before the first measures were found that could effectively control it. Italian governments and physicians led the way with measures to tackle the conditions that led to plague: filth, bad housing, dirty water and poverty. Hospitals were built to isolate plague victims; organisations were set up to clean streets and empty latrines; guards at city gates and mountain passes stopped plague spreading; even spy networks were set up across Europe and parts of Asia and Africa to report on any new plague outbreak. The Italian peninsula was thus the first region to rid itself of plague by about 1650, providing an example for other countries to follow.[24] Even though the cause of plague remained a mystery and no cure was known, the Black Death did lead to the creation of a system that could stop it spreading – quarantine.

It was obvious that plague could be caught from infected people. Doctors and priests who visited the sick thus had exceptionally high death rates. Many cities tried strategies to stop the spread of plague by separating the healthy from the sick. For example, in the Italian city of Reggio, people with plague were taken out of the city into the fields and were only allowed back in the unlikely event that they recovered.[25] At this time, Ragusa (the beautiful city of Dubrovnik in Croatia) was a major seaport, trading with other ports around the Mediterranean. Naturally, this placed it at high risk of importing plague. The city's chief physician, Jacob of Padua, recommended setting up a place outside the city walls where sick people from the city were sent. Outsiders who wanted to enter Ragusa, but were suspected of being infected, also had to stay there.[26] These measures were still not enough to prevent new plague outbreaks. One of the problems was that people could be carrying the disease and be infectious before any symptoms were apparent. In 1377 the Great Council of the City therefore decided to create a stronger system with a thirty-day isolation period called a *trentino*, from the Italian word for thirty. The new laws stated that:

1. Visitors from plague-endemic areas had to stay in isolation for thirty days before they were admitted to Ragusa.
2. No one from Ragusa was permitted go to the isolation area. If they did, then they had to remain there for thirty days.
3. No one could visit the people in isolation to bring food, apart from those assigned by the Great Council to care for those being quarantined. Again, the penalty for unauthorised visits was to remain for thirty days.
4. Breaking the regulations carried a fine and a thirty-day isolation penalty.

At last, a system was in place that was able to prevent the spread of plague. Shortly afterwards, similar laws were introduced in Marseilles, Venice, Pisa and Genoa. The isolation period was also extended from thirty to forty days, so changing the name from *trentino* to *quarantino*, from the Venetian dialect word *quaranta*, which means 'forty'. Hence the name 'quarantine'.[27]

Unfortunately, when care with the quarantine regulations slipped, plague could still return: the final major outbreak of the second plague pandemic that started with the Black Death was in the French Mediterranean port of Marseille in 1720.[28] Marseille had been a major port for 2,000 years, since its foundation by Greek colonists, with much trade with the Levant, the eastern Mediterranean coast of what is now Lebanon, Syria and Israel. As such, Marseille had already been the entry point for the Black Death to France in 1348. The city rulers were therefore well aware of the danger of ships bringing disease from further east, so had set up elaborate quarantine procedures to minimise the risk, while maintaining the trade that was making the city rich. A newly arrived ship's crew and passengers first had to be inspected for signs of disease and the ship's log was checked to see whether it had recently visited any other ports known to have plague. Ships that seemed to have no disease but had been to a high-risk port were obliged to wait at islands outside the main port of Marseille. Ships suspected of being infected could be sent to a more isolated island for sixty days to see if any plague appeared. Finally, crews were admitted to the city to sell their goods and prepare for their next departure.

Despite these precautions, plague reached the city in 1720, repeating the usual pattern of starting from an infected ship, this time the *Grand Saint Antoine*, which had departed from Sidon in Lebanon, having previously called at Smyrna, Tripoli and plague-ridden Cyprus. After a Turkish passenger died on board, several crew members also fell victim, including the ship's surgeon. The ship was not allowed to enter the port of Livorno in Italy, so instead moved on to Marseille. The port authorities placed the *Grand Saint Antoine* under quarantine outside the city, despite pressure from city merchants keen to get their hands on the ship's valuable cargo.

Even though the ship was in quarantine, it only took a few days before the disease broke out in the city, possibly via flea-infested cloth unloaded from the ship.[29] The death penalty was ordered for any communication between Marseille and the rest of Provence, to try to keep the outbreak localised. A two-metre-high wall with guard posts that can still be seen, the *Mur de la peste*, was built to stop travel from infected areas. Even though the city had already built a public hospital with full-time doctors and nurses ready for plague, the numbers were far too great for them to cope. In any case, doctors who were able to treat the sick often favoured a course of emetics, diuretics and laxatives; death from dehydration typically followed.[16] Plague pits were rapidly filled with bodies and thousands of corpses lay around the city. Fifty thousand of Marseille's total population of 90,000 died over the next two years, with a similar number of casualties in nearby French regions. Plague did not spread further, however, showing that quarantine systems could control outbreaks. The quarantine and inspection system for docking ships was later strengthened.

Yunnan province is in south-west China, bordering Burma and Vietnam. In the late eighteenth century millions of Han Chinese from elsewhere in China moved to Yunnan to work as miners in the rich yet plague-infested mountains of the province. While Yunnan already had occasional localised cases of plague, the combination of the increased number of people living near infected rats, large movements of people and expanding towns triggered a new epidemic in the 1850s. At this time, the Qing dynasty was starting to lose control of the country. Fighting between Han and Muslim Chinese, and the horrific Taiping Rebellion, in which a self-declared brother of Jesus Christ, Hong Xiuquan, fought the Qing in the bloodiest civil war in history, created ideal conditions for the spread of disease. Opium traders may have brought plague to coastal cities, such as Canton (Guangzhou), where 60,000 people died in a few weeks in 1894, and Hong Kong, where 100,000 died in a few months. Plague reached India in 1896, most likely on a ship from Hong Kong. As usual, it began in port cities and then moved to rural areas across the whole region. In total, 12 million Indians died over the next thirty years. The British colonial rulers struggled to control the epidemic with quarantine, isolation camps and travel restrictions. From East Asia, plague was then taken around the world to places as far away as San Francisco, Australia, South America, Russia and Egypt, before being brought under control. This third plague pandemic gave scientists the opportunity to investigate the cause of plague, using their new science of microbiology.

Alexandre Yersin was born in Switzerland in 1863, though he later took French nationality. He worked with Louis Pasteur in Paris, helping him create his rabies vaccine, and with the German microbiologist Robert Koch. One could not get a better education in bacteriology at the time. Pasteur and Koch were pioneers in developing and promoting the germ theory of disease – that specific microorganisms are responsible for infection. Pasteur had shown that the transformation of wine and beer into vinegar was due to microorganisms and suggested that other microorganisms could cause disease. Koch was a German physician who played a leading role in discovering the causes of many infectious diseases, notably tuberculosis and cholera. His methods were later used to discover the causative organisms of many other diseases, including typhoid, diphtheria, tetanus, leprosy, gonorrhoea, syphilis, pneumonia and meningitis. Koch didn't just discover the causes of these diseases, but also proposed a set of postulates to be used to prove whether a particular microorganism caused a specific disease:

1. The microorganism must be present in every case of the disease, but not in healthy organisms.
2. The microorganism must be isolated from the host with the disease and grown in pure culture.
3. The specific disease must be reproduced when a pure culture of the microorganism is introduced into a healthy susceptible organism.
4. The microorganism must be recoverable from the experimentally infected host and shown to be identical to the original causative agent.[30]

In 1894 Yersin and Japanese bacteriologist Kitasato Shibasaburō were sent to Hong Kong to investigate the plague. They worked independently, but both used Koch's postulates as their strategy to identify the cause of plague. Kitasato was also a former pupil of Koch and had helped him to develop antitoxins for tetanus and diphtheria while working with him in Berlin. After only a few months' work in Hong Kong, both Kitasato and Yersin succeeded in taking bacteria from bubo pus of plague-victim corpses and growing them in broth cultures. When injected into mice, the bacteria replicated rapidly and the mice died. Kitasato and Yersin both announced the isolation and culture of the plague bacteria in June 1894. Even though Kitasato got there first, his cultures are suspected to have been contaminated with an additional bacterial species, while Yersin's characterisation was more thorough. The plague organism was therefore named after him in 1970 as *Yersinia pestis*.

For at least a thousand years people had suspected a connection between rats and plague. Sure enough, Yersin also noticed that the streets of Hong Kong had many dead rats and wondered whether they were also dying from plague. Paul-Louis Simond was another veteran of the Pasteur Institute in Paris. In 1897 he was sent to Bombay to continue Yersin's work. Simond found tiny fluid-filled blisters on the legs and feet of plague patients that were full of plague bacteria. He suspected that these were where the victims had been bitten by fleas that had recently fed on infected rats, so transmitting the plague from rat to human. He noticed that the fleas were exceptionally thick on rats that had just died.[31]

Simond devised a clever experiment to test his hypothesis. Firstly he caught a plague-infected rat from the house of a plague victim (bravely risking catching plague from a flea bite himself), to which he added some extra fleas from a cat to make sure it was highly infested with the parasites. The rat was placed in a large glass bottle. Once it was suffering from the last stages of plague, Simond hung a wire cage containing a healthy rat above the sandy floor of the bottle. The caged rat could not have any direct contact with the sick rat, the wall of the bottle or the sand. The sick rat died the next day. Simond left its corpse for twenty-four hours so the fleas would be compelled to leave it and look for a new home. An autopsy confirmed that the dead rat was full of *Y. pestis*. Five days later the second rat in the cage became ill and died, also from plague. Simond knew that the disease must have been transmitted from rat to rat by fleas jumping up to the rat in the cage. He was understandably thrilled, writing, 'That day, 2 June 1898, I felt an emotion that was inexpressible in the face of the thought that I had uncovered a secret that had tortured man since the appearance of plague in the world.'

Simond also correctly deduced that plague could be prevented by tackling not just infected people, but also rats and parasites.[32] Now we understand that a major outbreak of plague in humans is preceded by an outbreak in the rodent population. Once the rats start dying in large numbers, infected fleas that have lost their rodent hosts seek other sources of blood, just as in Simond's experiment.

The tragedy of the discovery of the plague bacterium is that it took so long. Microscopes that were capable of seeing bodies as small as bacteria had been available since the seventeenth century and the idea that diseases are spread by germs had been around even longer. For example, Swiss physician Felix Platter had carefully argued in his publications of 1597 and 1625 that plague and syphilis were spread by contagion and that infection by germs was an essential condition for disease.[33] Such ideas were never properly followed up experimentally for 200 years, even though the tools were available.

We now know a great deal about why a *Y. pestis* infection is so damaging, how it manages to evade and subvert our immune system, and how it evolved.[34] In particular, analysis of DNA sequences in bacteria such as *Y. pestis* is an excellent tool to compare different strains of the organism and its evolution. Bacteria normally have one copy of each gene. When they reproduce, they simply divide in two, with each having the same DNA as their parent. Bacteria can also reproduce in less than an hour under favourable conditions, giving a vast number of generations per year. Each time its DNA is copied there is a chance of changes being introduced in the sequence, with these changes being passed on to all that cell's descendants. We can therefore track how strains of bacteria spread, as each strain has a unique DNA sequence. This makes DNA-sequence comparisons extremely useful in understanding the origin and spread of plague. If we are lucky enough to find well-preserved samples, we can also sequence ancient DNA, directly analysing the bacteria that killed hundreds or thousands of years ago.

At the height of the Black Death in 1349, 200 people were dying per day in London, far too many to be buried in churchyards. Instead, burial grounds were used outside the city, such as in East Smithfield, east of the Tower of London, near the River Thames. Archaeologists from the Museum of London excavated the site in the 1980s. They found 558 burials, with most aged five to thirty-five, showing that, unusually, plague killed healthy young people, not just the elderly or infants, as with most diseases. Bodies were laid east to west, in accordance with Christian custom, with most in mass graves piled five deep and covered with charcoal to try to absorb the foul fluids oozing from the bodies.

In 2011, ancient DNA from forty-six teeth and fifty-three bones from the East Smithfield site was analysed. *Y. pestis* DNA was found in five of the teeth. The results were compared to DNA sequences from seventeen modern strains of *Y. pestis*, one of which lived in a vole, and the bacterium's close relative *Y. pseudotuberculosis*, which lives in soil. The Smithfield strain was shown to be closely related to all the modern strains associated with plague, showing that the Black Death strain was the ancestor of all present-day pathogenic strains of *Y. pestis*. Black Death has thus never really gone away (though it may have mutated). This raises the question of why it was so lethal in the past compared to now. A plague outbreak is not just due to a pathogenic organism acquiring some mutations that make it especially deadly; other conditions are also needed, such as suitable human hosts that have not evolved resistance, climate, animal populations, ease of spread of disease, living with rats and fleas, social conditions and interactions with other diseases. Europe just before the Black Death was also overpopulated relative to the food supply, with frequent famine, leaving the population malnourished and less able to resist a new disease (as we saw in Siena and will discuss further in Chapter 11).[35]

In 2013, DNA studies of two 1,500-year-old teeth from plague victims found in a German cemetery also found traces of *Y. pestis*, confirming two things: that the plague of Justinian was indeed bubonic plague, and that it had spread north, beyond the borders of the Byzantine Empire. While the role of *Y. pestis* had long been suspected from reports by ancient historians, others had speculated that it was a different disease entirely, perhaps influenza or anthrax. The two new DNA sequences were compared to a database of sequences from 131 *Y. pestis* strains from the Black Death pandemics. The two Justinian samples were closely related to each other, but substantially different from the Black Death strains. The Justinian strain is now extinct in people, as far as we know. The Justinian plague and the Black Death therefore started from two separate events where the bacterium moved from rodent to man. This would help to explain why the symptoms of the plague were slightly different each time. *Y. pestis* may also have been living in different species of rat.

The closest relative of the Justinian strain is currently living in marmots in mountains in Kyrgyzstan in Central Asia.[36,37] The ancient Silk Roads, which link China and the West, run through Kyrgyzstan. About 1,500 years ago, the Justinian strain jumped from rodent to man and then travelled along the Silk Roads, perhaps with Attila and his Huns, before eventually catastrophically exploding through the people of the Byzantine Empire.[38]

Modern methods for sequencing DNA in ancient biological samples has now shown that we have been afflicted by plague for many thousands of years before Justinian. Six thousand years ago, densely populated towns of up to 20,000 inhabitants appeared in Ukraine, Moldova and Romania, known as the Trypillia culture, named after a present-day town in the region. These were the biggest settlements that Europe had ever seen, supported by novel technologies of pottery, animal-drawn ploughs, wheels and copper-based metallurgy. People farmed wheat, barley, lentils, cattle, sheep, pigs and goats. Trading networks connected populations thousands of miles apart, though what languages they used across this vast area is unknown.

Though they did not know it, building large towns linked by traders set the stage for catastrophe. The Trypillia culture collapsed about 5,400 years ago. Towns were abandoned, burned to the ground and the population crashed, staying low for the next 1,500 years. Speculation on the cause of this Neolithic decline had centred on environmental ruin, cutting down forests, climate change, overexploiting farmland or attacks by invaders.[39] Recent ancient DNA work suggests, however, that the collapse of Neolithic culture was also due to plague.

Five thousand years ago seventy-eight people were buried in a mass grave in the Neolithic settlement at Frälsegården, Sweden. Considering the low population in Sweden at that time, this was a large number of people to be buried all at once. The absence of injuries on the skeletons suggests that they were killed by an epidemic, rather than a massacre. DNA in teeth found in the Frälsegården grave was therefore sequenced in 2019 to search for possible pathogens. An ancient strain of *Y. pestis*, named Gok2, was found in two twenty-year-olds, one male and one female. Sequence analysis of the Gok2 strain showed that it was unique to the Bronze Age.[40] Several other *Y. pestis* strains appeared and spread after Gok2 in Siberia, Estonia, Poland and Armenia,[41] coincident with the decline of Neolithic populations in Europe. Before the invention of technology that could analyse ancient DNA, we were largely relying on written records describing symptoms to identify plague as the cause of disease. The Justinian plague was therefore previously thought to be the first plague epidemic. Now, ancient DNA sequencing can detect traces of plague in bodies within cultures that left no writing. It seems likely that the Trypillia culture was another victim of a devastating plague epidemic.

The figure below shows a family tree of *Y. pestis* strains over the past 6,000 years. Gok2 and the Bronze Age lineage are the strains that caused the Neolithic decline. All became extinct more than 3,000 years ago. Below these we see modern lineages of plague that appeared thousands of years ago and are still around today. The Justinian plague was caused by two strains called DA101 and A120 – both now extinct. The bottom branch, which split from the Justinian plague 2,000 years ago, includes all other modern *Y. pestis* strains, including the Black Death.

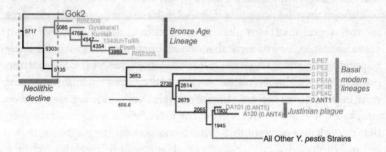

Ancient Y. pestis *strains. Numbers show the number of years before the present day.*[40]

DNA-sequencing technology is revolutionising archaeology. Whereas previously we had to use items such as pottery to identify peoples of the past, we can now analyse their DNA sequences directly to track population movements, ages and relatedness.[42] Combining these ancient DNA discoveries from both humans and *Y. pestis* with archaeology tells a story of how the Neolithic civilisation might have collapsed.[40] The Trypillia mega-settlements had high population densities and close contact with animals. Overpopulation and over-farming were causing a crisis from malnutrition and famine, weakening people's ability to fight off disease. At this time, the first case of a new strain of plague appeared, when a flea that had been feeding on an infected rat in the settlement jumped to a human. This was not the first time that someone had caught plague from a rodent. However, now it was able to spread within a few weeks to tens of thousands of people, as they were all living close together. Terrified people fled the settlement using their well-trodden trade routes, so spreading the disease across Europe and Asia. The mega-settlements typically only lasted 150 years before being abandoned, burned and rebuilt for reasons that we do not know. Perhaps these were drastic measures to try to stop plague. This massive depopulation paved the way for later migrations of people from grasslands in the east, speaking proto-Indo-European, the ancestor of nearly all European languages. Once the plague had destroyed the Neolithic culture, it became extinct in humans. Later plague epidemics therefore began with a new transmission from rodents.

Plague is still found in many parts of the world as a natural infection of rodents and their parasites. In the USA a few human cases develop each year following contact with infected wild rodents or their fleas, or, occasionally, other infected wild animals (bobcats, coyotes and rabbits) and domestic animals (cats and dogs). While most are isolated cases, epidemic plague can still happen if rats living with humans and their fleas become infected. In Africa, Asia and South America, people in rural areas can become infected from rodents; epidemics are then possible if they move to urban areas, particularly when social order is breaking down due to war, sanitation is failing and many people are on the move. Plague can be successfully cured with antibiotics. However, some strains of *Y. pestis* are now showing antibiotic resistance. Occasionally, a bacterium will have a mutation that means that it is not killed by an antibiotic – perhaps it has an enzyme that can break down the chemical structure of the drug or a transport protein that can pump the drug out of the cell. When this happens, all the other bacteria will be killed by the antibiotic and the mutant survivor will replicate, creating a new population in which the antibiotic does not work. This is natural selection in action; every antibiotic will lose effectiveness eventually. The fact that new, lethal strains have jumped from rodents to humans at least three times implies that it can readily happen again. Total elimination of the disease is unlikely to ever take place, due to its presence on every continent except Australia and Antarctica, and in many different species of rodent host.

Plague vaccines are available but are generally only given to people at particularly high risk – most obviously health workers or researchers working with live *Y. pestis*. Developing a plague vaccine has followed two strategies. First, vaccines made from dead cells were produced by inactivating *Y. pestis* by heating or with chemicals. These vaccines were safe and gave immunity against bubonic plague but were ineffective against pneumonic plague in animal models. Second, new non-lethal strains of *Y. pestis* could be developed by growing colonies for long periods and then using them as a vaccine. These types of vaccines work well against both bubonic and pneumonic plague, but they always carry the risk that introducing live bacteria could allow new colonies to replicate in people. Many fatal cases have been seen in laboratory animals and in non-human primates after vaccination with live vaccines, though none so far in people. We still need a better plague vaccine.[43] Research in this area is not easy, as it is hardly ethical to deliberately infect people with plague – hence, we are short of subjects to test potential cures on.

Plague is currently not a major cause of death. From 2010 to 2015 only 3,248 cases were reported worldwide, which led to 584 deaths, with the Democratic Republic of the Congo, Madagascar and Peru being the highest-risk countries. We cannot be complacent about the deadliest infectious disease ever to afflict humanity, however. As *Y. pestis* is living in many rodent species around the planet, it is not possible to make the bacterium extinct. People will always be bitten by fleas. Bacteria evolve fast and new deadly strains could appear. We know that *Y. pestis* can be converted into new strains that are antibiotic resistant by genetic manipulations in the laboratory[44] and that antibiotic resistance is beginning to appear in the wild.[45] Potentially, a new strain, deliberately created to be resistant to antibiotics, could be used for biological warfare, returning us to something resembling the horrors of the siege of Caffa in 1346.

Despite the impressive powers of modern medicine, we remain at risk from epidemics. New strains of deadly bacteria and viruses can easily evolve to be resistant to antibiotics and other therapies. Thanks to air travel, they could spread around the planet and kill far faster than we could devise and implement any cure or vaccine. The coronavirus outbreak of 2020 is only the most recent example of this inevitable outcome. After all, from the point of view of bacteria and viruses, 7.9 billion people is simply a vast potential food source.

5

The Milkmaid's Hand

Smallpox is a highly contagious and often fatal infectious disease spread by coughing and sneezing. Sharing contaminated clothing or bedding can also lead to infection, as poor Esther Summerson discovers in Charles Dickens's novel *Bleak House*, when, through an act of charity, she catches it. Thirty per cent of people who caught the disease died. Survivors usually had permanent scarring, once the extensive blisters had healed. Parts of lips, ears and the nose could also be lost. Blindness was common, as a result of corneal scarring. Smallpox still has no cure, though you can only ever get it once.

Smallpox is caused by the *Variola* virus, which most likely evolved from an African rodent virus and transferred to humans about 10,000 years ago, when agriculture started in north-eastern Africa.[1,2] Scars resembling those of smallpox have been found on the faces of mummies from the time of the eighteenth and twentieth Egyptian dynasties (1570–1085 BCE), including the head of Pharaoh Ramses V.[3] What seems to be smallpox was described in 1122 BCE in China and is mentioned in ancient Sanskrit texts from India at around the same time.

Smallpox reached Europe about 1,500 years ago, though at first it was just one of many childhood illnesses. In the early seventeenth century, for unknown reasons, it became endemic in adults as well.[4] In the eighteenth century in Europe, 400,000 people died annually from smallpox, and one-third of the survivors went blind.[2] The fatality rate varied from 20 to 60 per cent in adults and was even worse in infants, approaching 80 per cent in London and an astonishing 98 per cent in Berlin during the late 1800s.[2] Wealth and power were no defence: Louis XV of France, Mary II of England, Peter II of Russia, the Chinese Shunzhi Emperor and Maria Theresa of Austria all died of smallpox. Josef Stalin caught it as a seven-year-old. When ruling the Soviet Union, he had photographs altered to hide his scars. Similarly, Queen Elizabeth I of England caught smallpox at the age of twenty-nine. Afterwards, she made heavy use of make-up, wigs and flattering painters to hide her scars and hair loss.

An ancient way of preventing smallpox was variolation, where the smallpox virus was deliberately given to non-immune individuals. A blade was used to transfer fresh matter from a ripe pustule into the arms or legs of the recipient to give them immunity. Variolation seems to have been independently discovered several times in Europe, Africa, India and China.[2] In 1670, traders from Circassia, west of the Caucasus mountains north of Iran, introduced variolation to the Turkish Ottoman Empire. Families in Circassia were often keen for their daughters to get a position in the sultan's harem in Istanbul to live a life of indolent luxury and perhaps be the mother of the next sultan, so they practised variolation to avoid smallpox scarring. This helped give women from the Caucasus a reputation for beauty.

Lady Mary Wortley Montagu was the wife of the British ambassador to the Ottoman Empire in 1717. After observing variolation, she had her young children successfully treated in the same way. After Lady Montagu's return to England, the process was tested on six prisoners who had been sentenced to death. The lucky prisoners were all unharmed when deliberately infected by smallpox and were granted their freedom. Variolation then became widespread in England and in a few other European countries, such as Russia, where the Empress Catherine the Great and her son Tsar Paul I were treated by a visiting English physician in the late eighteenth century. The French King Louis XV died of smallpox in May 1776; one month later, his successor and grandson Louis XVI was inoculated.[2]

While variolation was a success, a better alternative was still needed, as it had two major flaws. First, the insertion of live smallpox virus was a risky procedure: about 2 per cent of recipients of the live virus died and other diseases could be transferred via blood. Second, while individuals who had received the treatment were better off, the rest of the population was not, as they could catch smallpox from these new carriers. A better idea was to administer a mild disease that could give protection against a different, more deadly one.

In eighteenth-century England, milkmaids had a reputation for beauty and sexuality,[5] and were frequently used as artists' models, as their work seemed to make them immune to smallpox and its subsequent scarring. See *Landscape with Milkmaid* by Thomas Gainsborough as an example. In 1796 a milkmaid called Sarah Nelmes came to Edward Jenner, a country doctor from Gloucestershire, with a rash on her right hand. Sarah told Jenner that one of her Gloucester cows called Blossom had recently been infected with cowpox. Jenner knew that milkmaids often developed blisters on their hands after working with cow udders that were infected with cowpox. Sarah had most pustules on the part of her hand that handled Blossom's udder.[6] It was widely believed that milkmaids never got smallpox due to exposure to cowpox, but Jenner resolved to test the old wives' tale directly. He extracted some pus from the blisters on Sarah's hands, which he proceeded to inject into eight-year-old James Phipps, the son of his gardener, giving him a mild case of cowpox. Phipps was then deliberately injected with smallpox on multiple occasions. Fortunately, he was unharmed.

Jenner followed up this promising result on a hundred other children and himself, again with complete success. In 1798, Jenner published his findings in a book entitled *An Inquiry into the Causes and Effects of Variolae Vaccinae*[6] and named his procedure 'vaccination', after the Latin word for cow: *vacca*. Cowpox pus was tricky to collect in quantity, transport and keep active, so he developed ways to preserve dried material that could be sent to doctors at home and abroad. The British government rewarded Jenner with the huge sum of £30,000 (equivalent to about £4 million today). Even Napoleon, not normally the greatest fan of the British, sent tributes and presents to Jenner.

Jenner was not the first person to try vaccination – it seems that at least six people had used cowpox to protect against smallpox before Jenner's first trial in 1796, though none had much impact. First of all may have been a farmer from Dorset in south-west England, called Benjamin Jesty.[7] Jesty knew two milkmaids who had attended relatives who were suffering from smallpox, but who escaped the disease themselves. To protect his family, and displaying outstanding confidence, he inoculated his wife and young sons using a knitting needle and material from a neighbour's cows that were infected with cowpox. He did not treat himself, as he knew that he had already had cowpox. After the treatment, pustules appeared on the boys' arms, while Mrs Jesty's arm also became inflamed, making her ill. Nevertheless, all recovered and never caught smallpox, despite later exposure decades later. Jesty's actions were not well received in Dorset, and he became a target for scorn, derision and abuse. Understandably, he was reluctant to get publicity for his idea. However, in 1805, upon hearing of Jenner's work and how he had been rewarded, the Rector of Swanage, Andrew Bell, wrote to the Original Vaccine Pock Institute in London, telling them that Jesty was the first vaccinator. This led to Jesty travelling to the Institute in 1805, where he was honoured by having his portrait painted.[8]

Jenner was taken more seriously than Jesty due to his professional training and credentials as a doctor. Most importantly, he was the first to get vaccination used extensively, thanks to his widely translated book, prolific correspondence and efforts to distribute the vaccine. Publication is critical in science – discoveries are of no use if no one hears about them. Jenner's rather lovely house in Gloucestershire is now a museum,[9] with the hut where he used to vaccinate local children still standing in the garden.

Vaccination was rapidly adopted in Spain, with thousands of people treated by the end of 1801. The Spanish were also keen to use vaccination in their vast territories in Central and South America, where up to half of infected people were likely to die and quarantine was unenforceable. Unfortunately, vaccine preparations degraded during long voyages in tropical weather, so a new method for getting cowpox across the Atlantic was needed. The solution they adopted was to transmit the vaccine in human bodies, specifically orphan boys aged three to nine. Every ninth or tenth day, material from pustules was used to transmit the vaccine to a previously uninfected pair of boys. This chain kept the vaccine active and viable for the duration of the two-month voyage. The expedition arrived in Caracas, Venezuela in 1804, to scenes of wild celebration. Fresh recruits were vaccinated, and the party divided, so that the vaccine could be brought to Mexico, Peru, Chile and Cuba. After immunising over 100,000 people in Mexico, mostly children, Dr Francisco Xavier de Balmis led a mission across the Pacific to the Philippines, using twenty-six Mexican boys as vaccine carriers. In China, Balmis brought the vaccine to the Portuguese colony of Macao. On the same day in 1805 that British and Spanish sailors were killing each other at the Battle of Trafalgar, Balmis teamed up with the British East India Company to save lives by setting up a vaccination centre in China, before returning to rewards and honours in Spain. All in all, within ten years of Jenner's discovery, the smallpox vaccine had travelled the world, thanks to the work of dedicated men like Balmis, government and societal support, and the help of a few dozen young vaccine carriers.[10, 11]

Bavaria was the first nation to make vaccination compulsory in 1807. Smallpox variolation was made illegal in Britain in 1840 and vaccination compulsory. Despite this, a few cases persisted into the twentieth century, due to vaccination being performed incorrectly or infected ship passengers bringing smallpox back into Britain at ports. Vaccination programmes were the responsibility of individual countries, so could be erratic or even non-existent, allowing the virus to persist. What was needed was a coordinated plan across the world to tackle the disease. In 1959 the World Health Organization instigated a plan to rid the world of smallpox. At first the campaign was short of funds, personnel, commitment and vaccine. Smallpox was still common in 1966, causing regular outbreaks in South America, Africa and Asia.

The WHO Intensified Eradication Program began in 1967 using better quality freeze-dried vaccine in much larger quantities, new types of needle, a surveillance system to detect and investigate cases, and mass-vaccination campaigns. By this time, smallpox had already been eradicated in North America (in 1952) and Europe (1953), leaving South America, Asia and Africa (smallpox was never common in Australia). By 1971 smallpox was eradicated from South America, followed by Asia (1975), and finally Africa (1977). Rahima Banu, a three-year-old girl from Bangladesh, was the last person in Asia to have active smallpox in 1975. Her case was reported by an eight-year-old girl. Rahima was kept in isolation, with guards posted outside her home round the clock until she was no longer infectious. Everyone on the island where she lived, within a 1.5-mile radius of her home, was vaccinated immediately. Each house, area where people might congregate, school and healer within five miles was visited by a member of the Smallpox Eradication Program team to check for any more cases. None were found, and Rahima made a full recovery.

Ali Maow Maalin, a hospital cook and health worker in Merca, Somalia, was the last person to have naturally acquired smallpox, caught when he accompanied two patients on a ten-minute journey from the hospital to the local smallpox office in 1977. Somalia was an especially difficult place to work at that time, as much of its population was nomadic. Huge measures were used to contain the potential outbreak in Merca: 161 people that Maalin had been in contact with were identified, forty-one of whom had not been vaccinated. All were treated, along with their families, and monitored for six weeks. Merca Hospital was closed to new patients, its staff were all vaccinated, and existing patients were kept inside. Residents of the part of town where Maalin lived were vaccinated, and searches were carried out through the town to look for any additional cases. The police prevented anyone leaving town, and vaccinated new arrivals who had not been recently immunised. Overall, 54,777 people were vaccinated in the two weeks following Maalin's diagnosis. The last person to die was a six-year-old girl named Habiba Nur Ali, who had been part of the family group that Maalin met. The containment efforts worked, and on 17 April 1978 the WHO was able to declare, 'Search complete. No cases discovered. Ali Maow Maalin is the world's last known smallpox case.' Two years later and nearly 200 years after Jenner, the WHO announced that the world was free from smallpox, perhaps the single greatest achievement in international public health.

In 2018, the US Food and Drug Administration (FDA) approved the first drug to treat smallpox in humans, called TPOXX.[12] However, given that smallpox has now thankfully vanished, why would a drug company bother to develop a cure for it? Because, horrifyingly, smallpox might return. First, because the DNA sequence of the virus is in the public domain and, using modern chemical technology, it is quite possible to synthesise and mass-produce the virus – a common theme in thriller literature. It may even be possible to engineer it to be even more deadly. And, secondly, because the virus still exists. We know it is stored in the US Centers for Disease Control and Prevention in Atlanta, Georgia, and in its Russian counterpart (VECTOR) near Novosibirsk. Perhaps other secret stocks exist. The virus might accidentally infect a worker at these centres (as happened in

Birmingham, England in 1978, when a lab worker died after accidental exposure to the virus) or even be released deliberately. Finally, an intact virus might be present in frozen corpses in the Arctic. A close encounter with a recently thawed body might cause re-infection. All of which goes to show we can never be totally complacent about a disease that has already killed hundreds of millions of people.

For a drug to be approved, it is normally necessary to show that it works in infected humans, compared to a control group given a dummy pill. As no human has had smallpox for forty years, and it would not be ethical (to say the least) to infect anyone deliberately to see whether the drug works, this drug has never been tested on people. The FDA therefore took the rare step of approving TPOXX when it had only been shown to work in monkeys and rabbits infected with related monkeypox and rabbitpox.

The smallpox story is of immense importance for several reasons. Most obviously, a horrific disease that killed 400 million people in the twentieth century is now extinct. The success of the WHO eradication programme showed that if the entire world cooperates, it is possible to wipe out a lethal disease. Smallpox remains the only disease for which this has been achieved, though we are close with polio, which is now only present in Afghanistan and Pakistan.[13] Finally, it proved the value of the strategy of vaccination, where exposure of someone to a mild form of a disease or to parts of an infectious microbe or virus stimulates the production of antibodies so that the body is ready to fight off future infection. Once a vaccine has been developed, mass-producing and administering it is cheap, easy and highly effective.

Despite the brilliance of Jesty's and Jenner's work, it remained a one-off for more than fifty years. The idea of catching one disease to prevent getting another didn't seem to generalise beyond cowpox and smallpox. It was not until the 1870s that the French microbiologist Louis Pasteur further developed the technique by using killed or weakened pathogens to protect against anthrax and rabies. By far the greatest inventor of vaccines was the American microbiologist Maurice Hilleman. His team developed more than forty vaccines, mostly while working for American pharmaceutical company Merck, including eight of major importance, still used today for measles, mumps, hepatitis A, hepatitis B, chickenpox, meningitis, pneumonia and *Haemophilus influenzae* bacteria. His strategy was usually to grow a virus in cultured cells until it had mutated to produce a weakened, non-dangerous version that was still able to generate an immune response. Hilleman's vaccines currently save over 8 million lives a year. In total, he saved more lives than any other person of the twentieth century.

Table 10 (below) shows some data illustrating how effective vaccination is, comparing death rates before and after vaccination was introduced for ten diseases in the USA. The colossal benefits are obvious. Still, some people continue to oppose vaccination, sometimes even by publishing fraudulent scientific papers for financial gain,[14] aided and abetted by scaremongering newspapers.[15]

How generally applicable is the vaccine concept? Can we invent vaccines against any disease? We have already found dozens of highly effective vaccines and continue to find more, like those for Ebola in

TABLE 10 *Deaths from infectious disease before and after vaccination in the USA, 2017.*[16]

Disease	Pre-vaccine deaths per year in the twentieth century	Deaths per year in 2017	Percentage decrease
Diphtheria	21,053	0	100%
H. influenzae	20,000	22	>99%
Smallpox	29,005	0	100%
Congenital rubella syndrome	152	2	99%
Measles	530,217	122	>99%
Mumps	162,344	5,629	97%
Whooping cough	200,752	15,808	92%
Polio	16,316	0	100%
Tetanus	580	31	95%
Rubella	47,745	9	>99%

2019[17] and Covid-19 in 2020. The technology is well established – many of the vaccines that are used today are decades old.

Unfortunately, some diseases are especially difficult to vaccinate against. Sometimes immunity is short-lived, whereas we are looking for the effect of a vaccine to last for a lifetime, or decades at least. Some pathogenic organisms mutate very rapidly, to a point where new strains are no longer recognised by the antibodies generated by a vaccine. Bacteria and viruses can replicate in hours, giving thousands of generations per year in which to pick up mutations. Viruses that use RNA instead of DNA as their genetic material (like HIV) mutate more easily. Hence, the parts of the organisms recognised by antibodies can acquire changes, purely by chance, that allow them to evade the immune system.

The influenza virus is a prime candidate to produce another great epidemic that could dwarf the impact of Covid-19. It mutates every year, changing the surface proteins where antibodies bind, thus evading vaccination. The most widespread disease event in history took place between the spring of 1918 and early 1919. An astonishing 50 million died in this brief time, with hundreds of millions becoming sick. The infection swept the whole planet in three waves, with the first cases possibly originating in Haskell County, Kansas in early 1918. This influenza pandemic was known as the Spanish flu, though American flu or Kansas flu would have been more accurate names. One month later it had reached Western Europe, brought by the American army, now being transported in large numbers to European battlefields. By June it had spread remarkably quickly as far as China, Australia, India and Southeast Asia. In June, half a million German soldiers were ill with the new strain of flu, ending any chance of continuing their advances on the Western Front. After years of poor diet, their resistance was lower than the comparatively well-fed Allied troops, and 175,000 German civilians therefore died of Spanish flu during the final few months of the war. In August a new wave appeared in France, which soon reached places as distant as Alaska, Siberia and the Pacific Islands. What was particularly nasty about this strain was that it was especially severe for young adults, such as soldiers. Normally infants and the elderly are worst affected by epidemics. With Spanish flu it was the opposite, perhaps because the older generation had acquired some resistance from earlier flu outbreaks.[18] The war made the epidemic worse by facilitating its travel around the world by sea and by spreading infection in large crowds, regularly gathered in army camps, or for rallies and speeches.

So how did the Spanish flu originate? Modern sequencing methods have revolutionised our understanding of viral evolution. Fast mutation of the virus makes it possible to compare different strains, so we can see how it spreads year by year. Thousands of flu RNA genome sequences are now available. The flu virus affects chickens and pigs, as well as humans. What seems to have happened is that in about 1905 a strain of flu called H1 jumped from birds to humans. H1 wasn't a big problem, but in 1917 the human H1 picked up some new variants of genes from an N1 strain in birds. It was this new H1N1 strain that was deadly. Humans then passed H1N1 on to pigs and H1N1 mutated again to a less lethal form a few years later, making the Spanish flu epidemic short-lived.[19]

A second crisis like Spanish flu in 1919 was narrowly averted in 1957, when another influenza epidemic broke out in Hong Kong, infecting 250,000 people. Maurice Hilleman took charge, suspecting that a new strain of flu was responsible. He got hold of blood samples infected with what became known as Asian flu. His team purified the Hong Kong virus and tested it with antibodies obtained from people's blood from elsewhere around the world. Almost none of the antibodies from the global blood samples could recognise the new virus. A new worldwide flu epidemic was therefore likely to happen, as very few people had immunity against the new strain. With worldwide travel and the high infectivity of flu, it was only a matter of time before it broke out from Hong Kong.

Hilleman sounded the alarm. A new vaccine needed to be developed urgently. He therefore sent the virus to several vaccine manufacturers, so that they could grow the virus in chicken eggs. In time, the virus adapted, picking up mutations that made it more at home in chickens and less suited to humans. Eventually the virus developed into a strain that was not dangerous when given to humans. However, antibodies generated against this chicken strain in people were also able to recognise the original Asian flu virus. The chicken strain of the virus was therefore the vaccine that they had been searching for. When Asian flu reached the USA in 1957, the manufacturers had already made 40 million flu vaccines, so could protect the most vulnerable people just in time. By the end of 1958, 69,000 people had died of Asian flu in the USA. Without the swift work of Hilleman and his teams, the number would have been far higher.[20] New strains of flu are sure to strike again. If we are unable to create, make and distribute new vaccines quickly enough, many millions of deaths will follow.

Vaccination relies on prior exposure to a pathogen generating immunity to future infection. With some organisms this simply doesn't work. For example, gonorrhoea is caused by *Neisseria gonorrhoeae* bacteria and can be cured by antibiotics, though resistance is a growing problem.[21] Someone can catch gonorrhoea over and over again, even if they have been infected previously. The human immune system cannot generate immunity against *Neisseria gonorrhoeae*: the surface of the bacterium that is recognised by antibodies is highly variable, and the gonorrhoea bacterium sneakily interferes with the normal course of an immune response. Pathogens often have cunning ways to hide from our immune systems. They might suppress the immune response, so they are not cleared, allowing them to replicate. Therefore, while vaccination is undoubtedly a marvellous way to prevent many deadly infections, it cannot deal with all of them. The war between people and infectious disease will never end.

6

Typhus and Typhoid in the Slums of Liverpool

Crowded cities have been hubs of disease from the start of civilisation. Access to clean water for drinking, cooking and washing, and disposal of human waste are particular problems for city dwellers reliant on rivers and rain. While water acquisition and disposal might be manageable for cities with populations of no more than a few tens of thousands, relying on natural watercourses could become hopelessly inadequate when city population densities and absolute numbers began to rise rapidly. Typhoid and typhus, in particular, became widespread when poor, undernourished people from lower socioeconomic backgrounds were packed in slum housing in the first industrial cities.

Britain was the first country to undergo the Industrial Revolution, transforming the country with steam power, machine tools in factories, and new methods to produce iron and chemicals. Britain thus stands as an excellent historical example of how premature death soared as a result of industrialisation, and how infectious diseases like typhus and typhoid were slowly brought under control. The problems that first arose in Britain often show up in other countries undergoing the same switch from an economy based on agriculture to one based on industry. The cities of Liverpool and Manchester in Lancashire are particularly informative as they became the most advanced manufacturing and port cities in the world in the first half of the nineteenth century.

The first precise census in the UK was undertaken in 1801, recording data on the numbers of people, occupations, baptisms, marriages, burials and houses. The total population was 10,942,646, with 30 per cent living in towns and cities.[1] Most people worked on the land, as they had always done, though dramatic changes in the ways they lived had already started to take place.

The textiles industry was a main driver in Lancashire. New inventions to increase the production of cotton and wool products enabled a switch from the work being done by hand in people's homes (literally a cottage industry) to mechanised mills. Iron production using coal instead of wood was developed in Coalbrookdale in Shropshire, culminating in the construction of the first cast-iron bridge across the Severn in 1779. Water power in the first factories was replaced by coal-powered steam engines.

Prior to the Industrial Revolution, families often spun yarn and wove cloth to make their own clothing or to sell. These traditional practices could not compete with the new manufacturing methods being set up in cities like Manchester. With work in the countryside collapsing, people poured into the cities. Manchester expanded from 75,000 people in 1801 to 645,000 in 1901. West of Manchester, the city and port of Liverpool grew at an even greater rate. Facing the Atlantic, Liverpool was ideally located to trade with North America and the West Indies and to export the products of Manchester and other industrial cities. The world's first wet dock, capable of handling a hundred ships, was built in Liverpool in 1715. Liverpool became a major centre for the slave trade, starting with one slave ship in 1699, then increasing to 40 per cent of the world's slave trade a hundred years later. The population increased from 4,240 in 1700 to 80,000 in 1800, making it the second largest city in Britain after London, a position it held for sixty years until overtaken by Glasgow. A canal was built to link Liverpool to Manchester in 1721, followed by the world's first railway between cities in 1830. By the mid-nineteenth century Britain dominated world trade, with Liverpool taking a leading role. While this boom generated great wealth and power, it also created enormous health and social problems.

From 1801 to 1901 the population of Liverpool leapt again from 82,000 to 704,000. The largest increase was in the late 1840s, when vast numbers of people travelled across the Irish Sea to escape the horrors of the Irish Potato Famine. Nearly 300,000 Irish people arrived in the year 1847 alone, making the city 25 per cent Irish-born by 1851 and creating the distinct Scouse accent. The British government at the time thought it had no obligation to provide for the health, education and general well-being of its citizens; government's two principal functions were to defend the realm and to administer justice. Housing the enormous numbers of desperate people moving to the new cities for work was not in its remit. Local government also had little concern for public health measures, such as providing sewerage and drinking water. In 1848 *The Economist* criticised attempts to improve public sanitation: 'Suffering and evil are nature's admonitions; they cannot be got rid of; and the impatient attempts of benevolence to banish them from the world by legislation ... have always been more productive of evil than good.'[2]

The need for housing was filled by exploitative slum landlords, who housed families in appalling conditions. In Liverpool in 1800, 7,000 people were living in cellars, never meant for habitation, and 9,000 in enclosed 'courts' (small houses built off dark, narrow courtyards) with little or no sanitation. Sewers, if they existed, were designed only to drain rainwater from the surface, rather than remove human waste from households. This instead went into buckets or cesspools in basements to be emptied by night-soil men (usually women) who carried carts slopping with human waste to the countryside to sell as fertiliser. The night-soil men required payment, something that the slum inhabitants often did not have. Privies were often simply emptied into the courts or streets, where children played. Cellars, where families might be living, were often deep in raw sewage.

In 1847 William Duncan was appointed as Liverpool's (and Britain's) first medical officer of health. A single part-time post to deal with the health needs of the entire city was deemed all that was necessary. Duncan believed that disease was spread by foul air. While mistaken, this belief did correctly point him in the right direction of improving sanitation and cleanliness to improve public health. After surveying the slum housing, Duncan reported that Liverpool was the unhealthiest town in England. As many as 55,000 people lived in court housing, at an average of more than five people per dwelling. Fifty or sixty people could sometimes be found sharing a single four-room house. Another 20,168 people were living in 6,294 cellars with no water, sanitation or fresh air. Only four miles of sewers served twenty miles of working-class streets. He described one cellar with a well of sewage four feet deep, above which was the family bed.[3]

Rural life 200 years ago was hard and often desperately poor, but it was still a great deal healthier than life in the city. Bread was the staple food, with any kind of meat a rarity. A typical evening meal might be dumplings made from flour and water – nothing else. In contrast, the rich lived mainly on meat, especially beef or lamb. Dairy products and green vegetables were looked down on, while root vegetables were simply fodder for peasants.[4] Malnutrition was therefore rampant. In 1843 social reformer Edwin Chadwick reported the following average ages of death in Liverpool, Manchester and the rural county of Rutland (Table 11, below).[5] While it was good to be rich (and this is still true), it was more important for your health to live in the countryside rather than in an industrial city. Even farm labourers in Rutland lived longer than the gentry in Liverpool.

These data do not, of course, mean that all working-class people only lived to be fifteen. Rather, the shockingly low life expectancy (comparable to the plague- and famine-ridden fourteenth century) was driven by the death of children, with more than 20 per cent dying before their first birthdays.

People in the first industrial cities were certainly dying young, but what were they dying of? Overwhelmingly, it was infectious disease. Major killers were: tuberculosis, scarlet fever, pneumonia, cholera, typhoid, smallpox, measles, whooping cough, typhus and childbed fever. Table 12 (opposite) shows the numbers dying from these diseases from 1840 (the first year in which data was accurately recorded) to 1910. Cholera is excluded from the table, as it appeared in

TABLE 11 *Life expectancies in England in 1843.*

Area		Life expectancy (years)	
	Professionals	Tradesmen	Labourers
Rutland	52	41	38
Liverpool	35	22	15
Manchester	38	20	17

TABLE 12 *Deaths from infectious diseases[6] and life expectancy in England and Wales, 1840–1910.[7]*

Disease				Year				
	1840	*1850*	*1860*	*1870*	*1880*	*1890*	*1900*	*1910*
Smallpox	10,876	4,753	2,882	2,857	651	16	85	19
Typhus				3,520	611	151	29	5
Typhoid	19,040	15,435	14,084	9,185	7,160	5,146	5,591	1,889
Scarlet fever	21,377	14,756	10,578	34,628	18,703	6,974	3,844	2,370
Whooping cough	6,352	8,285	8,956	12,518	14,103	13,756	11,467	8,797
Measles	9,566	7,332	9,805	7,986	13,690	12,614	12,710	8,302
Pneumonia	19,083	21,138	26,586	25,147	27,099	40,373	44,300	39,760
Tuberculosis	63,870	50,202	55,345	57,973	51,711	48,366	42,987	36,334
Childbed fever	3,204	3,478	3,409	4,027	3,492	4,255	4,455	2,806
Life expectancy (males)	40	40		41	44	44	48	51
Life expectancy (females)	42	42		45	47	48	52	55

four severe epidemics and was otherwise absent in most years. Typhus and typhoid, which have similar symptoms, were not distinguished until 1869.

Table 12 shows that smallpox and typhus were almost eliminated by the start of the twentieth century and that scarlet fever and typhoid were heading the same way. The situation was even better than the raw numbers suggest, as the population had expanded rapidly over this period, so deaths per person were falling even faster. This is reflected in substantial increases in life expectancy of eleven years for males and thirteen for females.

How did the Victorians succeed against infectious disease? Smallpox, typhus, typhoid and childbed fever were all tackled successfully in the nineteenth century, though using different strategies.

Typhus is caused by infection with bacteria called *Rickettsia* and its relatives. It is spread from person to person by body lice, a human parasite. Lice lay eggs in clothing, commonly in seams, which feed on blood once hatched. Without human blood, they die. If a louse feeds on a human who carries *Rickettsia*, then the louse is infected. Bacteria grow in the louse's gut and are excreted in its faeces. The disease can be transmitted to an uninfected human when the lice move to a new host who scratches the itchy louse bite and rubs the faeces into the wound. Symptoms start one to two weeks after infection and include headaches, fever, cough, rash, severe muscle pain, chills, low blood pressure, stupor, sensitivity to light, delirium, and death in 10–40 per cent of cases without treatment.

Typhus thrives in the worst depths of misery and degradation, where infestation with lice is common, such as in prisons and in war. Malnutrition, overcrowding and a lack of hygiene pave the way for typhus. During Napoleon's disastrous retreat from Moscow in 1812, which wiped out the largest army ever assembled in Europe at that time, typhus killed more of his soldiers than the Russians. They were especially vulnerable to disease as they were hungry, cold and exhausted on their long march back.

Antibiotics and a typhus vaccine were not available in the nineteenth century. Instead, typhus could be tackled by abolishing the squalid conditions in which people lived, sharing lice living in their dirty clothing. In 1847, for example, nearly 60,000 people in Liverpool contracted typhus, as thousands of Irish people poured into the city. Victims were housed in large sheds, warehouses and hospital ships. Some had become infected on the packed ships that brought immigrants across the Irish Sea, while others caught the disease in their overcrowded and unsanitary new living quarters.[8] If their only accommodation was a patch of floor in a filthy cellar, there was little chance of being able to wash clothes.

The first washhouse for the poor of Liverpool was opened in 1832 by Kitty Wilkinson, an Irish immigrant. She had the only boiler in her neighbourhood, so invited those with clothes or sheets suspected to be infected to use it, charging a penny a week. Boiling and using chloride of lime killed bacteria and cleaned the clothes and bedding. Her views on the importance of cleanliness in combating disease were supported by the public, who made donations to fund a public bath and washhouse in Liverpool. Huge demand led to more washhouses and baths opening shortly after. Poor women of the city now had places where they could clean clothes each week. Kitty became known as the Saint of the Slums.[9] By the end of the nineteenth century, diseases of filthy clothes such as typhus were nearly eradicated.

The connection between lice infestation and typhus was first made by French bacteriologist Charles Nicolle.[10] He realised that patients were no longer infectious if they had had a hot bath and a change of clothes, so reasoned that it was their clothing, or, more accurately, the parasites living in it, that was spreading the disease. In 1909 he infected a chimpanzee with typhus and was able to transmit the disease to a healthy chimp using only lice. While Nicolle did not succeed in creating a vaccine, his discoveries led to delousing stations being set up on the Western Front in the First World War to eradicate lice from soldiers' uniforms using insecticides. Life was grimmer on the Eastern Front, where soldiers would try to burn lice eggs in the seams of the filthy uniforms that they had to wear for months on end. Here, during the last two years of the conflict, and during the Bolshevik Revolution and Russian Civil War, approximately 2.5 million deaths from typhus were recorded.

After the First World War, Rudolf Weigl, a Polish biologist, developed a vaccine by extracting and grinding up the guts from infected lice into a paste – a dangerous procedure, as it had a high risk of infecting those who were working on it. Weigl himself caught typhus, though he recovered. After the invasion of Poland by Germany in September 1939, and then the breaking of the Nazi-Soviet Non-aggression Pact, the Germans allowed Weigl to keep working at his institute, so that he could mass-produce his vaccine for Wehrmacht soldiers fighting against the Soviet Union. Weigl despised the Nazis, so he and his team secretly made a less effective version of his vaccine for the German army while smuggling 30,000 full-strength doses to the Jewish ghettoes of Warsaw and Lwów.[11] Ten years later, American Herald Cox invented a safer vaccine by growing *Rickettsia* in egg yolks.[12] Nowadays, typhus is readily treated with antibiotics.

Typhoid was long confused with typhus, as its symptoms are quite similar. Indeed, the name typhoid means 'resembling or characteristic of typhus'. The causes, transmission, pathology and treatment of these diseases are different, however. Typhoid is caused by *Salmonella* bacteria, caught by drinking or eating contaminated food or water, rather than from lice-infested clothing. People with acute illness can contaminate the surrounding water supply through faeces, which contain a high concentration of the bacteria. Bacteria in water can then spread to food. It is also possible to be a carrier of the infection without symptoms. Typhoid in cities such as Liverpool was therefore a disease of dirty water. Given the vile conditions in court housing, it is hardly surprising that typhus and typhoid were common.

Despite the lack of any good treatments for disease, substantial reductions in their death rates were made in cities such as Liverpool.[6] After William Duncan published his analysis of the appalling living conditions in Liverpool slums in the 1840s, action began to be taken. In 1846 Liverpool Town Council (Liverpool was not officially granted city status until 1880) passed an Act for the Improvement of the Sewerage and Drainage of the Borough of Liverpool. For the first time, regulations were set out for minimum standards for the construction of dwellings. Living in cellars or building houses without drains or privies was banned. Public sewers, which had previously been intended to cope only with the drainage of rainwater, were also allowed to be connected to house drains. Armed with these new powers and his position of medical officer for health, Duncan began to improve housing. By 1851 he had used inspections and the law to move inhabitants from 10,000 cellars. From 1847 to 1858 the Liverpool sewage system expanded from 30 to 146 miles. The council bought out three private water companies so that they could improve the supply for washing, cooking and sewers. Immediate success was apparent, because when cholera returned in 1854, it was far less deadly than five years before. The pioneering and tireless work of Dr Duncan had transformed Liverpool, setting an example of how life for the poor should be improved.

Today, vaccines for typhoid are available for people living or travelling to high-risk areas. They are often ineffective, however, as various strains of the bacteria exist and vaccines do not protect against all of them;[13] treatment with antibiotics might therefore also be required. Encouragingly, the typhoid-causing strain of *Salmonella* can only live in humans, unlike most bacteria. This raises the possibility of totally eradicating the *Salmonella typhi* strain, if we can only remove it from every human host. Currently, India has the highest number of cases of typhoid. The WHO is driving a vaccination programme in high-incidence areas, following the example of smallpox. While this is useful, it will not be enough by itself to eliminate the disease, as stopping its spread from infected people is also needed. Nevertheless, we have successfully reduced infectious diseases like typhoid and typhus to shadows of what they once were.

7

The Blue Death

Cholera, the most terrifying disease of the nineteenth century, entered Britain for the first time in 1831, brought by ship to the north-east port of Sunderland. While cholera had tormented people in India for thousands of years, it was only when it reached Europe that the key steps were taken to reveal its cause. From 1816 cholera had spread from Bengal in seven great waves. The first took four years to cross India, then fanned out, getting as far as Java, the Caspian Sea and China before fading away by 1826. As travel increased throughout the world, the second pandemic of 1829–51 made it further, killing miners in the California Gold Rush, pilgrims in Mecca and survivors of the Potato Famine in Ireland. The most recent pandemic ended only in 1975, though still around 100,000 people get the disease every year, with a few thousand dying. The worst outbreak in recent times followed the earthquake of 2010 in Haiti, which devastated the capital city of Port-au-Prince. In its aftermath about 700,000 people contracted cholera, and nearly 10,000 died.[1] Cholera had always been greatly feared and not just for the numbers of deaths it caused. Even in 1832, at the height of the epidemic, it caused only 6 per cent of the total deaths in the UK, with tuberculosis at number one. What was frightening was the high mortality rate and the short time – perhaps only twelve hours – between good health and death. Before 1831, it was known to be only a matter of time before it made it to Britain. When the inevitable happened, the medical and popular press terrified the public with stories of the unstoppable and deadly new disease.[2]

We now know that cholera is caused by a bacterium called *Vibrio cholerae*. Its normal home is salty water and it is particularly fond of living on shells of crustaceans, such as crabs and shrimps. *V. cholerae* can therefore enter humans via drinking infected water, or by consuming undercooked or raw shellfish. We swallow vast numbers of bacteria all the time, but nearly all are exterminated in our strongly acidic stomachs. *V. cholerae* is tougher than the average bacterium, however, and a few can survive the stomach long enough to pass into the interior space, or lumen, of the small intestine. This is normally another hostile environment for bacteria, due to the presence of bile acids and our own natural antibiotics. To escape the lumen, *V. cholerae* penetrates a thick, viscous layer of mucus before reaching the epithelial cells that line the intestine. There it finds a new home by attaching itself to those cells. Very few of the bacteria manage to make it through all our lines of defence, but those that do start to replicate, forming colonies in the epithelial layer, all descended from a single cell.[3]

V. cholerae can thrive for a short time within the lining of our small intestines, but within a few days our immune systems will recognise the invaders and mobilise to kill them. The bacteria therefore need to get out. They do this by releasing a protein toxin[4] that enters the epithelial cells. Normally the concentrations of molecules inside our cells are tightly regulated, so that our organs and tissues function in an optimal way. The cholera toxin is able to hijack our regulatory systems, however, by locking a chloride transporter protein into a permanently activated state. Chloride, sodium, potassium and bicarbonate are pumped out of the cells and into the intestinal lumen, making it very salty.[5] Salts have a strong affinity for water, so water is pulled into the lumen, at up to two litres per hour and twenty litres per day. This enormous amount of fluid pouring into the intestine has only one place it can go, so explosive diarrhoea is the result, carrying large quantities of water and salt out of the body, along with some *V. cholerae*, ready to infect someone else.[6] Production of a colossal amount of diarrhoea is simply part of the lifecycle of *V. cholerae*, as it seeks new bodies of water in which to live. Whether its temporary human host lives or dies is neither here nor there to the bacteria.

Faeces are normally brown, as they contain dead red blood cells. The bad smell is molecules containing sulphur. In contrast, the diarrhoea from cholera is white and very runny, resembling water that has been used to cook rice, and can also smell of fish. Stomach cramps, nausea and vomiting also occur, adding to fluid loss. As the dehydration takes hold, victims experience irritability, lethargy, sunken eyes, loss of saliva, dry and shrivelled skin, and (unsurprisingly) extreme thirst. Blood turns acidic, urine production stops, blood pressure falls and the heartbeat becomes erratic. Losing salts in the blood causes muscle cramps and shock, as blood pressure becomes dangerously low. Patients scream and thrash as their muscles spasm, before they collapse exhausted.[7] Lack of blood means a lack of oxygen, which can be lethal. In the final stages, skin turns bluish-grey, giving rise to the name 'the Blue Death'.

Of course, none of this science was known in the mid-nineteenth century. Debates on the origins of epidemics and how they spread were frequent at the time, with more than 700 works on cholera alone published in London between 1845 and 1856.[8] Most widely accepted was the 'miasmatic theory', which claimed that disease originated from bad air, generated from foul substances like corpses or sewage. Continual exposure to contaminated air eventually tipped the body into disease. This not unreasonable belief helped drive improvements in sanitation, as we saw in the previous chapter, where providing clean streets and houses, fresh air, clean water and sewage systems improved both the air and the health of the people. Politicians liked the miasmatic theory, as it meant that there was no need to introduce unpopular quarantine measures for incoming ships to British ports.[2]

Not all doctors were convinced by the miasmatic theory, however. In 1850 the British General Board of Health published a report on the cholera epidemic of 1848–9,[9] which had killed millions in Asia, Europe and North America, including more than 50,000 in England. The main conclusion was the usual recommendation of sanitary improvements: cleaner streets and houses, purer air and better waste disposal. In an addition to the report, however, a Scottish doctor on the board called John Sutherland showed that water was likely to play a key role. Using data from an outbreak of cholera in Hope Street, Salford, he pointed out that cases only occurred in houses that used a particular water pump. Similar evidence was available from an epidemic in Bristol. Sutherland therefore proposed that contaminated water made cholera more likely, though he hung back from saying that it could be the sole cause. In his view, 'deficient and poisonous water' was one among several predisposing causes (like inadequate diet, overwork, poverty, inadequate housing, poor ventilation and alcohol).[2]

One man went further, however, with his conviction and determination to show that contaminated water was the main means for spreading cholera. This was John Snow, a physician from York, who was already well known for advocating the use of anaesthetics, such as ether and chloroform. In 1853 he had administered chloroform to Queen Victoria when she gave birth to her eighth child, Prince Leopold. He also used it in 867 tooth extractions and the removal of 229 breast tumours. Chloroform is not the ideal anaesthetic – it is too easy to cause unconsciousness or even death if too much is given – but it is still preferable to no anaesthetic at all.

Snow's other main professional interest was cholera. He had first encountered the disease in Newcastle when working as a young medical apprentice, before moving to London in the 1830s. In 1849, John Snow published *On the Mode of Communication of Cholera*.[10] Based on observations of numerous cases that he had seen, he became convinced that cholera was a waterborne disease, with the 'cholera poison' entering the body through the mouth, before multiplying in the stomach and intestines. The poison was also found in the diarrhoea of cholera patients, which contaminated the water supply.[2] Disease could therefore be prevented by rigorous washing and stopping the transmission of the poison from sewage to drinking water. Still, he needed stronger arguments to convince his colleagues and the authorities. If he could show that the victims of an outbreak were all connected to a single water source, then his theories would be vindicated.

Snow's opportunity came five years later. On the night of 31 August 1854, what Snow called 'the most terrible outbreak of cholera which ever occurred in the kingdom' broke out in a poor district of London called Soho. Snow knew the area well; it was a ten-minute walk from his home in central London and he used to live even closer, where he had got to know many of the locals. Snow began to visit the sick at their homes – a courageous move, since if cholera really could be spread by bad air, he was sure to fall victim to it. Presumably, he avoided any offers of a drink of water on his house visits.

Over the next three days, 127 people in or around Broad Street would die, with most houses affected. One week later, nearly all the survivors had fled the district and more than 500 were dead. By this time, however, Snow was sure he knew the reason: there was 'some contamination of the much-frequented street pump in Broad Street'. Snow took a sample of the water on 3 September and saw that it contained 'small, white, flocculent particles', though this was hardly convincing in itself. One resident told him that the water had recently changed its taste. Snow requested a list of names and addresses of the dead from the General Register Office. Eighty-nine people were on the list and when he checked their addresses, he immediately saw that nearly all deaths had taken place close to the Broad Street pump. Snow could also explain some anomalies in his theory: relatives of five victims who lived far from Soho told Snow that they always travelled to get the Broad Street water, as they liked the taste. Two children who died went to school near Broad Street, so could have easily stopped for a drink on the way. A nearby workhouse was barely affected, despite being close to the pump; Snow found that it had its own well. On the evening of 7 September, Snow presented his evidence to the local board of guardians. The next day the handle of the Broad Street pump was removed. There was one more death on 12 September; by 14 September there were none.[11]

One week later the outbreak was over, though Snow continued to gather evidence for his infectious water theory. One puzzle was that a woman in Hampstead and her niece in Islington had died from cholera despite neither having visited Soho for a long time. Snow spoke with the widow's son and discovered that she used to live in Broad Street and liked the taste of the well water so much that she had a servant fetch her a bottle of it every day. The last bottle had been collected on 31 August, and both ladies had drunk from it when the niece was visiting. Secondly, none of the workers in a brewery on Broad Street had died from cholera. Snow found that they were given free beer all day, so never touched the Broad Street water. If cholera was caused by bad air, then the brewery and workhouse would not have been spared.

Snow recorded his findings on a map of the district, annotated with the locations of the pumps and a black bar for every death from cholera (see map overleaf). The way the deaths clustered around the Broad Street pump was plain.

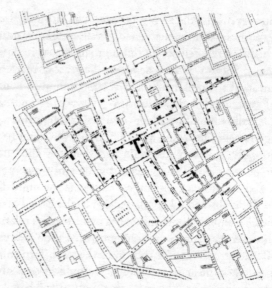

John Snow's cholera map.[10] *Each black bar marks a death. The brewery and workhouse are marked, as are several other pumps. The Broad Street pump is in the centre.*

In 1854 a local vicar called Henry Whitehead published his own account of the epidemic called *The Cholera in Berwick Street*. Whitehead favoured the miasmatic theory and did not mention the Broad Street pump at all. In 1855, Snow finished his book *On the Mode of Communication of Cholera*[10] and gave a copy to Whitehead. Whitehead was not convinced, so decided to carry out his own investigation, with the aim of proving Snow wrong. He spoke with many people in the area, some of whom he already knew as his parishioners. For every person who had died of cholera, he recorded their name, age, house layout, sanitation arrangements, whether they had drunk water from the Broad Street pump and the exact hour of the onset of the disease.[12]

To Whitehead's surprise, his data only confirmed Snow's reasoning. In June 1855 he produced a report called *Special Investigation of Broad Street*,[13] writing (to his great credit), 'Slowly and I may add reluctantly,' he concluded that water from the Broad Street pump 'was connected with the continuation of the outburst'. Furthermore, Whitehead managed to identify the likely original source for the epidemic. A five-month-old girl called Frances Lewis, who lived at 40 Broad Street, had been taken ill with diarrhoea on 24 August and died on 2 September. Her nappies had been tipped into a badly built cesspool, just three feet from the Broad Street well. Infected water could have easily leached from the cesspit into the water supplying the pump. Frances's father, Police Constable Thomas Lewis, caught cholera on 8 September, dying eleven days later, leaving Sarah Lewis a widow with two children.[14] How baby Frances became infected in the first place remains a mystery.

John Snow might have convincingly demonstrated that cholera was transmitted by water, but there were still big gaps in his chain of reasoning. Most importantly, he had no idea what the supposed cholera poison actually was. Unknown to Snow, an Italian doctor called Filippo Pacini had also been investigating cholera during a parallel outbreak in Florence in 1854. Pacini performed autopsies on cholera victims, finding tiny comma-shaped cells in the walls of the intestines. He correctly proposed that these cells were the cause of cholera,[15] and named them *Vibrio cholera*. The idea that minute bacterial cells could cause disease was highly controversial at the time. In a series of papers from 1865 to 1880, Pacini developed his ideas on cholera, correctly describing the disease as massive loss of fluid and salts due to the bacteria affecting the intestinal mucosa, the layer of the intestine that surrounds the lumen. Pacini understood that the *Vibrio bacillus* was the causative agent of cholera and that the disease was contagious.[16] As a therapy for severe cases, he recommended an intravenous injection of saltwater. Sadly, Pacini's work went unnoticed (not least because it was in Italian). Mainstream opinion was still wedded to the miasmatic theory. At an international conference on sanitation in 1874, representatives of twenty-one governments voted unanimously that 'ambient air is the principal vehicle of the generative agent of cholera'.[17]

Pacini's work was repeated thirty years later by Robert Koch, who we already met in the story of the discovery of the cause of plague. By 1883, Koch was famous for discovering the bacteria that cause anthrax and tuberculosis, so was given the resources to head a team to investigate cholera epidemics in Egypt and India. Like Pacini, he found a species of bacteria in the intestinal mucosa that was only present in cholera victims. While this was suggestive, Koch knew that the definitive experiment would be to isolate the organism, grow it in culture, then infect an animal with his cultured bacteria. Causing cholera in a human would have been even more decisive, but medical ethics had moved on from when Jenner deliberately infected a boy with the smallpox virus. Koch at first struggled to grow a pure culture of the bacteria, but later succeeded in Calcutta, where his team had travelled, following the disease. Koch reported that the *bacillus* was comma-shaped, always found in cholera patients, never found in patients without cholera, even if they had diarrhoea, and was abundant in the white diarrhoea caused by cholera. He still could not get the bacteria to induce cholera in any animal, though he correctly suggested that none was susceptible to the disease. This reasoning (and Koch's authority) was convincing enough for his conclusions to be accepted by the Germans in 1884, though not at first by the French or British.[17] Pacini had died the year before and Snow a quarter of a century earlier in 1858, so neither lived to see their work vindicated by Koch.

Fortunately, the present-day treatment for cholera is simple, cheap and reliable. The fluids and salts lost through the diarrhoea must be rapidly replaced. Best is to use a pre-packaged oral rehydration solution, which contains sugar and salts in water. This can be drunk in large amounts to treat any severe diarrhoea. If just drinking fluids is insufficient, an intravenous drip can also be used. As long as the rehydration therapy is given quickly, fewer than 1 per cent of patients will die. A course of antibiotics might also help fight off the bacteria,[18] though normally your immune system can do this by itself. High death tolls from cholera should only occur when the healthcare system has collapsed.

Snow's work not only persuaded authorities of the critical importance of providing clean water, but it also illustrated the power of careful use of data. His analysis of the Soho cholera outbreak and his decisive demonstration that a single water source was entirely responsible is now seen as a classic pioneering study in epidemiology, the study of how and why disease occurs in different groups of people. Epidemiological information is now central to our understanding of every disease. It can be used to develop strategies to prevent illness, and to manage disease outbreaks, by seeing which types of patient are most vulnerable, for instance. We shall later see a classic use of epidemiology in uncovering the link between smoking and lung cancer.

8

Childbirth

Childbirth has always been a risky and painful procedure for humans, not only because the baby may get stuck in the birth canal, but also because of the chance of infection. In particular, childbed fever, caused by bacterial infection during or shortly after childbirth, became a major killer for women in seventeenth-century Europe, when births began to take place in disease-ridden maternity hospitals. Brilliant work by the Hungarian Ignaz Semmelweis not only showed how to stop new mothers catching childbed fever, but also demonstrated the immense value of cleanliness, especially for doctors, who were frequently transmitting infections from patients to new mothers. Current routine use of personal protective equipment, antiseptics and sterile environments can be traced directly to Semmelweis's pioneering epidemiological work in Vienna.

About 5 million years ago our ancestors became bipedal, walking upright on just two limbs, leaving our arms for other purposes. Why we (literally) took this step remains a puzzle, as very few animals walk this way. A 2010 review by German evolutionary biologist Carsten Niemitz on reasons for the evolution of the upright posture reported that at least thirty hypotheses had been put forward. These ranged from being able to see further; freeing hands for purposes other than walking; reaching high-growing food; changes in habitat, such as lakes, forests or savannas; and regulating body temperature.[1]

Whatever the positive reasons were, walking upright on two legs created numerous problems. Running is faster with four legs than two, making escaping predators and hunting more difficult. Injuries from falls are more likely, as the head is at a greater height and balancing is harder. An upright stance needs more energy to maintain it. Joints that were previously optimised for quadrupeds became highly stressed. The curses of back pain and arthritis thus emerged. Most importantly, childbirth changed from something that animals manage with little difficulty on their own to a lengthy, painful and dangerous experience.

A baby's head has very little leeway when it makes the journey through the pelvis. The bones in a baby's skull have not yet fused, so the head can be squashed, making the passage easier. Babies are therefore born with diamond-shaped soft spots on the tops of their heads, which close completely through bone growth in the first eighteen months of life.

The passage for a baby through the female pelvis is so tight because the shape of the pelvis is a compromise between the shapes needed for upright walking and for childbirth. During childbirth, a baby has to follow a more complicated trajectory than in other primates, rotating and adjusting its head and shoulders through the birth canal and the narrowest parts of the pelvis. Women giving birth therefore need help, unlike all other animals, which give birth alone. Newborn babies are especially helpless compared to those of most animals. A horse is on its feet and walking within only thirty minutes of birth.[2] In comparison, human babies take a whole year before they are able to walk. Babies are born small, vulnerable and totally dependent on adults, as if they continued to grow *in utero*, their heads would be too large to pass through the birth canal. Additionally, a nine-month-old foetus is taking so much energy from its mother that further growth inside her is not possible.

As the journey through the birth canal is so tricky, there is always a chance that a baby will get stuck, especially if it is coming feet first (breech). Most breech babies these days are delivered by Caesarean section. In the Middle Ages, if a baby could not be delivered, then there were three choices: do nothing, when both mother and baby could die; try a Caesarean section (without anaesthetic), where the mother would almost certainly die; or kill the baby to save the mother by crushing its head, then pull it out, sometimes after cutting the body into pieces as well. Midwives at the time carried sharp hooks, called crochets, for this purpose.

Forceps became widely used in the eighteenth century, saving the lives of many babies and mothers. Forceps had been invented in the sixteenth century by the Chamberlen family of surgeons, who specialised in midwifery, working in Paris and London. Disgracefully, they kept their invention secret, to give themselves a competitive advantage in the midwifery business. The Chamberlens put on a remarkable performance to keep the secret of the forceps. After being summoned to the home of a rich woman in labour, they took a large, seemingly heavy box from their carriage into the house, to convince watchers that they were about to use some kind of complicated contraption. The Chamberlens then locked themselves in the room where the baby was to be delivered, blindfolded the labouring woman so she could not see what they were up to, and rang bells and made other noises to deceive listening relatives. Once a baby had been successfully delivered, the tools were packed away and smuggled back to the carriage, leaving spectators none the wiser as to what they had really done. These measures worked – the secret of the forceps was kept in the family for more than a century.[3]

Forceps can occasionally harm the baby or mother, particularly in the hands of an inexperienced or incompetent doctor. The gentler ventouse, a cup-shaped suction device, that is stuck to the baby's head and looks like a miniature sink plunger, has therefore largely replaced forceps.

Babies had traditionally been delivered in the home, aided by formally untrained, though experienced women, where death of the mother following successful childbirth was quite rare. Death from childbirth in Europe became much more likely when the medical profession began to be involved, a few hundred years ago. Previously, Christian doctors showed little concern about suffering in childbirth, seeing it as punishment of women for the sin of Eve in the Garden of Eden. For example, Charles Meigs, nineteenth-century lecturer in obstetrics in the School of Medicine, Philadelphia, strongly opposed using anaesthetics in childbirth, arguing against the morally 'doubtful nature of any process that the physicians set up to contravene the operations of those natural and physiological forces that the Divinity has ordained us to enjoy or to suffer'.[4] Here, Meigs is using the word 'us' to mean women. Presumably he would have had a different opinion if he had had to give birth himself.

The seventeenth century saw the establishment of maternity hospitals in many European cities. Despite their good intentions (such as making forceps available), sending women to hospital to give birth caused a huge increase in deaths, following infection from what was known as childbed fever. Immediately after giving birth, the site where the placenta was attached is an open wound, highly vulnerable to infection from bacteria. In the maternity hospitals, doctors and midwives were transmitting infections from mother to mother on their dirty hands, clothing and instruments. The first cases were recorded in the Hôtel-Dieu hospital in Paris in 1646. The death rate for new mothers then soared, with one in four dying being commonplace. One midwife in 1830 and 1831 was reported to have delivered thirty women, of whom sixteen died.

Childbed fever was an exceptionally cruel disease, striking mothers after they had passed the dangers of the birth itself. Millions of families were destroyed, and many young children ended up in an orphanage as a result. The first symptoms of childbed fever in a new mother were shivering, a rapid pulse and a high temperature. Most cases developed the agony of peritonitis, with intense pain in the abdomen, comparable to a burst appendix. If the disease appeared shortly after the birth, death rates could be as high as 80 per cent. Perhaps half a million women died from childbed fever in England from 1700 to 1900, making it, after tuberculosis, the second highest cause of death in women aged fifteen to forty-four at that time.[5]

The first publication suggesting that childbed fever (also known as puerperal fever) was caused by doctors was by Scottish physician, Alexander Gordon, in 1795, who noticed that childbed fever only occurred when a new mother was visited by a practitioner or nurse who had recently visited another patient affected by the disease. He even bravely and honestly admitted, 'I myself was the means of carrying the infection to a great number of women.'[6] These highly controversial (at the time) claims were picked up by American professor Oliver Wendell Holmes. In his 1843 essay, 'Contagiousness of Puerperal Fever', he presented a large amount of evidence to show that doctors were the mode of transmission of the deadly infection from patient to patient.[7] He urged physicians who had come in contact with puerperal fever cases to purify their instruments, burn the clothing they had worn during the delivery and stay away from pregnant women for at least six months.[8] Hands should routinely be washed with chlorine solution and clothing changed regularly, all novel practices at the time, when a doctor would frequently visit a patient wearing a coat covered in dried blood. Holmes's publication was not popular among the medical profession. Many were outraged by the suggestion that they might be harming patients.

The most convincing data for the malign effect of doctors in childbirth came from the work of Ignaz Semmelweis, a Hungarian working in Vienna General Hospital from 1846.[9] The hospital had two maternity clinics, providing free care to poor women. Both hospitals used the same standard of facilities and types of practice, and since they admitted women on alternate days, had no difference in the type of patient. The only difference was that the First Clinic was used for training medical students and the Second Clinic for training midwives. Which clinic you got to use had a huge effect on the likelihood of catching childbed fever – 10 per cent mothers in the First Clinic were dying, while the death rate in the Second Clinic was less than 4 per cent. This was well known in Vienna. Women entering labour would beg not to be admitted to the First Clinic and some would even choose to give birth in the streets instead.

Semmelweis was amazed that street births were safer for women than using the First Clinic and he resolved to find out why. The two clinics provided an excellent environment for assessing the effects of doctors without the confounding effects of any other differences, as the types of patients being admitted were identical. When one doctor died with puerperal-like symptoms after being accidentally stabbed with a scalpel that had been used in an autopsy, Semmelweis realised that this meant that it was material from the dead body that was carrying the infection. Medical students were frequently handling corpses as part of their training, then going with dirty hands straight to women in labour. Semmelweis therefore introduced a rigorous policy of handwashing in chlorine solution after autopsies. It worked. The mortality rate dropped as much as 18 per cent to less than 5 per cent per month. Some months even had no deaths at all.

Semmelweis did his best to promote cleanliness by publishing his conclusions[9] and writing to colleagues across Europe. Sadly, his views were treated with scorn by doctors, who took personal offence at his claims and ridiculed the idea that invisible particles could cause disease. This hostile reception helped drive him out of his job and into an asylum, where he died. It was only twenty years after his death, when his work was rediscovered, that his reputation changed to one of an unjustly forgotten genius.[5]

Final endorsement of the importance of cleanliness in childbirth did not come until acceptance of the germ theory of disease in the late nineteenth century and the value of antiseptic techniques in surgery, which helped make Caesareans routine. Midwives were also required to undergo formal training. In 1902 the Midwives Bill was passed by the British Parliament. It stated that from 1910, no woman should attend a birth unless certified, having attended a course of lectures, passed oral and written examinations, and attended a required number of births. These measures, together with general improvements in sanitation and nutrition, at last successfully reduced death rates from childbed fever (Table 12, page 93) and lowered infant mortality rates from thirty-nine per 1,000 in 1840 to twelve per 1,000 in 1903.[10] The total defeat of childbed fever came from the introduction of sulphonamide drugs in the 1930s, followed by penicillin. These were able to kill the bacteria that were the true cause of the disease. Within twenty years, childbed fever had almost completely disappeared. Death in childbirth is now thankfully very rare.

9

Deadly Animals

About a million people are killed each year by animals, mostly by them spreading infectious diseases, adding up to just over 1 per cent of total deaths.[1, 2] Of these, more than 80 per cent are killed by mosquito-borne diseases. A few other invertebrates are also important disease vectors: sandflies spread leishmaniasis; kissing bugs (so-called because they bite your face while you sleep) cause Chagas disease; tsetse flies cause sleeping sickness; freshwater snails cause schistosomiasis (bilharzia). Some animals can kill by poison: notably snakes, but also scorpions, bees and jellyfish. A few large animals are dangerous – crocodiles take about 1,000 people per year; hippos, elephants, bears, buffalos, lions and tigers are also best not provoked. Dog bites can give rabies, and hitting animals on the road, particularly deer, causes accidents. Some of our deepest fears are of animals, yet these are often misplaced: in 2016, wolves killed only ten people worldwide, sharks six and spiders none.

As well as animals that hurt us by biting or stinging, some harm us by taking up residence in our bodies. Even today it is not unusual to carry some form of parasite, though most cause little harm. One-third of us are living with *Toxoplasma gondii*, for instance, which can cause toxoplasmosis in people with weakened immune systems.[3] France comes top for *Toxoplasma gondii* infection at 86 per cent, thanks to their love of undercooked steaks. The British style of cookery yields an infection level of only 22 per cent, as the parasite can rarely survive a good charring.[4] There is often a fine line between being a burdensome parasite and being a beneficial symbiont, like gut bacteria that help us digest food. It is generally not in the interest of a parasite to make its host ill. A sick host would provide less food or even die, so the parasite loses its happy home. Nevertheless, some parasites do cause disease, specifically single-celled protozoa, such as the *Plasmodium* species, helminths (worms), and blood-sucking arthropods, such as ticks, fleas, lice and mites. These bugs attach to or burrow into the skin, where they can stay for months. Sometimes this can cause disease by itself, like scabies, but more importantly, the arthropods act as disease vectors, transmitting typhus, Lyme disease, plague, leishmaniasis and Chagas disease, among many others. Understanding the relationship between the parasite and the disease-causing microorganism allows us to tackle the disease by targeting weak points in its lifecycle.

Guinea worm provides a nice example of current success in the field of parasitology, as a very rare example of an infection that we are close to completely wiping out. The guinea worm is a species of roundworm (nematode) that until recently affected millions of people, mostly in Africa. As usual with human parasites, it has a rather disgusting life cycle. The roundworms live as larvae in water within small crustaceans called copepods (water fleas). If infected water is drunk, the copepods are killed by stomach acid, releasing the larvae. These penetrate the stomach and intestine wall, and then start to live and grow within the abdominal cavity. Inside the body, the adults mate, the males die, and the females grow for about a year. Once the worms have reached a metre or so in length, and are as thick as spaghetti, they travel downwards through the body, causing intense pain, giving rise to its name of the 'fiery serpent'. The worm induces a blister on the skin, typically on the foot, from which it will emerge over several weeks. To try to relieve the pain, people will often put their blisters in water. This contact with water will trigger the worm to release thousands of larvae, ready to be ingested by copepods, thus completing the cycle.[5] While not often fatal, guinea worm infection causes months of suffering, and disability that can be permanent.

From 1981, the World Health Organization, together with UNICEF, the US Centers for Disease Control and Prevention (CDC), the Carter Center, led by former US President Jimmy Carter[6] and others, developed and implemented a strategy for eliminating guinea-worm disease. Several features of the disease made it a good target for eradication: diagnosis is easy (you can see the worm); larvae only live in water; measures to stop the disease are simple and inexpensive; and governments of countries where the disease existed were all on board. Breaking its life cycle at any point should be sufficient to get rid of the guinea worm. This can be done in two ways: either stop people drinking water contaminated with the copepods or prevent the new larvae entering the water supply. Water that is suspected to contain copepods can be filtered using nylon mesh to make it safe. Copepods are often visible as swimming white specks. In addition, when the worm is emerging through a blister, the foot or leg is put into a bucket of water that can be safely disposed of later, by emptying it onto dry ground where the larvae will die. The water supply is thus not contaminated.

Since the 1980s, the guinea-worm eradication programme has shown enormous success. The plan started with mapping every location with guinea-worm disease and reporting each case. Communities at risk were enrolled on the new strategy using village-based health workers. In 1985, about 3.5 million new cases occurred in twenty countries. In 1989, 892,055 cases were reported, though data from Chad, the Central African Republic, Senegal and Sudan was missing. In 2020, only twenty-seven cases were reported from nineteen villages in six countries (Cameroon, Ethiopia, Mali, Chad, Angola and South Sudan).[7] From 3.5 million to twenty-eight is a spectacular 99.999 per cent decrease. Guinea-worm disease is therefore on the verge of being the first parasitic disease to be totally eradicated, and the second human disease altogether, after smallpox.[7] The work is being done without any medicine or vaccine that can cure or prevent the disease. All that is needed is to cut the worm's life cycle, but to do it thoroughly, in every location thought to be at risk. Ending guinea-worm disease would be an outstanding achievement and points the way to how international teams can tackle carefully chosen diseases at low cost, provided that all affected parties are firmly committed to the programme. So far, so good, but what about the insect that kills more people than all other animals combined?

In 1513, Spanish explorer Vasco Núñez de Balboa became the first European to cross the Isthmus of Panama and reach the Pacific Ocean. Balboa raised a sword in one hand and a standard of the Virgin Mary in the other, waded into the sea, and in magnificent conquistadorial style, claimed possession of the entire ocean and all adjoining lands in the name of the Spanish sovereign. If you took this seriously (and the Spanish very much did so), then King Ferdinand now owned half the planet. Balboa's discovery of an unexpected ocean to the west of the Americas naturally made the Spanish wonder whether a strait existed that would allow a ship to sail between the Caribbean and the Pacific without having to travel thousands of miles around the southern tip of South America. Further exploration found no such waterway, so in 1534 Ferdinand's successor, Holy Roman Emperor King Charles V, directed surveyors to investigate whether a suitable site existed for the construction of a canal to link the two oceans. The surveyors reported back that such a project was sadly not possible, with sixteenth-century expertise at least, and the project was put on hold for more than three centuries.

The first serious attempt to build a canal through the isthmus was by the French, led by Ferdinand de Lesseps, following his success in building the Suez Canal in 1869. The Suez route was easier than Panama, even though the distance was longer, as it traversed flat terrain. De Lesseps had therefore built a sea-level canal between the Red Sea and the Mediterranean that did not need locks. The French started work at Panama in 1882, at first attempting a sea-level canal, even though this required cutting through extensive elevated and rocky terrain. After six years' work, the project collapsed in 1888, undone by inadequate equipment, a lack of funds, construction problems and corruption. The greatest opponent of the canal, however, was disease. Panama was a prime habitat for the mosquito, which carried malaria and yellow fever. Infection debilitated construction crews so they were unable to work. Some 20,000 workers died between 1882 and 1888. De Lesseps' company went bankrupt and digging stopped. In the resulting scandal, he and other company executives (including Eiffel of the tower fame) received prison sentences for fraud, though these were later overturned.

The collapse of the French Panama Canal project was just one of countless disasters caused by the mosquito. Mosquitoes themselves cause no direct harm, other than an annoying itch and inflammation at the site of a bite. They readily transmit disease, however, since they feed on human blood. Zika, dengue, chikungunya and yellow fever are all major viral infections transmitted to humans by the *Aedes aegypti* mosquito. After feeding on an infected person, viruses replicate in the mosquito gut before spreading to other tissues, notably the salivary glands, ready to infect a new victim. Though originating and most prevalent in Africa, mosquito-borne diseases have spread around the world. Dengue cases have risen eightfold in the last twenty years, for instance, with more countries reporting their first outbreaks.[8] Over half the world's population live in areas where *Aedes aegypti* is present.

Most important in Panama was yellow fever, an African disease that was transported to North America and Europe in the last few hundred years, probably on slave ships. Typical yellow fever symptoms are a few days of fever, muscle pain, headache, loss of appetite, nausea and vomiting. A second more deadly phase is possible within twenty-four hours of recovering from the first symptoms. Fever returns and the liver and kidneys malfunction. Jaundice appears, giving the characteristic yellow skin. Urine turns dark and there is abdominal pain with vomiting. The mouth, nose, eyes and stomach can bleed. Half of the patients who enter this second toxic phase die within ten days. At present, about 30,000 people die each year from yellow fever, mostly in Africa.[9] While we have no antiviral drugs for yellow fever, we do have a highly effective vaccine, where a single dose gives lifelong immunity. The Eliminate Yellow Fever Epidemics (EYE) Strategy, launched in 2017, aims to eradicate the disease. Led by the WHO, the EYE partnership works with forty at-risk countries in Africa and the Americas to prevent, monitor and deal with yellow fever outbreaks. Populations are vaccinated, outbreaks contained, and the spread of the virus around the world is curtailed. The plan is for more than 1 billion people to be protected against the disease by 2026.[10]

More important than any other mosquito-borne disease is malaria. There had been speculation that mosquitoes were somehow responsible for malaria for thousands of years. It wasn't hard to notice that the insect that you had finally managed to splatter on the wall was full of blood, and that the blood was yours. For example, in the first century BCE, a Roman agriculturist called Columella wrote, 'A marsh always throws up noxious and poisonous steams during the heats and breeds animals armed with mischievous stings which fly upon us in exceeding thick swarms … whereby hidden diseases are often contracted…'[11] The Roman Emperor Nero ordered swamps near Rome to be drained, as they were so unhealthy. Unfortunately,

Western medicine then took a wrong turn, blaming disease on miasmas and imbalanced humours in the body, which held medicine back for nearly 2,000 years. Nonetheless, in 1717, Italian physician Giovanni Lancisi wrote about 'the harmful effect which the insects of the swamps, by mixing their injurious juices with the saliva ... inflict upon us', also proposing draining marshes.[12] Still, experimental proof was lacking, and views like these flew in the face of conventional wisdom, so met much opposition.

We now know that malaria is caused by four main *Plasmodium* species called *falciparum, vivax, ovale* and *malariae. Plasmodium* species have a complicated life cycle, inhabiting various organs in two hosts. Malaria begins when a female *Anopheles* mosquito, feeding on a human, injects thread-like forms of *Plasmodium* that were living in her salivary glands into the blood. These travel to the liver, where each thread replicates to create tens of thousands of descendants in the form of a cyst. The human victim has no symptoms during this incubation period and is unaware that they are infected. Eventually the cyst ruptures, releasing parasites, which invade red blood cells to feed on the oxygen-carrying haemoglobin protein. These develop into forms called schizonts, each containing eight to twenty-four parasites. Mature schizonts can settle in various organs, such as the brain or placenta, with disease symptoms dependent on which organs are affected.[13] Schizonts eventually rupture, releasing the next generation of parasites into the bloodstream, ready to infect a fresh batch of red blood cells. This rupture triggers fever, sweating and chills, rather like flu, often happening in waves, giving symptoms every few days. After a mosquito feeds on infected human blood, the parasites form a cyst within the insect gut. This cyst releases spores that colonise other sites in the mosquito's body, including salivary glands. The next time the mosquito feeds on a human, these spores get injected, so completing the cycle.[14]

Severe malarial symptoms arise from organ failure or blood abnormalities, depending on which part of the body is affected. Malaria can cause seizures, loss of consciousness and coma; severe anaemia is due to loss of red blood cells; kidneys can fail; lungs get inflamed; spleens enlarge; blood sugar levels plummet, and so on. Patients then need urgent medical treatment. Relapses can take place years later, when dormant liver cysts reactivate. Long-term problems can persist, such as speech difficulties, deafness, kidney disease, rupture of the spleen and blindness. Malaria is especially dangerous during pregnancy, for both mother and baby.[15]

After the acceptance of germ theory in the 1870s, the mindset was right to try to find a microorganism responsible for malaria. Figuring out all the steps in the three-way dance between mosquitoes, *Plasmodium* species and humans took many decades.[16] The blood stage was first detected by Charles Laveran, a French army doctor working in Algeria. In the blood of malaria patients, he saw crescent-shaped bodies that contained a small dot of pigment. These were never seen in healthy people. Laveran went on to describe four distinct forms in blood that we now know are distinct stages of the parasite life cycle. Italian Camillo Golgi then connected the rupture of blood schizonts with the release of malaria parasites and the onset of fever.[17]

This was indeed progress, but it wasn't clear how this understanding could be translated into a way of preventing or curing the disease. However, in 1897 in India, British bacteriologist Ronald Ross discovered parasites of a form of bird malaria in the stomach of a mosquito species. At the same time in Rome, Giovanni Grassi and colleagues discovered a parasite of human malaria in an *Anopheles* mosquito. The key role of mosquitoes in acting as a disease vector, transmitting a disease-causing microorganism between species, was thus revealed. Crucially, this gave a target that technology of the time could deal with: we could reduce mosquito populations by getting rid of the places where they liked to live, like pools of standing water.

The idea that yellow fever was also transmitted by the mosquito was first proposed by the Cuban doctor Carlos Finlay in 1881. Epidemics of malaria, yellow fever, cholera and others were an enormous problem for Cuba in the nineteenth century. Finlay had noticed how the areas susceptible to yellow fever coincided with where mosquitoes lived, so he studied how they fed.[18] His presentation to the Royal Academy of Medical, Physical and Natural Sciences in Havana was not well received. The idea that a tiny insect could kill a fully grown person was too radical to be taken seriously. Finlay therefore set out to get further evidence to test his hypothesis by using hundreds of volunteers, who allowed themselves to be bitten by infected mosquitoes. Even though this was the most direct way to prove his ideas (albeit highly dangerous), the results were still unconvincing.[19] With hindsight, we now know that his experiments failed as the incubation time that Finlay was using – the number of days between a mosquito becoming infected and biting a new victim – was too short.[20] A vital clue on incubation came a few years later from the work of Henry Carter, who served as quarantine officer in American ports on the Gulf of Mexico. He found that the time between infection of a human and the first appearance of yellow fever symptoms was about five days. Introducing a quarantine period of seven days for ships coming from Mexico or Cuba to the USA therefore prevented the entry of yellow fever.[20] Carter followed this up by studying yellow fever cases in isolated farmhouses, seeing how long it took before a visitor to the farmhouse would contract the disease.

Vindication for Finlay came with the help of the US Army. During the ten-week Spanish–American War of 1898, American forces had invaded Cuba. Yellow fever and malaria spread rapidly among the troops, until 75 per cent were unfit for service and the army had to be withdrawn. Fewer than a thousand American soldiers had been killed in combat, but more than 5,000 had died of disease, especially of yellow fever. Despite these setbacks, the USA won the war and took over the country. After establishing a US military government, a Yellow Fever Commission was set up to find a solution. With the help of Finlay, the commission retested his mosquito idea using longer incubation periods, this time with success. After several years of experimental work, and the early deaths of some team members, the following conclusions were reached:

1. Yellow fever is not transmitted by bedding or clothing.
2. It is transmitted through the bites of mosquitoes that have previously taken up blood from persons sick with the disease.
3. The specific mosquito culprit is identified – now called *Aedes aegypti*.
4. Females that have fed on an infected person, and that bite healthy individuals up to ten days later, do not transmit the infectious agent. An interval of twelve days or more is needed.[20, 21]

This new knowledge was rapidly turned into practice in Havana by Major William Gorgas, chief sanitary officer of the city. He ordered the isolation of yellow fever patients in buildings, with screens over doors and windows to keep mosquitoes out. Teams of soldiers searched the city, attacking mosquitoes, both as flying adults and as larvae living in water. Within five months, yellow fever was eliminated from Havana. Even though no one knew what the infectious agent actually was, knowing a weak point in its life cycle meant that the disease could be stopped.

This success came just in time for the American Panama Canal project. The Americans now knew that the reason why so many died during the French attempt to build the canal was that the Panama isthmus swarmed with malaria- and yellow fever-infected mosquitoes. Sending tens of thousands of construction workers to such a region with no protection from the insects, as the French had done, was sure to end in disaster. The American government was determined that the same thing would not happen to their workers. In 1904 they therefore sent Gorgas to inspect the area and come up with a plan of action. Before any construction crews lifted a shovel, Gorgas set to work to eliminate the mosquito from the canal zone. All bodies of slow-moving or stationary water were treated with insecticide to kill mosquito larvae. Containers for standing water, where mosquitoes might breed, were removed. Swamps were drained and clean water systems built, so there was no need to collect rainwater. Windows of buildings to be used by crews were covered with wire screens. Health workers searched buildings for mosquitoes and their eggs. The entire US supply of sulphur was burned to decontaminate rooms. Any workers who did become sick were quarantined. By 1906, after less than two years' work, yellow fever was gone from the canal zone and malaria much reduced.[22]

Now construction work could take place in much safer conditions – for some workers, at least. Protected housing was not provided for black workers, who were mostly from the West Indies. They had to live in tents outside the mosquito-controlled areas. As a result, the death rate during the project was ten times higher for black workers than white, with 4,500 dying, compared to only 350 whites.[23] On top of disease, many still died in accidents, such as landslides and dynamite accidents.

The American design featured colossal locks near the Pacific and Atlantic Oceans. Raised ships would cross a vast artificial lake, created by a new dam, and go through a gigantic cutting through the highest land on the route. High rainfall would keep the water level in the elevated portion of the canal topped up. After overcoming these enormous challenges, the canal opened in 1914, 401 years after Balboa first made the journey on foot. Today some 15,000 ships make the fifty-mile crossing each year. As well as being one of the greatest feats of engineering ever attempted, the project also demonstrated and publicised how disease could be prevented.

Malaria and yellow fever are just two of the many diseases that are specific to tropical regions. Once Europeans began to trade and colonise more southerly regions, starting with the Portuguese exploring the African coast, they were hit with a devastating set of diseases to which they had little resistance. Malaria, dysentery and yellow fever were the worst, but there were countless others, many of which were spread by insects, lice and snails. On the coasts of West Africa, 50 per cent of a newly arrived company could expect to die within a year,[24] making these regions essentially uninhabitable by non-natives. Even worse was that ships exported diseases from their homelands. Malaria was the most important case. At its peak in the nineteenth century, over half the world's population was living in environments with malaria-infected mosquitoes, reaching as far north as Montreal and Scandinavia. In these areas, about 10 per cent were dying from malaria, with many more infected and suffering from long-term sickness. Malaria thus peaked at killing 5–10 per cent of the world's population at that time.[25] (The widely reported factoid that the mosquito has killed over half the people who have ever lived is false. It may have originated in an 2002 article in *Nature*.[26])

From this peak, malaria began to be driven back by targeting the mosquito. The building of the Panama Canal was an example of how this strategy could work. Malaria disappeared from Europe in the first half of the twentieth century, thanks to changes in land use and agriculture, getting rid of the environments that mosquitoes loved, like marshes, and building better housing. After the Second World War came the insecticide DDT. Spraying DDT on walls inside houses was successful in India, the Soviet Union and other countries. By 1966, the use of DDT, bed nets, and removing mosquito breeding sites had removed the threat of malaria from more than 500 million people.[27, 28] Sub-Saharan Africa was a much tougher prospect, not least because mosquitoes were far more widespread, so someone living in the worst-affected parts of Africa was 200 times more likely to be bitten by an infectious mosquito than someone in Asia.[28]

Our second weapon against malaria was drugs to kill the parasite. Drugs can not only help the patient, but also prevent them being a reservoir of disease for someone else. One effective drug is artemisinin, found in sweet wormwood and used by Chinese herbalists for more than 2,000 years. The active chemical was isolated by Chinese scientists in 1972, after Vietnamese Communist leader Ho Chi Minh asked China for help against malaria during the Vietnam War. Team leader Tu Youyou gained China's first Nobel Prize for Physiology or Medicine for discovering artemisinin; she is also the first Chinese woman to receive the award. Quinine, found in the bark of the cinchona tree, which grows wild in the Andes, has been used for 400 years. Most production was from trees grown in Java. Problems with supply from East Asia during the First World War incentivised German chemists to come up with an alternative. Workers at IG Farben discovered many promising compounds in the 1930s, notably chloroquinine. DDT and chloroquinine became the front-line compounds in the WHO's attempt to eradicate malaria after the Second World War. Unfortunately, it didn't take long for resistance to chloroquinine to appear in new strains of the parasite.[17] Dozens of other antimalarial drugs have followed, though none are 100 per cent protective. Resistance, side effects and lack of effectiveness are common. Best is not to get bitten by an infected mosquito in the first place.

Descriptions of diseases that sound much like malaria are nearly as old as writing. The Chinese canon of medicine, the *Nei Ching*, written nearly 5,000 years ago, links malaria-like symptoms to swollen spleens. Clay tablets from the Assyrian emperor's library in Nineveh in Iraq describe the disease, as do Indian writings of the Vedic period (1500–800 BCE) and an Egyptian medical papyrus from 1550 BCE.[17] *P. falciparum* infection has been found in Egyptian mummies that are more than 5,000 years old.[29] Homer, Plato, Chaucer and Shakespeare all mention malaria.

Diseases that have been with us for 5,000 years are older than most, but our troubled relationship with malaria actually goes back far longer. The ancestors of mosquitoes appeared about 150 million years ago. Ancestral malaria parasites then adopted life cycles in which they lived in the insects and the animals on which they fed – a wide range of reptiles, birds and mammals. *Plasmodium* parasites are particularly common in primates, our order of mammals.[25] At some point in the last 10,000 years, mosquitoes transmitted *P. falciparum* from gorillas to humans.[30] *P. vivax* has been living with humans, chimps and gorillas for even longer.[31]

As humans have been living with malaria for tens of thousands of years, it has had profound effects on our DNA. One example is a DNA variant called Duffy-negative.[32] The Duffy gene, named after the patient in whom it was first found, encodes a protein on the surface of red blood cells that *P. vivax* uses to enter cells. Duffy-negative people lack this protein on red blood cells, so the parasite finds it much harder to enter them, blocking a key step in its life cycle and preventing *P. vivax* malaria, or at least reducing its severity. Being Duffy-negative is thus highly desirable in regions where *P. vivax* is common.[33] The map below shows that the likelihood of being Duffy-negative is close to 100 per cent in sub-Saharan Africa and near zero in most other parts of the world. Malaria caused by *P. vivax* is therefore rare in sub-Saharan Africa, though common in southern Asia and Latin America. Before the great movements of populations that began 500 years ago, the Duffy-negative gene was non-existent in the Americas. If a population has the Duffy-negative gene there now, it is a reliable sign of Black African ancestry. We see it in African Americans, West Indians and South Americans in varying proportions, where they are descendants of people brought over in slave ships from Africa.[34]

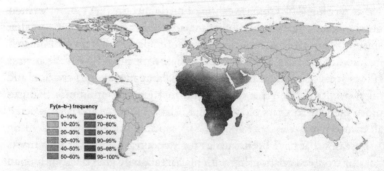

Global distribution of Duffy negativity.[34] We carry two copies of the Duffy gene in our DNA, so this is the probability of neither copy expressing a functional Duffy protein.

Why are people in India and Southeast Asia not Duffy-negative as well? This would protect them from *P. vivax* malaria. What seems to have happened is that about 100,000 years ago, our species lived only in Africa and was commonly infected by *P. vivax*, as with other great apes. About 50,000 years ago, a small group of modern humans left East Africa, travelling around the Indian Ocean coast to reach Arabia, Persia, India and Southeast Asia. They brought a strain of *P. vivax* with them. The Duffy-negative gene[35] began to spread in Africa 30,000 years ago, eventually becoming so abundant that *P. vivax* malaria was virtually eliminated in that continent,[36] leaving it today as a disease of Asia and Latin America. Non-Black Africans are still at risk from *P. vivax* in Africa, however. In 2005, a thirty-two-year-old Caucasian male caught a *P. vivax* infection from a mosquito that seemingly fed on him after biting an infected ape, when he was working for eighteen days in Central Africa.[37]

Being Duffy-negative may come at a cost. The Duffy protein does a lot more than helping *P. vivax* enter red blood cells: it works as part of the immune system,[38] so lacking it might affect the severity of numerous diseases. Duffy-negative people (who virtually all have substantial African ancestry) may be more susceptible to cancer, for example.[39, 40, 41] Unless you live in a place where *P. vivax* is rampant, it is probably best overall to retain the Duffy protein on your red blood cells.

Being Duffy-negative is also of no use against the more deadly form of malaria caused by *P. falciparum*. At-risk populations have therefore evolved various other mutations that help protect against it. Unfortunately, the most widespread antimalarial mutations also cause sickle-cell disease, thalassemia or glucose-6-phosphate dehydrogenase (G6PD) deficiency. Sickle-cell disease can cause pain, infection and stroke, with life expectancy lowered by decades; thalassemia causes anaemia, heart problems, bone deformities and a damaged spleen;[42] people with G6PD deficiency are susceptible to attacks triggered by broad (fava) beans, when they are hit by jaundice, anaemia, shortness of breath and kidney failure. The Greek sage and mathematician Pythagoras banned his followers from eating beans. We can guess that Pythagoras was G6PD deficient. Sickle-cell disease, thalassemia and G6PD deficiency are thus all serious, yet widespread, genetic conditions. Still, they are better than malaria. They persist because the mutations confer resistance to *P. falciparum* via their action on red blood cells. Malaria is such a debilitating condition, and so common, that these damaging mutations have spread across Africa, Asia, the

Mediterranean and the Middle East, despite the harm that they cause. While these mutations are nature's way of fighting disease, we need something better.

Today, the mosquito remains the deadliest animal in the world, with malaria killing half a million people in 2017, mostly young children who have not developed any immunity. We are making progress, though, with the death toll halving in the last fifteen years. Malaria has been eradicated from many places where it used to be endemic, like the USA and Europe. For example, the National Malaria Eradication Program began in 1947 in the USA, following encouraging results from similar projects in and around military bases. Thirteen states in the south-east USA were targeted. Five million homes were treated with DDT, and mosquito-breeding sites were drained and sprayed with insecticides. In 1949 the USA was declared free of malaria as a significant public health problem; only monitoring was then necessary.[43]

Will we ever totally eradicate malaria and other mosquito-borne diseases? We have done so for many countries. Success against guinea worm and smallpox shows that international cooperation against disease can work. Many factors make tackling malaria in Central and West Africa especially challenging: multiple species of insect and *Plasmodium* can transmit and cause disease. Wiping out one mosquito species might simply mean that another, which is just as bad, takes over. Poor government and lack of funds have hindered previous malaria-control programmes. We need to help impoverished communities that can be hard to reach and have little access to health systems. While traditional methods against malaria and mosquitoes remain valuable, like bed nets, window screens and removing standing water, we also need new technologies. Better drugs, insecticides and diagnostic methods need to be continually developed. In the last ten years, new innovations, and more political and financial commitment, have seen the number of malaria deaths worldwide decrease by 44 per cent from 2010 to 2019.[44] Each year more countries are declared malaria-free. Entirely novel approaches might also be valuable. An antimalarial vaccine on trial in Burkina Faso is showing encouraging early results.[45]

A more radical idea is to create genetically engineered mosquitoes and release them to spread desirable genes into the population.[46] So-called gene-drive technology would mean that the new gene is preferentially found in offspring. For example, mosquitoes might be modified so that they cannot be infected by *P. falciparum*, potentially ending the worst form of malaria for ever. Then we would need to release a small number of these genetically modified mosquitoes so that their new genes eventually take over, generation by generation. Alternatively, we might add genes that prevent mosquito reproduction, to push them towards extinction. Gene drives are a tool of immense potential power. While we have selected and created mutated animals in the lab for a hundred years, gene drives give us the power to reach out and genetically modify every animal on the planet. After a decade of discussing the ethics and risks of releasing genetically modified mosquitoes,[47] the first trial has begun, targeting *Aedes aegypti* in Florida, using genes that kill female offspring when larvae, rather than gene drives.[48] While this might seem like a promising idea, there are deep concerns: once GM mosquitoes are released, there is no way of getting them all back and there may be unexpected consequences to ecosystems. The new genes could mutate or might jump to additional species. The evolution of resistance in the mosquito to such damaging genes is also inevitable.

If we commit to fund the programmes, it is not unrealistic to aim to eradicate malaria, dengue and other mosquito-borne diseases worldwide within a few decades. Widespread and long-lasting diseases like malaria damage a country's wealth, as well as health. Eliminating them would allow escape from years of debilitating disease. Malaria-eradication programmes are expensive, but the long-term financial return on such an investment would therefore be huge.[49] These enormous benefits would benefit billions of people, transforming nations in Africa, in particular.

10

The Magic Bullet

What general lessons have we learned from the ongoing, but largely successful war against infectious disease? Until the widespread availability of antibiotics after the Second World War, doctors could do little about any infectious disease. In fact, as we saw in the case of childbed fever, encounters with the medical profession could be downright dangerous. The incidence of many infectious diseases showed huge decreases in Victorian times; typhoid deaths decreased by 90 per cent from 1840 to 1910 in England and Wales, for example (Table 12, page 93). These gains took place before mass vaccination or effective drugs were available. While medical knowledge was certainly growing, such as understanding the circulation of the blood or human anatomy from dissections, it took centuries for this to be translated into actual medicines. Smallpox was the only disease that had a vaccine until the late nineteenth century. The biggest medical advances by this date were in preventing infection, rather than curing disease. Antiseptic techniques began to be used in surgery. The invention of anaesthetics, together with antiseptics, meant that patients now had a fair chance of surviving surgery. Before anaesthetics, surgeons took considerable pride in being able to amputate a limb as fast as possible, even if their victims invariably died afterwards from shock and infection. Life expectancy in the UK rose from the high thirties to the low fifties in the nineteenth century.[1]

As we have seen, politicians in the first half of the nineteenth century believed in *laissez-faire*, that is, abstention by government from interfering in the workings of the free market. If enough people wanted medicine, clean water, sewers or housing, then private companies would spring up to provide them. Attitudes changed when national and local governments started to fund the public services that we enjoy today. These measures were generally justified by reducing the financial and health costs to the tax-paying wealthy, rather than on humanitarian grounds and the public good. Nevertheless the general public, and particularly the poor, benefited enormously.

While knowing that disease was caused by polluted water did not immediately lead to cures, it did point to the importance of sanitation to prevent disease. Victorians might have been terrible doctors, but they did know how to build; countless roads, railway lines, bridges, canals, viaducts, sewers, pipes and reservoirs from this time are still in use. Water-filtration plants were built, first simply passing water through sand; water purity was later improved further by chlorination. Clean water for cooking, cleaning, toilets and drinking transformed millions of lives for the better, with sewers safely taking the dirty water away to be treated. Slums built to house thousands as cheaply as possible were slowly demolished and replaced with better-quality housing. Standards of nutrition also improved at this time. Strong bodies provided with adequate calories and a well-balanced diet are better able to fight off infections.[2] Milk was sterilised by pasteurisation, rather than being carried from farms to cities in churns that were breeding grounds for bacteria that caused tuberculosis and other diseases. The importance of a mix of carbohydrates, fats and proteins was understood. The great increase in national wealth in the Victorian period improved living standards and diet for nearly everyone.

The pioneering work of John Snow, Ignaz Semmelweis, Robert Koch, Louis Pasteur and many others made a powerful case for the acceptance of germ theory, which claims that infectious disease is caused by transmission of disease-causing microorganisms. Disease is therefore spread by microorganisms in water and not by foul air. It was easy to be misled in a hot summer by the fumes coming off a sewage-laden stream, especially when drinking water from a pump looked clear and tasted fine. Nevertheless, good-looking water could still be deadly if it contained the wrong germs, like those for typhoid and cholera. The realisation that disease was spread by infectious microscopic germs immediately led to powerful conclusions.

- Cleanliness can prevent the spread of disease.

- Doctors should wash and change into clean clothes between patients, so that they don't transmit germs, rather than treating them with hands that had recently been inside infected people or corpses.
- Hospital bedding should not be soaked in dried blood or pus.
- Wash clothes and bedding regularly.
- Avoid contact with human waste and bodily fluids.
- Wash yourself regularly.

These are basic hygiene measures that we drum into children, but only became commonplace in the nineteenth century. Additionally, if we understand that disease can be spread by animals like mosquitoes and rats, then getting rid of their habitats and reducing their contact with people will stop disease. Thus we drain the swamps where mosquitoes breed and drive vermin out of our homes.

Germ theory rationalises how vaccination and inoculation work. Once our bodies have been exposed to a microorganism, they are able to fight it off if they see it again, as our immune systems will be primed to recognise it as a dangerous invader. Perhaps dead microorganisms, parts of them or similar microorganisms might be all that is needed to trigger an immune response. If so, we have a vaccine. No complex tools or any knowledge of how the immune system works is necessary. All we need to be able to do is to grow the disease-causing microorganism, then kill it, fragment it or modify it until it is no longer lethal, but can still generate an immune response.

If we can identify and grow disease-causing microorganisms, then we can experiment on finding ways to kill them. In 1907 Paul Ehrlich, a German-Jewish former colleague of Robert Koch, began a search for chemicals that might kill bacteria, but not human cells. Ehrlich's dream was his concept of the 'magic bullet' – a drug that would kill its target organism while leaving all other cells untouched, analogous to firing a machine gun into a melee on a battlefield and only hitting the enemy soldiers. He knew that this would not be easy. For over 99 per cent of chemicals, there is little variation in their effects on cells: cyanide kills everything, for instance, so it doesn't make a great drug. Ehrlich did not know whether selectively killing just one group of cells was even possible.

Ehrlich came to his magic bullet idea from his earlier work on staining cells with dyes. Hundreds of new dyes were available to him from the rapidly growing chemical industry. He had found that by adding a range of dyes to cell preparations, he could get different cell types to light up in distinct colours when viewed through a microscope. In this way, he was able to discover new kinds of cells. He therefore reasoned that if cells varied in how they bound to dyes, then perhaps they might also have different affinities to molecules that could kill them. These molecules would be a magic bullet if they selectively went for the disease-causing microorganisms.

Ehrlich's plan to find his magic bullets was to start with a chemical that had some activity in killing his target, not worrying too much if it was not ideal. It might show some unwanted toxicity to human cells, for instance. This starting molecule was called a lead compound. Lead compounds could then be modified chemically to improve their ability to work as a drug, increasing their activity against the target cells, while reducing their toxicity. What Ehrlich was doing was linking the world of chemistry to the world of biology by seeing how altering the structure of a chemical alters its effect on an organism.

Ehrlich tried his approach with African sleeping sickness, known to be caused by infection by trypanosome parasites and spread by bites from tsetse flies. His starting point was a compound called Atoxyl. It had been tried in 1905 as a drug for sleeping sickness with some success, though prolonged use eventually caused blindness by damaging the optic nerve. Ehrlich and his team first determined the exact structure of Atoxyl. With this knowledge, they could synthesise hundreds of different versions of the structure to try to improve it. Best was compound number 418, which not only killed trypanosomes, but also showed low toxicity in mice.[3] In 1907 they tried it on humans. Though it often had some bad side effects, on the whole it was helpful for the worst types of sleeping sickness.[4]

Encouraged, Ehrlich then turned to syphilis. In 1905 Fritz Schaudinn and Erich Hoffmann discovered that syphilis was caused by infection by bacteria called *Treponema pallidum*.[5] Hoffmann suggested to Ehrlich that he should see whether anything in his library of compounds developed for sleeping sickness might be good for syphilis. Ehrlich handed the project to his Japanese colleague Sahachiro Hata, who had been able to infect rabbits with *Treponema pallidum*. After a heroic effort, Hata found that compound 606 worked, killing *Treponema pallidum*, while leaving the rabbits unharmed. This was arsphenamine – truly the magic bullet that Ehrlich had been searching for.[4]

After further animal tests to check that arsphenamine really worked and was safe, Ehrlich ran a clinical trial on patients with syphilis. Success led to immense demand, so Ehrlich teamed up with the Hoechst company to manufacture and sell the drug under the name Salvarsan. A modified version with fewer side effects called Neosalvarsan followed in 1914. Salvarsan and Neosalvarsan remained the drugs of choice for syphilis until the introduction of penicillin thirty years later. Ehrlich's drugs based on Atoxyl were the only synthetic antibiotics that we had until the discovery of a new class of drugs in the 1930s called sulphonamides. A modest, though brilliant man, Ehrlich said of his discovery of Salvarsan, 'For seven years of misfortune I had one moment of good luck.'[6]

The pioneering work of Koch, Hata, Ehrlich and others established the way in which drugs can be discovered. The scale and sophistication of drug discovery has increased enormously over the last hundred years, but the overall scheme still follows the plan that Ehrlich conceived and put into practice with sleeping sickness and syphilis. Following his vision has given us thousands of effective drugs, saving billions of lives and increasing life expectancy by decades over the last century. Though we keep getting better at preventing and tackling infections, new diseases are sure to arise. We will always need our magic bullets.

PART III

YOU ARE WHAT YOU EAT

The deviation of man from the state in which he was originally placed by nature seems to have proved to him a prolific source of diseases.

Edward Jenner, *An Inquiry into the Causes and Effects of Variolæ Vaccinæ*, 1798[1]

11

Hansel and Gretel

In his famous and influential book of 1798, *An Essay on the Principle of Population*, an English clergyman called Thomas Malthus argued that population levels are controlled by resources.[1] Malthus claimed that if the means of subsistence (basically food) in any country can easily support its inhabitants, then the result will be a population increase. The food supply will then need to be divided among a greater number of people, so how the poor live becomes worse, with many reduced to severe distress. By distress, Malthus meant:

> The power of population is so superior to the power of the earth to produce subsistence for man, that premature death must in some shape or other visit the human race ... sickly seasons, epidemics, pestilence, and plague advance in terrific array, and sweep off their thousands and tens of thousands. Should success be still incomplete, gigantic inevitable famine stalks in the rear, and with one mighty blow levels the population with the food of the world.[2]

Efforts to increase agricultural production can only have a temporary benefit, as 'ultimately the means of subsistence become in the same proportion to the population as at the period from which we set out'. The ultimate check on human numbers is therefore simply running out of food, so famine is 'the last, the most dreadful resource of nature'. Intermittent famine is an inevitable part of the human condition. Mankind is in a trap. Malthus was one of the world's greatest pessimists, arguing that whatever we try, 'The superior power of population cannot be checked without producing misery or vice.'² But was his claim that population is limited by food supply right?

We have very good records on life in Western Europe for the past thousand years, so we can look at this long period to see how famines happened and how they were eventually overcome. From 1250 to 1345, immediately before the Black Death, famines in Europe were frequent.² Europe was in a vulnerable state where lack of food was endemic, as the demands of the population were on the brink of exceeding the food resources available. Malnutrition reduces the ability to fight off disease, so the plague of the late 1340s arrived at a particularly bad time. In contrast, for about two centuries after the Black Death, when the population had crashed, famines were rare. By 1550 the population had expanded to pre-Black Death levels and famines became common again. Famines therefore cluster in periods when regions have reached their maximum possible populations, which in the Middle Ages was about 20 million people in France, 14 million in Italy and 5 million in England. When at these levels, any substantial decline in food production could generate famine.

One frequent trigger for famine was prolonged bad weather, leading to harvest failures. In the spring of 1315 heavy rain started in northern Europe, 'most marvellously and for so long', according to the Abbot of Saint-Vincent, near Laon in France. The rain did not stop until mid-August, in a vast area from France and Britain in the west, across Germany and Scandinavia, to Poland and Lithuania in the east. One account reported rain for 155 days in a row. Bridges broke; mills and whole villages were swept away by floods; sodden wood and peat would not burn; quarries and cellars flooded. Straw and hay could not be dried, so there was no fodder for livestock over the winter. Underfed cattle and sheep were too weak to fight off disease. The staple food of wheat would not ripen and rotted in the fields. It was a struggle to evaporate sea water to make salt, needed to preserve food and make cheese. Worst of all was the damage to fields: crops could not be planted or harvested in saturated land, and precious topsoil was washed away, reducing many previously fertile fields to clay or even bare rock.

One year's failed harvest, though a serious matter, did not usually cause famine. King Edward II of England first tried to buy grain from Louis X of France. When he found out that the French had been hit just as badly by the rains, he arranged shipments from Spain, Sicily and Genoa in southern Europe. While measures such as these might be expensive, they were usually enough to avert catastrophe, provided that the next year's harvest was reasonable.

Next year's harvest was not reasonable. The rains returned in 1316, following the same disastrous pattern as the previous year. Now peasants were eating their seed corn and their breeding animals, ruining their prospects for years to come. The rains did not return to normal until the summer of 1317, but the people were too weak to work properly, and they had eaten their work animals and seed corn. In addition, during the winter of 1317–18, the weather turned very cold. Thousands of malnourished animals froze to death or died from disease. It was not until 1325 that the food supply returned to previous levels. In all, 10–25 per cent of the people in northern Europe died.[3]

A second common cause of catastrophe is natural disasters, such as earthquakes, tsunamis or volcanoes. In addition to generating deadly lava flows, toxic gases and rains of boulders, volcanoes are quite capable of causing famine thousands of miles from the eruption, and months or years later. Iceland is a major site for volcanoes with this power. When one erupted in 1783, more than 20,000 people died in Britain, making it the greatest natural disaster in modern British history.[4]

The longest mountain range on Earth runs down the middle of the Atlantic Ocean. Here, the plates are moving apart, like two gigantic conveyor belts moving in opposite directions, and molten rock rises at the split forming the Mid-Atlantic Ridge. In this way, Europe and Africa move apart from the Americas at a rate of a few centimetres per year, fast enough to create the Atlantic Ocean in only 120 million years or so. At Þingvellir in Iceland, the ridge rises to the surface with a rift valley in the centre, where you can see exactly where the plates meet. This makes Iceland one of the most volcanically active countries on Earth. When oceanic crust melts, it forms runny lava that pours out of volcanoes like rivers, unlike volcanoes that form on continents, which have sticky lava that plugs vents, and hence are more likely to explode. In June 1783, the Laki volcano in southern Iceland began to erupt. It didn't stop for eight months. The lava flows, fountains and explosions from 130 vents along a 23-kilometre length of fissures and cones ejected 15 cubic kilometres of lava, making it the biggest eruption of its type since 934 CE (which was also in Iceland). For comparison, in a period of eight months Laki expelled as much lava as one of the currently most active volcanoes on Earth – Kīlauea on Hawaii – has in the last one hundred years. In addition, nearby Grímsvötn, Iceland's most frequently active volcano, was also active at the same time.[5]

Twenty villages were destroyed by lava flows from Laki. Our best accounts are from the Reverend Jón Steingrímsson, who wrote an eyewitness description of the Laki eruption and its effects on his people called A Complete Treatise on the Síða Fires. Steingrímsson was believed to have performed a miracle one Sunday in July 1783. During his service, a lava flow threatened to destroy his church. Despite the danger, he decided to go ahead with the service, expecting that it would be the last ever for the church (and himself). During his preaching, the lava river stopped, and the church and congregation were saved.

More importantly than the lava, Laki also pumped out vast amounts of toxic hydrogen fluoride and sulphur dioxide gases. Sulphur dioxide reacts with water to form sulphurous acid and sulphuric acid, which kill plants, and damage lungs and skin. Worse is hydrogen fluoride. As well as being a corrosive, acidic gas, it leads to fluoride being incorporated into grasses, which are eaten by livestock, poisoning them from fluoride overdoses. The Laki eruptions killed 60 per cent of the grazing livestock in Iceland, as well as most of the crops, while more than 10,000 people, a quarter of the Icelandic population, died in the resulting famine.[6]

Most of the sulphur dioxide reached the upper atmosphere and circulated around the northern hemisphere. The toxic haze killed thousands in Western Europe. Crops were damaged by acid rain. Weather was affected, with the high-altitude droplets blocking sunlight, causing low temperatures for several years. Disruption of normal weather patterns further south meant droughts in India and little rain in the highlands that feed the Nile River. Egypt was totally dependent on the Nile flooding annually to fertilise and irrigate its fields. When the Nile floods failed, the disastrous harvest meant that one-sixth of the population of Egypt died.[7] In total, as many as 6 million people were killed by the effects of the eruption, firstly by inhaling toxins, as in the UK, and then later from famine.

What happens in a famine? When harvests fail, and the usual products are unavailable, people will turn to an astonishing variety of alternative things to eat. First will be foodstuffs that might not taste good but are still nutritious. Folk wisdom, particularly in the elderly, can tell us what can be eaten in hard times, how to recognise famine foods and how to cook them. As things get worse, people will consume more or less anything to try to fill their bellies. These famine foods include, but are very much not limited to: sugar beets, flower bulbs such as crocuses, irises and tulips, potato peelings, nettles, wild berries and currants, beechnuts, acorns, wild fungi, tree leaves, nuts, crab apples, dandelions, cats, rats, dogs, zoo animals, earthworms, sparrows, tarantulas, scorpions, silkworms, grasshoppers, grass, seaweed, sawdust, dung, tree bark, leather, locusts, thistles, peanut hulls, horses and animal feed.[8, 9] It was even reported that in the Chinese famine of 1959–61, starving children would hang around bus stations hoping to find vomit to eat on the floor of arriving buses.[9] Needless to say, this was not the healthiest of diets. Eating rotten food and carrion, coupled with bodies unable to resist infection causes gastrointestinal disease and diarrhoea. Thus, many deaths in famine come from disastrous choices in food.

When a family was faced with starvation, members might try to sell their children to someone who is better able to feed them. This practice was legalised in Japan from 1231 to 1239, in response to the Kangi famine, the worst in Japanese history.[10] Cannibalism is frequently reported in the worst famines, though hard evidence for this is often shaky. Survivors are reluctant to admit to the desperate and illegal measures they used to survive, though cut marks on cooked bones can be a giveaway. In the 1315 Great Famine, an Irish chronicler reported that people 'were so destroyed by hunger that they extracted bodies of the dead from cemeteries and dug out the flesh from the skulls and ate it; and women ate their children out of hunger'.[11] In Poland, 'in many places parents devoured their children and children their parents'. Some ate the bodies from gibbets after executions by hanging. Parents might swap children, as it is easier to eat someone else's child than your own. For similar reasons, the last body part to be eaten is generally the head.

In the well-known German folk tale *Hansel and Gretel*, a starving woodcutter and his new wife decide to leave their children in the forest as they can no longer feed them. The children find a wonderful house made of gingerbread where they are caught by a witch who wants to eat them. Hansel is kept in a cage and fattened up, while Gretel has to work for the witch. Luckily, the children fool the witch and manage to kill her by pushing her into an oven. They find her treasure and return to their father. Fortunately, their stepmother has died, so they live happily ever after.

This vile story features all the common horrors of famine in just a few short pages, namely: obsession with food, the death of a parent, poverty, child abuse, slavery, starvation, murder, abandoning children and cannibalism. Strangely, it has been considered to be a bedtime story suitable for young children for hundreds of years. The tale of Hansel and Gretel may have originated in Germany in the Great Famine of 1315, when desperate families did indeed leave their children to starve, and resorted to cannibalism (though it may be much older, as similar stories are found around the Baltic and not just in Germany).

How does extreme hunger affect people? The body can survive with no food at all for about eight weeks, depending on its fat reserves and the conditions. If it is very cold or you must perform physical work, you need more calories to maintain your body temperature. How does the body adjust to prolonged starvation?

After eating carbohydrates, your blood glucose levels rise before being transported to the liver. There, the glucose molecules are joined together to make a starch-like polymer called glycogen. During the first stage of starvation, the glycogen is broken back down into glucose to provide energy. Once this is used up, blood glucose levels are maintained by breaking down fats and proteins. Fats are split into glycerol and fatty acids. Fatty acids can be used as a source of energy, particularly by muscle, leaving the remaining glucose for organs that need it more, like the brain. This switch from glycogen to fats is what happens when marathon runners hit the 'wall'. During a marathon, a well-trained runner will find the first eighteen miles or so not too challenging. However, quite suddenly energy will drain away and pain set in with every stride, from toes to hips. However much you stuff yourself with carbohydrate in the few days before a marathon to maximise your glycogen stores, you can only make enough to power yourself for three-quarters of the distance (for most people, anyway).

In the second phase of starvation, which typically lasts for several weeks, fats are the main energy source. The liver metabolises fatty acids into ketone bodies that can be used as an alternative source of energy for the brain. Ketone bodies are turned into acetone, which smells bad on the breath.

Once the fat reserves have gone, proteins are used as the main source of energy. Muscles are the biggest store of protein, and we can manage without them to some extent, so these go first. Weakness naturally sets in. Once muscles have gone, proteins critical for cellular function are broken down instead, causing more serious symptoms. People are now more vulnerable to infectious disease, as their immune system loses effectiveness. Additional signs of starvation are flaky skin, changes in hair colour, dehydration, decreased need to sleep, headaches, sensitivity to noise and light, disturbances of sound and vision, and a swollen belly. Body temperature, heart rate and respiration all drop, as the body tries to minimise its need for energy. The immune system is now functioning very poorly, and unable to withstand infectious disease. If a fatal infection is avoided, death finally comes from heart failure.

A fascinating, though ethically dubious study on the psychological effects of starvation was carried out at the University of Minnesota in 1944, led by American physiologist Ancel Keys.[12, 13] The study recruited thirty-six young men, chosen for their high levels of physical and psychological health, as well as commitment to the objectives of the experiment. The subjects were conscientious objectors, who volunteered as an alternative to military service in the Second World War.

For the first three months of the experiment, the volunteers ate normally, while their behaviour, personality and eating patterns were carefully monitored. During the next six months, the men were only allowed half of their former food intake and had to stay active, so lost about 25 per cent of their former weight. The six months of going hungry were followed by three months of recovery, when the men could eat normally again. Although individual responses varied greatly, most experienced big physical, psychological and social changes, which usually persisted even when they were in the re-feeding stage and beyond.

The volunteers developed a deep interest in food. While this is not surprising, this preoccupation often manifested itself in strange ways. Concentration lapsed as the men couldn't stop thinking about food. When they were talking, food became the main topic. Meals could be dragged out for hours, while others wolfed their food as fast as possible. The favourite reading matter became cookbooks, menus and articles on farming. Top entertainment was watching others eat. Some men began to collect food-related items that they couldn't use, such as coffee pots, ladles, spoons and pans. This progressed to hoarding useless non-food items, including old books and clothes they couldn't wear. Tea, coffee and chewing gum use rocketed, to the point where coffee had to be limited to nine cups a day, and gum to two packs a day.

During the three-month refeeding phase, most men went on massive binges, consuming a staggering 8–10,000 calories per day (triple normal). Many made themselves ill through overeating; others ate as much as possible, but still felt hungry even after a 5,000-calorie meal. Nearly all settled back to normal eating habits after a few months, however.

Starvation often caused emotional distress, including depression, occasional elation, anger, intolerance, anxiety, apathy and psychosis. One even chopped off two of his own fingers. This was despite the men being selected for their sound physical and mental condition at the start of the programme. Men began to avoid social contact, particularly with women, becoming progressively more withdrawn and isolated. They lost their sense of humour, of comradeship, their interest in sex and felt socially inadequate. One man said,

> I am one of about three or four who still go out with girls. I fell in love with a girl during the control period, but I see her only occasionally now. It's almost too much trouble to see her even when she visits me in the lab. It requires effort to hold her hand. Entertainment must be tame. If we see a show, the most interesting part of it is contained in scenes where people are eating.[13]

They lost energy, concentration, alertness, comprehension and judgement, though not overall intelligence, as well as showing the physical symptoms described above.

The study shows how humans when starved devote more and more resources to food. Things normally of major interest to young men, like socialising, particularly with women, are put aside in favour of an overwhelming obsession with food. Our ancestors undoubtedly went through many episodes of famine, and we are the descendants of those who were successful in surviving. These physical and mental changes are therefore likely to have evolved as necessary measures to get through times when food runs short, until it becomes available once more.

The Minnesota study was conducted in a safe environment. If subjects became a real danger to themselves or others, they could be taken out of the programme (though admittedly sometimes short of the correct number of fingers). In real famines complete breakdown of society often occurred. The intense stress of famine can bring out extremes in behaviour, often for the worst. Everything is put aside in the interests of survival. People lose shame and compassion for others; crime rockets, particularly theft of food or anything that can be quickly sold or exchanged for something to eat. In societies with slavery, slaves might be 'set free' when their masters did not want the responsibility of feeding them, or simply killed. In desperation, parents might sell their children into slavery or try to get themselves enslaved. Women turn to prostitution, as their bodies are all they have left to sell, though the demand for sex from starving men disappears. Suicides and child abandonment increase. The elderly and young children die first. Desperate people migrate from rural areas to cities, or to lands thought to have food.[9]

Malthus published his book arguing that human population is ultimately controlled by the food supply in 1798. Evidence up to that time showed that he was more or less right: after a run of poor harvests, people starve, disease and social breakdown ensue, and the population falls. With good harvests, more people live, especially infants, and the population rises. A permanent increase in food production, as a result of the introduction of new foods, new land being farmed or better transport, can only be a temporary fix. The population will rise to a new level to match the greater availability of food, and again be at risk of famine.

So it seemed in 1798. Returning to the relationship between population and famine, however, something odd happened after about 1650 in England, and about fifty years later in France and Italy. The population rose, but contrary to what Malthus would expect, there were no famines. Somehow, the link between overpopulation and vulnerability to famine had been broken.

The first country to end endemic famine was the Netherlands in the seventeenth century. In 1568, the Seven Provinces, predecessor of today's Netherlands, started the Eighty Years' War to achieve independence from Spain. In 1585 the Netherlands were split between the Catholic south, which eventually became Belgium, and the Protestant north, which became the Netherlands. The tolerant north benefited from an influx of talented and wealthy Protestants and Jews from Flanders, France, Spain and Portugal. The Dutch economy boomed for a hundred years, particularly in shipping, so by 1670 half of all the merchant ships in Europe were Dutch. Some of the wealth was spent on making the Dutch world leaders in art and science. This wealth and trade allowed the Dutch to escape famine.

In 1602 the Dutch East India Company (Verenigde Oostindische Compagnie, VOC) was founded as a corporation to trade with Asia. It took over from the Portuguese as the major player in European trade with Asia and became the world's largest commercial enterprise. The Dutch created the first stock exchange and central bank, vital tools in capitalism to finance their operations. Most of the VOC's trade was in the North Sea and Baltic, importing timber and grain, which was stored in Holland in vast quantities. These stockpiles allowed the Dutch to cope with a bad harvest. Their wealth could buy foodstuffs from abroad if necessary, transported by sea. They were also fortunate that the Netherlands was rarely a battlefield, unlike Germany, which had been ruined during the Thirty Years' War (1618–48). The Dutch were experts in land reclamation, building canals and dykes, and using wind power to drain lakes, creating new farmland. Even so, bad harvests could still happen, leaving the poorest in a vulnerable position. The Dutch developed a system of poor relief, where town leaders or churches gave to the poor – an early form of welfare state. About 10 per cent of households benefited.[14]

The Dutch and British were commercial and military rivals in the seventeenth century. Eventually the British concluded that if you can't beat them, join them, and in 1688 invited the Dutchman and Protestant William of Orange to be their king, instead of the Catholic James II. Agricultural production had started to increase from about 1600. This naturally led to a population increase, but as food production grew faster than the number of people, starvation was avoided. Food production in England doubled from 1600 to 1800, achieved by improving transport and reclaiming land, as well as introducing better ways to farm.

North of Cambridge in England lie the Fens, characterised by flat fields stretching to the horizon and few towns. Even the rivers run in straight lines. Dutch engineers led schemes to drain the Fen marshland in the seventeenth century, using their expertise in canals, dykes and windmills. The job was mostly complete by the early nineteenth century and provided new highly fertile farmland, now sunk below sea level in many places, just like Holland.

A medieval 'road' was not much more than a right of way, in practice often no more than a well-trodden path. It was not surfaced or fenced and had no signposts. When it rained, roads turned to mud, so that half the time wagons could not use them, and goods had to be transported by packhorse. Things began to improve in the eighteenth century with the start of the turnpike system, where travellers paid tolls at turnpike gates. The tolls were (supposedly) used to maintain better-quality roads. This new form of taxation was not entirely popular. Sometimes men would destroy the turnpikes and burn down or blow up the toll houses with gunpowder, particularly in Yorkshire. Nevertheless, the journey time from London to Manchester was cut from four and a half days in 1754 to just over a day thirty years later, as a result of the turnpike system. By the mid-1830s more than 20,000 miles of road was being run by Turnpike Trusts.[15] Internal tariffs, customs barriers and feudal tolls were steadily removed to facilitate trade. The Dutch and British also benefited from geography, as their cities were on the coast or rivers, easily accessible to shipping.

Francis Egerton, the third Duke of Bridgewater, owned coal mines in Worsley, ten miles west of Manchester. Coal was needed to power steam engines in industrial areas of the city, but its transport by river or packhorse was slow, unreliable and expensive. His solution was to build the Bridgewater Canal, featuring an aqueduct and tunnel. Canal boats pulled by a horse could carry more than ten times the load that was possible with a cart, halving coal prices in Manchester. The success of the Bridgewater Canal (which is still in use) helped trigger canal-building mania in Britain from 1770 to 1830, with more than 4,000 miles built. Canal mania was followed by railway mania from 1830. Rail passenger numbers jumped from 5.5 million in 1838 to 111 million in 1855.

Gentlemen farmers, such as the splendidly named Jethro Tull and 'Turnip' Townshend, began to take an interest in agriculture. They applied new scientific and enlightened thinking to experiment with crops, breeding livestock and technology. If the same crop is used repeatedly in the same field, the land can become exhausted of nutrients, making yields plummet. The traditional solution was to leave a field fallow for a year, when being unfarmed would allow it to recover. A better solution was to rotate crops, particularly peas, beans, turnips or clover, that were able to fix nitrogen from the air and reinvigorate the soil.

Contact with the Americas brought valuable new crops to Europe – potatoes, tomatoes, maize, beans, squashes, peanuts and cocoa. Access to a wider range of foodstuffs mitigated against the failure of one crop and gave a healthier, more varied diet. By the end of the eighteenth century, rice, tea, sugar (from cane) and potatoes were all a regular part of the diet of even the poorest.[16] Overexploited common land was taken over by new owners with more interest in taking care of it. Peasants took their produce to market, rather than primarily using it to feed their families. New machines, such as better ploughs and seed drills, improved productivity, while high-quality sodium nitrate fertiliser began to be shipped in from Chile. English agriculturist Robert Bakewell's selective breeding programmes led to greatly improved breeds of animals, doubling the average weight of cattle. Many breeds of horses, sheep and cattle farmed today are descended from his pioneering stock. Agricultural shows, first held in Salford near Manchester in 1768, allowed farmers to compete, entertain the public and exchange the best animals and crops.

These changes helped create great increases in agricultural output. In England, production of wheat, barley, peas, beans, oats and rye roughly doubled from 1650 to 1800. Food imports by sea also soared. England was fortunate that no major wars were fought in the country after the Civil War of 1642–51. At last, food production grew faster than the population for a sustained period, avoiding yet another catastrophic famine, as predicted by Malthus. When Malthus published his conclusions and forecasts in 1798, he was right about the past, but utterly wrong about the future. Even today, where the planetary population has reached an all-time high of more than 7 billion, famine has almost been eradicated.

While we can be grateful that few of us have personally experienced famine, we should bear in mind that from the onset of farming until the Agricultural Revolution, which began a few hundred years ago, periodic famines were regular occurrences. Long-term health effects of starvation would have affected the great majority of adults. Stunting and long-term susceptibility to diseases caused by famine could then have been the normal human condition. Again, the modern world, with abundant and varied food, despite the enormous world population, is very unusual. The effects on our bodies and minds of having survived famines have largely gone.

The traditional view of economists on why famine happens is a lack of food, usually due to harvest failure. In other words, not enough food is available compared to the number of people who need it. Market forces will then operate, so businesses will move in to meet the demands of the people who are now willing to pay more to eat. Authorities have no need to intervene by providing free food, as the free market will take care of this by itself. In fact, intervention is damaging, as it interferes with the perfect self-correction of the market. Robert Malthus and Adam Smith[17] were often quoted in support of these views. Smith's economic arguments were highly influential on policymakers, particularly in the British Empire. For example, when a famine was developing in Gujarat in India in 1812, the Governor of Bombay rejected a proposal for the government to lead on moving food into affected areas, as such matters ought to be left to free markets, quoting Adam Smith in support,[18] even though it is doubtful whether Smith would ever have supported starvation.

This simple approach of concentrating on the availability of food was demolished by the economist Amartya Sen in his book *Poverty and Famines: An Essay on Entitlement and Depravation*, first published in 1981.[19] By examining economic data for several famines, he showed that a decline in food supplies cannot explain famine in the present day. Instead, it is when people lose the ability to access food that famine takes place. More simply, desperately poor people can no longer afford to eat.

Amartya Sen was born in 1933 in India, then ruled by the British. As a nine-year-old boy, he witnessed the Bengal Famine of 1943, when 3 million people died. A Famine Inquiry Commission was set up to investigate why this happened. It concluded that the primary cause of the famine was 'a serious shortage in the total supply of rice available for consumption in Bengal', their primary staple crop. Sen's economic data showed that this standard explanation of the famine was false. The appalling loss of life was actually avoidable, as India had sufficient food for the people of Bengal. The problem was that rural labourers had lost their jobs in a time of rising food prices, and so starved. The British authorities did not take the action needed to avert the famine, as their main concern was saving India from a Japanese invasion, and the free market failed. This abject failure of so-called benevolent British rule was a powerful argument for Indian independence four years later.

Sen's conclusion was that social and economic factors, such as declining wages, unemployment, rising food prices and poor food-distribution, could lead to starvation within certain societal groups. Food might exist, but this is useless if people lose their ability to obtain it. Famines are therefore economic disasters, not just food crises, and Malthus's work does not apply to the modern world.

Shortly after *Poverty and Famines* was published, reports gradually came out on the appalling Chinese famine of 1959–61. This was the worst famine of the twentieth century, caused by communist dictator Mao Zedong's disastrous Great Leap Forward. China had done its best to keep the catastrophe secret, but after Mao died in 1976, it became clear that tens of millions had died. To Sen, this secrecy and the death toll were two sides of the same coin. China had neither a free press nor political opposition to sound the alarm. Chinese officials were too scared to report that Mao's policy was failing. In contrast, India has had no famines since it became an independent democracy in 1947, with a free press, in stark contrast to when it was ruled by the British, or various kings or emperors.[19] Sen argued that any similar famine in India would have caused outrage in the newspapers, creating demands for action, and would have brought down the government. The situation was completely different in China, where few people in the rest of the world had any idea what was going on.

In 1999, Sen wrote, 'there has never been a famine in a functioning multiparty democracy'. In a democracy, parties 'have to win elections and face public criticism, and have strong incentive to undertake measures to avert famines and other catastrophes'.[20] A more recent analysis shows that Sen was right. Democratic countries with effective governments and a lack of corruption do indeed avoid famine.[20] Of course, democratic countries are hardly perfect and many non-democratic governments do an excellent job in taking care of their citizens. Nevertheless, democratic governments must have the interests of their people at heart, or they would lose power.

As we have seen, famines in modern, industrial societies are not usually caused by harvest failures. Instead, modern famines are caused by governments, either inadvertently, through bad policy and incompetence, or as an effect of war. It is how we respond to the inevitable times of bad weather and harvest failures that counts. Examples of modern famines include potato famines in Ireland and Scotland (1845–9); the Taiping Rebellion (1850–73) in China; failed communist agricultural policies in the USSR, particularly Ukraine (1932–3); Mao's Great Leap Forward in China (1959–61); North Korea (1995–9); starvation in Holland, Indonesia, India, Greece, Warsaw and Leningrad in the Second World War; Bangladesh (1974); Ethiopia (1984–5); and South Sudan (2013–20) and Yemen during civil wars (2014–present).

Sometimes governments cause famine deliberately, as an instrument of war. Starving the residents of a city to compel them to surrender had been used for thousands of years in siege warfare. Even an entire country can effectively be placed under siege, as Germany was in the First World War.

At the start of the twentieth century, both Germany and Britain were heavily reliant on imports of food and raw materials from the Americas to feed their people and supply their industries. Both therefore aimed to cut off each other's supplies by sea, using either the British Royal Navy or the German U-boat fleet. The Imperial German General Staff were well aware that they were vulnerable to a long-term blockade that would stop their shipping. Their war plan was therefore to send nearly all their armies west to rapidly defeat France, then turn east to fight Russia, France's ally. They made few plans for a drawn-out war of attrition. Britain had a tiny army, so would be irrelevant in a quick war, if they decided to join in on the side of France and Russia.

While the German advance was initially successful, the French army managed to drive back the invaders at the Battle of the Marne, east of Paris. Both sides then dug in to build hundreds of miles of trenches. With military technology at that time greatly favouring the defenders, the Western Front remained static from late 1914.

The British war plan to defeat Germany relied on their navy, the most powerful in the world, while their allies, France and Russia, were to provide the armies. Planning for a blockade had been under way since 1904. Winston Churchill, First Lord of the Admiralty in 1914, said, 'The British blockade treated the whole of Germany as if it were a beleaguered fortress, and avowedly sought to starve the whole population – men, women and children, old and young, wounded and sound – into submission.'[21] The blockade stopped merchant ships entering the North Sea to trade with Germany, but it involved much more than just the Royal Navy. Neutral states were persuaded to join the coalition, or at least convinced (in one way or another) to stop trade with Germany and its allies. Thousands of analysts carefully studied the German economy to work out which of its imports were most critical, so that special efforts could be made to stop these. Spies and code-breakers identified any ships still trying to get to Germany, where big profits were available.[22]

A partial blockade was initiated at the outbreak of the war in August 1914, but it was not fully implemented until November, as the British were at first nervous about antagonising the neutral United States. When American opinion turned against the Central Powers upon reports of atrocities by the German army against Belgian and French civilians, the British were able to strengthen the blockade. Britain used its position as the world's largest trading nation to pressure neutral states to comply, by denying them use of coaling stations, detaining vessels for lengthy inspections, or simply offering a higher price than the Germans for their most-needed imports. Eventually the most important neutral trading partner for Germany was Sweden, which could continue to send food, iron ore and other commodities across the Baltic Sea, out of reach of the Royal Navy.[23]

Shortages of foodstuffs contributed to hundreds of thousands of wartime deaths in Germany, mostly by making the population vulnerable to disease. Losing Danish dairy products caused a critical deficiency of dietary fats. Potassium nitrate from Chile, used as fertiliser and for explosives, was no longer available, though the excellent German chemical industry did their best to compensate. The German government imposed controls on all aspects of the economy, prioritising the military. Agricultural production fell as farm labourers and horses went to the front.

From early 1915 potatoes had vanished from much of the country, followed by wheat. Civil unrest and crime grew, as allowances of food, fuel, clothing and detergents declined or disappeared altogether. In Stuttgart alone, within a three-month period in 1917, 273 children aged twelve to fourteen were convicted of theft. Every child had been attempting to steal food from farms.[24] By 1916 almost all foodstuffs and fuel were rationed, and their official prices controlled. Civilians had to spend hours queuing for goods that often ran out before they reached their turn. In Berlin the black-market price for meat soared twentyfold from the eve of war to the end.[25] In 1916 the potato harvest failed and people in the so-called 'Turnip Winter' were forced to live on the less palatable swede turnip (or rutabaga) that was normally only used to feed pigs. Toni Sender, a German woman, recalled the situation as follows:

The worst winter, that of 1917, when almost all food consisted in whole or in part of turnips … Bread made of flour mixed with turnips, turnips at luncheon and dinner, marmalade made of turnips – the air was filled with the smell of turnips and it almost made you vomit! We hated turnips and had to eat them. They were the only foodstuff obtainable in abundance.[26]

Food and clothing provided inferior alternatives, such as caffeine-free 'coffee' that included ground acorns, and shoe soles made of wood instead of leather. The illegal black market thrived, and theft, riots and strikes grew, all driven by a lack of food. The situation was just as bad in Vienna and Budapest, major cities of the Germans' ally Austria-Hungary. Some blamed Poles and Jews, following ancient tradition, as well as the government. Morale fell in the army, as their rations and food quality also declined, and the soldiers were well aware of how their families were suffering at home. In 1917–18, the average German ate less than 1,500 calories per day, down from 1,700 calories in 1916 and 4,020 calories in the pre-war years, when most people were manual workers. The average civilian's body weight had decreased by 15–20 per cent by the end of 1917.[27]

By November 1918, Germany had had enough. Their final offensives in spring 1918, using soldiers newly available after the defeat of Russia, had made impressive gains, but from August 1918 the army was suffering defeat after defeat from the Allied armies, which now included a large and rapidly growing American contingent. Their people had been hungry for years and were desperate for the war to end. The German leaders knew that the war was lost, so signed an armistice on 11 November 1918. Even though the fighting had stopped, the blockade cruelly continued, used as a weapon to pressure German leaders to sign the vindictive Versailles Treaty that made Germany accept blame for the war. The blockade finally ended completely on 12 July 1919, eight months after the Armistice.

Twenty-five years later, in the Second World War, Churchill again sought to win the war indirectly by killing the inhabitants and destroying the cities of Germany – this time using bombing from the air. The Americans joined them. In addition, in 1945 their fleets of advanced Boeing Superfortress bombers dropped mines into the Inland Sea between the major Japanese islands, crippling Japan's transport of food. The Americans were not hypocrites – the campaign was code-named Operation Starvation.

While the numbers are uncertain, the 1914–19 blockade of Germany undoubtedly killed many hundreds of thousands. Official British post-war statistics said that 772,736 Germans starved to death,[28] while the German Board of Public Health in December 1918 reported that 763,000 German civilians died from starvation or diseases caused by the blockade.[29] In addition, about 100,000 more would die in 1919, even though the fighting had ended. A 1928 academic study put the death toll at 424,000.[30] Such statistics are often suspect for political reasons. During the war, British propaganda said that the Germans were living on glue, while the Germans tried to persuade the Americans that the blockade was having little effect. Neither was true. Once the war was over, these positions were reversed, as the British downplayed their role in killing civilians, while some Germans exaggerated the famine's effects to justify fighting their old enemies.

Cases of tuberculosis, pneumonia and other lung conditions soared in Germany. Typhus returned, always a sign of the worst living conditions. Lack of vitamins caused rickets and scurvy, particularly in children. Long-lasting intestinal disorders became known as 'turnip disease'. Watered-down milk and questionable substances added to food to boost their bulk (such as sawdust and dirt) caused many disorders. Severe lack of soap, detergents and textiles meant that people were reduced to living in dirty rags, obviously another health hazard. Suffering from various ailments went on for years. Most pigs and cattle were killed, and those animals that survived were emaciated, so providing little milk and meat.

From 1872, the German Imperial Statistical Office began to collect data, including the heights and weights of nearly 600,000 schoolchildren measured between 1914 and 1924. This precious data set had been unexamined and unpublished until 2015, when Mary Cox from Oxford University found it after an extensive search in German archives and libraries.[31] Children born in 1910 showed evidence of malnutrition from the ages of six to thirteen, with 1918 being the worst year. All were shorter and lighter than pre-war children, and their short statures were maintained their whole lives. Adolescent growth spurts were delayed, particularly for boys. As children from different backgrounds went to different schools, it was possible to see that upper-class children were a few centimetres taller than middle-class children, who were in turn taller than working-class children. This could have been due to richer families acquiring more food from the black market, as factory workers, particularly in the arms industries, were supposed to get extra rations.

When the war ended, many charities and religious groups helped to provide food to poor German children. Herbert Hoover, head of the US Food Administration and future president, worked compassionately and heroically to arrange shipments of food and clothing, in the face of British and French opposition, saying that 'the United States is not at war with German infants'.[32] Hoover had much help with food aid from the Quaker American Friends Service Committee. The health of German children improved markedly as a result, returning to their mean pre-war heights and weights by 1923.

The blockade of Germany in the First World War, the Dutch Hunger Winter of 1944–5 and the Siege of Leningrad (1941–44) have been closely studied to see the effects of living through an episode of famine. Given the length of time since these events, we can track how people were affected throughout their whole lives. Results of such studies are sometimes contradictory and new work is published all the time. Certainly, lack of calories, protein, essential amino acids, vitamins and minerals in childhood stunts growth. Stunted growth is linked to poor achievement at school and behavioural abnormalities, which may last a lifetime.[33] Famine perhaps has its greatest effects on the unborn. When a mother is starving, the foetus adapts, via chemical modifications of its DNA, to be ready for a life short of food. Unfortunately, this change has the side effects of increased likelihood of cardiovascular disease, stroke, diabetes and hypertension.[34] The only certain long-term effect of the Great Leap Forward famine in China appears to be an increase in schizophrenia.[35] In contrast, young children who lived through the Ukraine or Dutch Hunger Winters were more likely to develop type 2 diabetes sixty years later.[36, 37] Why these two famines had such varying effects is not known.

How are we doing today at feeding the world? The Global Hunger Index (GHI)[38] gives a score for every country to track hunger, as follows:

First, for each country, values are determined for four indicators:

1. **Undernourishment:** the share of the population that is undernourished (has insufficient calories).
2. **Child wasting:** the share of children under the age of five whose body weight is too low for their height; i.e. too thin.
3. **Child stunting:** the share of children under the age of five who have low height for their age; i.e. too short.
4. **Child mortality:** the mortality rate of children under the age of five.

These measures are combined to give a single GHI for each country, on a scale from 0 (best) to 100 (worst). The graph opposite shows progress in the world and in six regions from 2000 to 2021. By every measure and in every region, the situation has greatly improved in the last eighteen years. Of course, much still needs to be done if no one is to go hungry, but this is still excellent news. Democracy is also spreading, consistent with Sen's ideas on the link between democratic governments and avoiding famine.

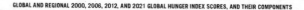

GLOBAL AND REGIONAL 2000, 2006, 2012, AND 2021 GLOBAL HUNGER INDEX SCORES, AND THEIR COMPONENTS

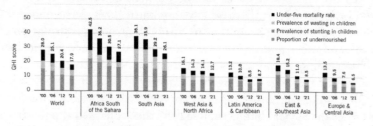

Global Health Index data from 2000 to 2021.

Only Venezuela has a worse GHI score in 2020 than in 2000, out of 107 countries. Still, there are more than twenty countries in a poorer state than Venezuela. Chad comes bottom overall, followed by Timor-Leste, Madagascar, Haiti and Mozambique. With chronic conflict and frequent drought, Chad is one of the only countries where more than 10 per cent of children die before the age of five.

Bad as Chad is, I would rather live there than North Korea. North Korea is by far the most repressive totalitarian state in the world, and the closest we have to the horrifying state described in George Orwell's *1984*. It is not at all easy to find out what life is like in North Korea. The state tightly controls all information. The people only have access to a single TV channel and are subject to hours of propaganda every day. They are told that their country is the best place on Earth and is a shining example to the rest of the world. Whether people actually believe any of this is impossible to say. Criticism of the regime is punished by a lengthy sentence in a brutal prison camp. Foreigners are often only allowed to visit the capital Pyongyang, where electricity and heating only work for a few hours each day. In the countryside, things are likely to be worse.[39]

In the mid-1990s foreigners noticed that Pyongyang now had many starving people, with hungry workers and orphaned children roaming the streets looking for food. This was a sign of a major famine, which is still deeply mysterious. No one knows how many died – estimates of the death toll vary from the low hundreds of thousands to several millions in a total population of about 25 million. North Korean officials have never even admitted that the famine happened and instead call the time the 'Arduous March'. Referring to famine or hunger in North Korea is forbidden.

To understand why this famine happened, we need to look at the history of North Korea. A communist government under the Kim family was set up in the late 1940s, controlling distribution of food and other goods. Political elites and the military got the best of everything, to buy their loyalty. Land in North Korea is not well suited for farming, but this didn't matter too much at first, as the Soviet Union supported its fellow communist state with aid, food and fuel. As the Soviet Union crumbled and then collapsed altogether, its support for North Korea sank and finally stopped completely. China helped instead to some extent, but this also ended in 1993 when China needed its grain for itself after poor harvests. In response, Kim Il Sung switched to a Marxist-Leninist philosophy of national self-reliance and isolation, or 'Juche'. North Korea had previously used cheap fuel from the Soviet Union to make chemical fertilisers. When this fuel was cut off, the fertiliser plants stopped working. Farmers were reduced to using human waste instead, so crop yields plummeted and parasitic infections spread. Food allocations to the people were cut and they were urged to eat only two meals a day. North Korea was now in a state that would have been recognised by Malthus as highly vulnerable to famine, where food production was barely meeting its people's needs, even in a good year for agriculture.

The years 1995 and 1996 were not good for agriculture. Rainfall in 1995 was the heaviest for seventy years, causing catastrophic flooding and destroying about 20 per cent of farmland. The state cut food allowances, and farmers began to hide their grain rather than hand it over for distribution. In a rare, desperate move, the North Korean leadership asked the international community for food aid. They did eventually respond, but much of what they provided was kept by the rulers or given to the military rather than starving civilians. North Koreans began eating grass and fleeing across the border to China. Nearly all the people suffered, but children were worst affected. A whole generation is thought to have physical and mental impairments from lack of food when young.

North Korea remains in a desperate state. The United Nations estimates that 40 per cent of North Koreans currently go hungry and lack basic healthcare and sanitation. More than 70 per cent of the population relies on international food aid to survive (despite Juche).[40]

We know how to avoid famine, though North Korea is a shining example of how not to do it. Firstly, information and freedom of speech is essential. Newspapers, television companies and other media outlets must hold governments to account, not just act as their cheerleaders. We can't do anything about a famine if we don't know that it is happening. Officials need to be able to report problems to leaders without fear of being punished for criticising the regime. Many international agencies and governments can and do help, but need to be aware of the situation, and be allowed access. The deliberate isolation and secrecy of North Korea is a major handicap in dealing with its problems.

Secondly, the government must care. Rather than looking after its people, the top priority of the North Korean regime is maintaining its own power. One way it does this is by spending a staggering 24 per cent of its GDP on the military – far more than any other country.[41] Keeping the military happy discourages interference from other countries and helps prevent the overthrow of the government in a military coup, though it deprives everything else (food and fuel, for instance) of sorely needed funding. North Korea is obviously not democratic, so the common people have no say in who is in charge. Rulers have little incentive to keep the people happy or even to feed them properly.

Thirdly, open borders are needed so that food can be brought in in times of crisis. Trade and transport also help generate wealth so that food can be purchased if needed. North Korea follows Juche, deliberately pursuing isolation with closed borders to keep its people ignorant, depriving it of funds and making imports and exports difficult.

Fourthly, modern methods of agriculture should be used to maximise food production. Severe fuel shortages mean that North Korea has regressed to using human labour instead of tractors, and sewage instead of chemical fertilisers. Mechanisation, up-to-date crops and fertilisers are needed, though the recent promotion of potatoes as an alternative to rice is a sensible move.

All places will suffer harvest failures from time to time, most often from natural disasters. When this happens in a country too poor to buy its way out of trouble, famine can still be prevented, thanks to better communications to alert us to the danger, cheap transport and food storage, aid from foreign governments and charities, antibiotics to deal with new infections, electrolytic fluids for rehydration and availability of emergency foodstuffs. For example, Plumpy'nut, a concoction of peanut butter and milk fortified with micronutrients and high in calories, is an excellent famine food for children.[42] These approaches work: even in sub-Saharan Africa, famines are now rare and minor compared to a few decades ago. We have switched from a situation where countries routinely teetered on the edge of starvation to one where we really can feed the world.

12

A Treatise on the Scurvy

Even though the constant threat of famine first came to an end in a few countries in Western Europe in about 1750, these remained far from being happy lands of plenty. For the poorest people, chronic malnutrition remained the norm. The emergence of the new science of chemistry in this period began to show what exactly our bodies were made from, and that if what we ate was out of step with what our bodies needed, disease could result. Food quality was not the same as food quantity. Instead, what exactly you are eating is of vital importance. Poor diet, particularly if it lacks essential micronutrients, causes disease in billions of people, even today.

The most basic measure of food quality is the number of calories it contains, which essentially tells us how much energy it provides. While many of us keep an eye on the number of calories we consume to avoid getting fat, people in the nineteenth century had the opposite problem. Most simply could not get enough, so were often hungry for days on end. At present, we are advised that a man needs about 2,500 calories per day to maintain his weight; for a woman it is about 2,000 calories per day. These values are relevant to our present-day lifestyles, where we have decent clothing and heating, travel to work by driving and have jobs that involve sitting. In the past, people typically had cold homes, as fires were an expense and a hassle; they lacked adequate clothing; and they had manual jobs in a field, mine or factory. This meant that their calorific requirements were a lot higher – perhaps 4,000 per day.

While the period from 1750 to 1900 saw the spectacular advances of the Industrial and Scientific Revolutions, and the expansion of

European power all over the globe, these brought little improvement to the health of the lower classes until the latter part of the nineteenth century. Hunger was common. We have data on the average number of calories per day per person in France and England from 1700. These values are remarkably low, being only about 2,100 in England in 1700, and even less in France. By 1850 both countries had increased to 2,400. For comparison, in 1965 the most malnourished country in the world was Rwanda. The energy value of the average diet there was the same as France in 1700. The English diet of 1850 had the same number of calories per person as present-day India. In addition, not only was the European diet short on energy, it was also lacking in meat and dairy products. Peasants were mostly living on cereals and root vegetables. High-fibre foods like these are low in calories per kilo.[1]

The primary use for the energy in our food is to maintain basic bodily functions, powering the heart, brain and lungs, as well as maintaining our internal temperature at 37° C. Energy is also needed to eat and digest food. It is only when these essentials have been met that people can use their energy supplies for other activities, notably work. In 1750, the average person in England had only about 800 calories per day available for work; in France, it was barely more than half that. The most malnourished 20 per cent therefore had only enough energy to do a few hours' slow walking per day.[1]

Small bodies need less food. Today, a typical male is 177 cm tall and weighs 78 kg. A body like this needs 2,280 calories per day simply to maintain its weight, without doing any work. A person this large 250 years ago would have starved. The meagre food supplies available at that time, on top of parasitic and diarrhoeal infections that took part of the food intake, meant that people had to be small and thin. Persistent lack of food in childhood and in the womb resulted in small adult bodies. Small bodies required less food and so could avoid starvation. Europeans in 1750 were severely stunted by modern standards. For example, in 1705 the average Frenchman was 161 cm tall (5 ft 3 in), weighed 46 kg and had a BMI of 18, a value that we would now consider to be worryingly low. In 1967 Frenchmen were 12 cm taller on average (reaching 5 ft 10 in) and a whopping 27 kg heavier. People now have 50 per cent larger bodies compared to those 200 years ago.

Shortness and stunting allowed survival in times when there was rarely enough to eat. But it came at great cost. The incidence of many chronic diseases grows with increased stunting. People's muscles, bones, hearts, lungs, and other body systems are all more likely to show long-term health conditions. Things began to change for the better in the late eighteenth century, first in the USA and England, then elsewhere in Europe. A little more food meant significantly more energy left over for work. More work could be used to improve living standards, so the population could finally climb out of a desperate existence on the edge of starvation. People now had the time and energy to work more productively and make better clothing and shelter. Taller, healthier people were better able to fight off chronic disease, parasites and other health conditions. A virtuous circle, where each generation was better off than the one before, kicked in.

Two hundred years ago, French chemist Antoine Lavoisier showed that the way we get energy from food is essentially the same as burning. In both processes, substances react with oxygen in the air to make carbon dioxide and water. Thus the energy value of a foodstuff (in calories) can be found by measuring the amount of heat it gives off when burned. Uncontrolled burning is accompanied by flame, sound and heat; in bodies, this energy is instead carefully channelled into useful processes, like building new molecules and keeping body temperature up.

Was there anything more to the value of a food than the number of calories it contained, though? In other words, as long as you had enough food, did it matter what form it took? Was it possible to thrive solely on a staple food, like rice or potatoes, or was it necessary to eat a range of foods, even if the total number of calories was the same?

By 1840, the new science of chemistry had advanced to the point where it was understood that everything is made of atoms, and substances have a formula, showing how many of each atom are present. For example, ammonia is NH_3, carbon dioxide is CO_2 and sulphuric acid is H_2SO_4. A formula like this is just a list of the elements present. What about food? Applying separation and analytical techniques to food revealed its basic parts: proteins, fats and carbohydrates. The Dutch chemist Gerardus Johannes Mulder concluded that all proteins had the formula of $C_{400}H_{620}N_{100}O_{120}S_{1 \text{ or } 2} P$.[2] These high numbers for each element show that proteins must be very complicated molecules. Even if the protein formula was correct (it isn't), working out how all these atoms were connected to each other with chemical bonds was well beyond the powers of nineteenth-century chemistry. Life therefore did seem to work by chemistry, but the molecules involved were fantastically complex.

Proteins were necessary for life, as dogs fed on a protein-free diet of sugar, olive oil and water died, apparently of starvation, even though they had all the calories they needed from the sugar and oil. Based on these kinds of results, Justus von Liebig, the influential German chemist, proposed in 1848 that proteins were needed to build all the chemicals within the body, while fats and carbohydrates were needed to provide energy. Thus, proteins, fats and carbohydrates – the 'Dietetic Trinity', plus a few minerals, like salt – provided everything the body needed.[3]

Von Liebig was wrong – you cannot survive just on proteins, fats and carbohydrates. Something else is essential in the diet, something found in abundance in citrus fruit, as shown by the appalling experiences of sailors on long sea voyages. We now know that this substance is vitamin C. The long and tortuous story of the discovery of vitamin C and its role in preventing scurvy shows how we came to understand the importance of micronutrients – substances that are essential in our diet, even if only found in tiny amounts.

The hideous disease of scurvy had been known since ancient times. Crusaders besieging castles in the Holy Land had often been afflicted with it, particularly during Lent, when they fasted. For example, during the Eighth Crusade in 1270, within the French army:

The disease worsened in the camp so much so that the dead flesh of the gums was removed by the barber to help soldiers chew and swallow their food. It was such a pity to hear the people in the camp from whom the barber was cutting the dead flesh; for they were shouting as loud as pregnant women do when giving birth.[4]

Scurvy only became of major importance, however, when Europeans began epic sea voyages. It could sometimes take years to make a round trip to India or the Spice Islands in what is now Indonesia, where extremely valuable goods were available. Similarly, military navies might need to be at sea for prolonged periods, chasing each other's fleets or maintaining blockades of enemy ports. Under such conditions, the dreaded scurvy was likely to strike. Scurvy featured bloody patches under the skin, joint pain, rotting gums and loosening teeth (making chewing agonising), extreme lethargy, softening of muscles and a foul stench. The disease progressed to pain in old wounds and bruises. Limbs then swelled and turned black. In the end, the patient was unable to move, and death followed.

On long voyages, sailors' staple diet was salty dried meat or biscuit baked from flour and water. Biscuit was rock hard when first baked. After a while, however, weevils and maggots would get into the biscuit and soften it so that it could be chewed, even by decaying gums. Maggot-infested biscuit was so vile that sailors would eat it in the dark.[5]

It is well known now that scurvy is readily cured or prevented by consuming fresh fruit and vegetables, with oranges and lemons being particularly effective. Strangely, this apparently simple fact was discovered and forgotten numerous times up to the start of the twentieth century. As far back as 1510, the Portuguese captain Pedro Álvares Cabral reported that afflicted sailors were cured by citrus fruits. Dutch and Spanish seafarers found the same, so the Dutch East India Company planted fruit trees on the Cape of Good Hope, where its ships routinely stopped. Nevertheless, many doctors persisted in insisting that scurvy was caused by foul air, too much salt, corruption of the blood, bad water, lack of exercise, infection, idleness or a discontented state of mind.

A Scottish ship's surgeon called James Lind is often given most of the credit for discovering that lemon juice prevents scurvy. Lind was appointed surgeon on HMS *Salisbury* in 1746. Scurvy was then a major concern for the Royal Navy, particularly after Commodore Anson's return from a four-year trip two years earlier, where only 600 of his 2,000 crew survived, the most killed by scurvy. Scurvy was killing far more ships' crew than the French or Spanish guns.

Lind set out to tackle the problem. He first read over sixty writers on the topic, finding most to be worthless. A new rigorous, rational approach was required, where he would 'propose nothing dictated from theory, but shall confirm all by experience and facts, the surest and most unerring guides'.[6] Severe scurvy broke out on the *Salisbury*'s second voyage, giving Lind his opportunity. He chose twelve men, all at a similar stage of the illness, and divided them into six pairs. For two weeks all were kept in the same accommodation and given an identical diet, other than a supposed cure. These remedies, given daily, were: two pints of cider; twenty-five drops of sulphuric acid (diluted with water, of course); vinegar; half a pint of sea water; two oranges and one lemon (until they ran out after only six days); or a strange concoction called the 'bigness of a nutmeg', made of garlic, horseradish, mustard and other ingredients. The results of Lind's trial were crystal clear. After six days, 'the most sudden and good effects were perceived from the use of oranges and lemons'.[6] The pair given cider was a little better, while the rest were worse. Scurvy could therefore be cured by citrus fruit.

Lind had hit upon what is still the gold standard way to perform an experiment – a clinical trial. If we want to see whether a new drug cures a disease, we study two groups of patients: one group gets the drug and the other gets a dummy pill (a placebo) that is identical to the drug as far as possible, including pill size, colour and taste. The patient groups must be matched as well, with the same distributions of sex, age, health conditions and so on. If we go to all this trouble, then any differences between the patient groups must result from the drug, since everything else is exactly the same. This is what Lind did on the *Salisbury*: the pairs of sailors differed only in whether they consumed the citrus fruit or not.

Previous confusion on the matter had arisen from too many things changing between voyages. For example, with hindsight, we can see that a voyage to South America might have escaped scurvy as it picked up fresh fruit in Madeira in the Atlantic on the way. However, a thousand things had also varied on that ship, not just what they ate for dessert for one week, so it was impossible to be sure that it was the oranges that made the crucial difference.

All scientific experiments try to follow Lind's strategy, using comparisons to control groups. This is part of the scientific method, in my opinion the best idea that anyone ever had. The scientific method is a way of generating accurate information about the natural world, a tremendously powerful idea that has given us the way we live today. We start with a hypothesis – for example, citrus fruit prevents scurvy. A hypothesis makes a prediction, in this case: treating scurvy with citrus fruit will cure the disease. Predictions are tested by experiment and observation, using control groups, just as Lind did. If the experimental results match the prediction, then we can be more confident that the hypothesis is right; if the prediction fails, then the hypothesis is shown to be false. Thus the hypothesis that sulphuric acid prevented scurvy was falsified when the pair of sailors taking this treatment fared no better than the control group that did not get the acid. Arguments from authority – 'I believe that the moon is made of green cheese because Professor Waffle says so and she is really clever' – do not count in science.

James Lind had made two discoveries of tremendous importance: oranges and lemon prevent scurvy and, more importantly, the clinical trial – yet he seemed not to have realised the value of what he discovered, was overcome with doubts, and never managed to break away from conventional tradition. In 1753, he published a *Treatise on the Scurvy*,[6] where the results of his great experiment were buried as five paragraphs in 358 pages, a golden nugget within a mass of junk. Instead of giving a clear message that lemon juice works, Lind obscured this simple and powerful conclusion with a host of other suggested therapies, including warm air, bleeding, drinking acids, mustard and even installing a machine that simulated the action of riding a horse. His great work concluded that scurvy was caused by faulty digestion, not a dietary deficiency.[7]

Even if fresh fruit prevented scurvy, making sure that sailors ate it regularly was not so easy, as the fruit quickly rotted. Lind's solution was to take on board what he called a 'rob' of oranges and lemons, made by boiling the juice for at least twelve hours until it was reduced to syrup. Rob stored in glass bottles could be kept for years. When mixed with water, Lind claimed that it was indistinguishable from freshly squeezed juice. In this way, sailors could obtain the benefits of citrus fruits throughout their voyages. This seemingly excellent idea unfortunately had a fatal flaw: boiling the juice destroys its vitamin C, a problem not noticed for 150 years.[8] James Lind had found the cure for scurvy but went on to recommend a remedy that didn't work. Now promoted to First Lord of the Admiralty, Anson took Lind's advice, but his captains found that his rob syrup was useless, thus discrediting the idea that citrus fruit was the solution for scurvy.

Forty years after Lind's trial, Gilbert Blane, physician to the West Indies fleet, went back to testing possible cures for scurvy. In 1793 HMS *Suffolk* sailed for twenty-three weeks to the East Indies without taking on any fresh food, conditions that would normally trigger an outbreak. This time, however, small amounts of lemon juice were given as a preventative measure, with higher doses when scurvy appeared. The success of this treatment (even though there was no control group) led to lemon juice becoming part of the daily ration throughout the navy in 1795. Scurvy was thus eliminated from the Royal Navy, just in time for the epic conflict with France that culminated in the crushing victory of the Battle of Trafalgar in 1805. Lemon juice allowed British crews to stay at sea for years without major outbreaks of disease, a decisive advantage. A somewhat sour French view of the conflict was therefore that 'we were defeated by a lemon'.[9]

That should have been the end of the matter. However, more blunders followed when, in 1860, the navy switched from using lemons grown in Sicily to limes from the West Indies. The names lemon and lime were used interchangeably for the different fruits at the time, so it was not anticipated that the switch might matter. Unfortunately, limes have only a quarter of the vitamin C content of lemons. No one noticed the problem at first, as steam-powered ships were now so fast that crews were not at sea long enough to get scurvy, even if they had little to no protection. Scurvy did reappear during polar exploration, where men might go for months or years without fresh food. Captain Scott's expedition to the South Pole in 1911 was afflicted by scurvy – one of the contributing factors that led to the death of the whole team on its return.[10]

A further clue to there being more to food than just proteins, fats and carbohydrates came from the single-grain experiment, carried out at the University of Wisconsin from 1907 to 1911.[11] Wisconsin is America's Dairyland, so an excellent choice if you are looking to do research on cows. Four groups of heifers were fed rations composed entirely of corn (maize), wheat, oats or a mixture of all three; all sets of rations were known to have the same energy and protein contents. The thinking at the time was that all these diets should therefore be of equal value, but the results showed otherwise. The cows all ate the same amounts, but those on the wheat diet struggled compared to the others: they gained less weight, did not produce healthy calves and gave less milk. Corn-fed cows thrived the most. Clearly, cows needed some additional nutrient that was missing in wheat.

Experiments along these lines led to the discovery of vitamins – chemicals essential for humans that cause disease if they are lacking in the diet. Only a tiny amount might be needed, but there cannot be none. Vitamin C itself was discovered by the Norwegians Axel Holst and Theodor Frølich. They first worked on a disease similar to scurvy called beriberi. Beriberi is the oldest known vitamin-deficiency disease, first reported in China nearly 5,000 years ago.[12] In the 1880s the Japanese doctor Kanehiro Takaki realised that the high incidence of beriberi among sailors in the Japanese Navy was due to their white-rice-based diet, which lacked sufficient nitrogen. Adding vegetables, barley, fish and meat to meals eliminated the disease by providing nitrogenous protein.[13] In 1897 in the Dutch East Indies, Dutchman Christiaan Eijkman had found that a disease similar to beriberi could be induced in chickens if they were fed solely on white rice. Symptoms went away if brown rice was fed instead. Eijkman wondered whether there was something toxic in polished rice counteracted by an antidote in the husk. We now know that beriberi was due to a lack of vitamin B_1 in white rice. B_1 is present in the rice husk, but this is removed when it is polished to make white rice.

Inspired by this work, Holst and Frølich decided to switch to studying beriberi in a mammal, rather than a bird. Luckily, they chose the guinea pig. Guinea pigs are one of the few species, other than our own, that cannot make its own vitamin C. Hence, when they fed guinea pigs on a diet consisting only of various types of grain, to their surprise, they did not develop beriberi, but scurvy-like symptoms instead. Scurvy had never been seen before in an animal. The guinea pigs were cured when given fresh cabbage or lemon juice, just like humans.[9, 14] For studying scurvy, the guinea pig therefore makes the ideal guinea pig.

So why does a lack of vitamin C cause scurvy? By far the most abundant protein in our bodies is collagen. It is a major component of skin, bone, ligaments and tendons, as well as muscle, blood vessels and the gut. The collagen structure resembles a rope made of three strands twisted round each other. Vitamin C is essential for the synthesis of collagen, as it adds extra oxygen atoms along the chains. These oxygen atoms form bonds along the strands to stabilise the rope-like structure. Thus, no vitamin C means missing oxygen atoms and a more fragile collagen. The symptoms of scurvy then flow from where collagen is needed. For example, the periodontal ligament connects the roots of teeth to their sockets in the jawbone. Weaker collagen means weaker periodontal ligaments and your teeth fall out.

Most animals can make their own vitamin C, with the exceptions of guinea pigs, some fish, bats, birds and primates (including humans). At some point in our monkey ancestry, the gene that makes the enzyme in the final step of vitamin C synthesis acquired mutations that made it non-functional. We can still see the remains of this gene in our DNA, in a highly mutated form that cannot work as an enzyme. These mutations were no problem for this ancient primate. It had plenty of fruit in its diet, so it could manage fine without the ability to make vitamin C. Present-day wild gorillas, for example, eat far more vitamin C than they can ever need, so never get scurvy. The gene for non-functional vitamin C was thus harmless in our distant ancestors and passed on down the generations. It was only when humans started living on bad diets, short of fruit and vegetables, that the lack of the enzyme became a problem.[15]

Vitamin C is, of course, just one of the vitamins. For thousands of years, people have been afflicted by diseases caused by lack of vitamins when they are on too narrow a diet.[12] A lack of vitamin D (and sunlight) causes soft bones and rickets; lack of vitamin B_3 causes the vampire-like condition of pellagra, with blistering of the skin in the sun, pale skin, a craving for raw meat, blood dripping from the mouth, aggression and insanity; and a shortage of vitamin B_{12} causes blood disorders and impaired brain function.

Vitamins form part of the larger class of micronutrients – substances that are essential in small quantities in our diet, in addition to the carbohydrates, fats, proteins and water that are needed in bulk. At present, the most prevalent micronutrient deficiencies worldwide are for iron, iodine, vitamin A, folate and zinc, mostly in sub-Saharan Africa and South Asia. Half of children under five in these regions have health problems due to the lack of one or more micronutrients; globally about 2 billion people are affected.[16, 17] Pregnant women and children are at most risk, as they have a greater need for specific micronutrients.

Vitamin A deficiency primarily affects children, causing loss of vision in low light (night blindness) and, eventually, total, permanent blindness. This is because vitamin A is needed to make rhodopsin, the molecule that absorbs light in the retina. It is also needed by the immune system. Iron is used to carry oxygen in haemoglobin in blood cells. Lack of iron causes anaemia, most often in women and infants. Young children with anaemia have retarded physical growth, reduced resistance to infection and slow intellectual development. Anaemia in pregnancy slows foetal growth and increases risk of death for newborn babies and mothers in childbirth. Lack of iodine is common in areas where soils are deficient in this element; it is the most common cause of intellectual disabilities, as well as miscarriage, stillbirth and birth defects. Zinc is needed for many enzymes to work; it promotes resistance to infection and development of the nervous system; lack of zinc increases the chance of premature birth. A few weeks after conception, a layer of embryonic cells forms a groove that folds and closes into the neural tube. This is the precursor to the brain, spinal cord and the rest of the central nervous system. Folate is essential for this process to complete successfully, so lack of folate causes neural tube defects, like spina bifida, where the neural tube does not close completely.

The good news is that all these deficiencies are easily treatable by consuming food rich in the required micronutrient or by food fortification. For example, vitamin A is abundant in liver, carrots, broccoli and cheese; and zinc is found in meat and nuts. Iodine can be added to salt; iron and folate can be added to flour. Supplement pills, powders or liquids can also be taken. Crops in many areas are deficient in zinc, as it is lacking in the soil. Using zinc-based fertilisers will then not only give healthier crops, but the total crop yields get a boost as well.

Bodies like the World Health Organization and the Centers for Disease Control and Prevention[18] are driving initiatives to end malnutrition. Measures to tackle a lack of micronutrients are cheap and highly effective. As with many other health conditions, once we understand the science behind the problem, high-tech solutions are often not needed: political will is more important. Alternatively, we can create improved strains of crops through plant breeding or genetic-modification technologies to increase the concentration of desired micronutrients in staple food crops. Golden Rice, which is enriched in Vitamin A, is the best-known example. Malnutrition is therefore an entirely avoidable problem. Dealing with it gives healthier babies and children, who grow up to become healthier adults, better able to contribute to the wealth and well-being of their countries.

13

The Body of Venus

Obesity is a major problem in nearly all countries. In 2016, 39 per cent of people worldwide were overweight, with no difference in prevalence between men and women.[1] This is a recent phenomenon. The maps below compare women's mean BMI by country in 1975 and 2016; the maps for men are very similar. In almost every country, the mean BMI has increased. In 1975 there were twice as many people underweight as obese; now more are obese than underweight, everywhere except for some parts of sub-Saharan Africa and Asia.

The gradual increase in amount and quality of food after the Agricultural Revolution, which started 300 years ago, coincided with better public health measures, generating bigger and longer-lived people. These measures drove economic growth, more productive work and more leisure time. Work became less physical, with machines replacing manual labour and more jobs requiring sitting, rather than working in a factory, boat, field or mine. The amount of energy we need to obtain food is now little more than that needed to walk to the fridge or drive to the supermarket, whereas previously, most of us had to be engaged in hard agricultural work all year to be able to eat. Reduced physical activity at work, together with plenty of easily accessible food rich in sugar, fat and complex carbohydrates, has led to an increased number of overweight and obese people since the Second World War.[3] People have not just grown in terms of weight – they are much taller now too. In 1860 the average Dutchman was only 164 cm in height. Now, they are 182 cm on average, making the Dutch one of the tallest nations on Earth.

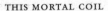

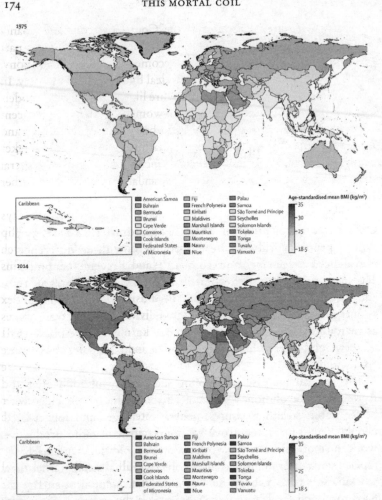

Age-standardised mean BMI in women by country in 1975 and 2014.[2]

Lack of food through most of history meant that being overweight used to be a desirable state. This was reflected in art and literature, from obese mother goddess figures in the Palaeolithic to the plump models of Peter Paul Rubens (1577–1643). The body of Rubens' Venus in his paintings reflected her wealth and high status: she obviously ate well and her white skin showed that she never had to work outside like a common peasant. Corpulent figures, like Cervantes' Sancho

Panza, Shakespeare's Falstaff and the Coca-Cola company's Santa Claus, used to be regarded as jolly and lovable.[4] Only in the latter part of the twentieth century did fatness become stigmatised, when bony, though tall, figures were presented as ideal by the fashion industry. In the seventeenth century obtaining a figure like one of Rubens' models was out of the question for almost all women; similarly, 99 per cent of women today cannot possibly get a body like a supermodel and nor should they. Being overly thin is harmful – it leads to a weaker immune system, likely nutrient deficiencies and low bone-mineral density, which in turn causes cardiovascular disease,[5] among other problems.

As we have seen, famine is now thankfully a rarity, and the days of chronic malnutrition and hunger are also largely gone. The flip side of this progress is that many people now consume too much food, leading to soaring rates of obesity and all the health problems associated with it.

The size of a person can be quantified using the body mass index (BMI), defined as weight in kilograms divided by height in metres squared. A healthy range is 18.5 to 24.9 kg/m^2, while obese is BMI > 30 kg/m^2. The BMI is a useful rough index of whether you are overweight, though not perfect. Some super-fit athletes come outside the healthy range, as they carry lots of muscle. While the USA and UK have (not entirely undeserved) reputations for overeating, neither country features in the top ten for BMI.[1] Instead, two regions dominate the list of the most obese countries: the Pacific and the Middle East.

The State of Kuwait lies on the Persian Gulf. Its wealth from oil attracts numerous foreign workers, so that 70 per cent of its 4.2 million people are expatriates, mainly from the Indian subcontinent or other Arab countries. Most live in the capital, Kuwait City. Health in Kuwait is generally good, with a life expectancy of seventy-eight years. The high number of migrant workers gives an unusual ratio of the sexes, with 60 per cent of the population male and only 40 per cent female.[6] Kuwait has the dubious distinction of being one of the most obese countries in the world, with 43 per cent of people obese and 70 per cent overweight. Fast food, sugary drinks and sweet dumplings called luqaimat are very popular. The hot climate discourages outdoor activity and encourages staying in air-conditioned environments.

Children tend to be driven to school, rather than walk in the heat. As a result, type 2 diabetes rates are soaring, especially in young people. One of Kuwait's answers to this problem is weight-loss surgery, such as sleeve gastrectomies, which remove a large part of the stomach to reduce the amount of food that can be consumed in a meal. Over 3,000 patients are now treated surgically for obesity in Kuwait each year.[7]

A reason why Kuwait and other Middle Eastern countries are struggling with obesity is their recent and sudden change in culture. For many centuries the people were nomadic, living from their flocks of animals and growing food to feed their own families. This somewhat precarious existence led to the beliefs that plump children are healthier and a rich diet is preferable. Overeating when possible makes sense if your life includes lots of physical activity and periods with food shortages; it is not suited to a modern, urbanised world with readily available junk food.[8]

Scattered across the Pacific Ocean lie Nauru, the Cook Islands, Palau, the Marshall Islands, Tuvalu, Tonga, Samoa and Fiji. These tiny island countries contain the most obese people on Earth.[9] As in the Middle East, the population has recently switched from a traditional diet of fresh fruits, vegetables and fish, to processed, high-calorie food imported from Australia, New Zealand and the USA. Ecological damage has adversely affected the islands' farmland, increasing the reliance on food imports.

Pacific Islanders typically have high bone and muscle mass, making them great rugby players,[10, 11] but with a marked tendency to put on too much weight. This may be partly due to natural selection. The Polynesians and Micronesians are part of the large Austronesian ethnic group, which originated in Southeast Asia around 4,000 years ago. From this homeland, they embarked on some of the most epic sea voyages of all time, following their invention of the outrigger canoe, the first technology enabling long-distance travel across oceans. Outrigger canoes have one or two extra floats or hulls, held by poles to the main hull, making them stable in rough seas while still being fast. They were developed from pairs of canoes lashed together. Most people in Taiwan now are of Han Chinese descent, but the indigenous Taiwanese people are Austronesians. From Taiwan, the Austronesians moved south to the Philippines, Indonesia and New Guinea, intermingling with the native populations. From there, they headed out into unexplored seas, eventually founding colonies halfway round the planet. They first inhabited the hundreds of tiny islands in Micronesia, north-east of New Guinea, 3,000 years ago. Hawaii was colonised 1,500 years later and then New Zealand. Heading west from Indonesia, they crossed the Indian Ocean to Madagascar at about the same time. The furthest east they seem to have reached was Rapa Nui (Easter Island), 2,000 miles west of Chile, though they may have also gone further to meet the people of South America or west from Madagascar to East Africa. While these people had no writing (except, remarkably, on Rapa Nui, where the islanders invented their own script that no one can now read), their common cultures, artefacts, languages and genetics tell the story of these amazing feats of exploration and settlement.[12]

It is this history that may have led to high rates of obesity and diabetes in Pacific Islanders. When setting off in an outrigger canoe into an unexplored ocean, the intrepid mariners could not have known when they might find land, or even whether they would find land at all. On many voyages the sailors would have run out of food and starved. The first to die would have been those lacking fat reserves. Surviving Pacific Islanders may therefore be descended from those who started sailing when fat. Over thousands of years, passing through numerous genetic bottlenecks where all the skinny sailors died, there was strong selection for a predisposition to obesity.[13] Travelling for weeks in an open canoe and rough weather could mean that the occupants were soaked with water the whole time. Even though the Pacific voyages were mostly in the tropics, they would still have been bitterly cold at times. Body types that were able to cope with these conditions and resist hypothermia may therefore also have been selected.

The Pacific Islanders' story is a special case of the thrifty gene hypothesis, first proposed by American geneticist James Neel in 1962 as an explanation of why obesity is so common in modern times.[14] Neel was puzzled how a disease like diabetes could have evolved, when it is clearly harmful, common and has some genetic basis. His suggestion was that genetic variants that lead to fat deposition were beneficial in the past, since they would give their owners an advantage in times of starvation. If the food supply cannot be trusted, it pays to put on weight during the good times, knowing that next year's harvest might be disastrous. Only in recent years, with abundant high-calorie food and no famine, is fat accumulation a problem. Obese people in the modern world are therefore prepared for famines that never happen.

Even though it is a plausible story, evidence for the thrifty gene hypothesis is unconvincing.[15] It is not at all easy to separate effects of culture, lifestyle and genetics when comparing populations, so attributing everything to a few genes is highly questionable. In addition, all of us, not just Pacific Islanders, are descended from famine survivors, where being fat was a survival asset. Only a few genes that fit the 'thrifty' description, and gene variants that have been selected to promote fat accumulation, have been found.[16] One is in Samoans.[17]

Another possibility to explain obesity is simply that mutations that predispose humans to get fat are no longer disadvantageous. They can therefore accumulate in our DNA without penalty. Mutations that affect weight will always occur randomly from time to time. In wild animals there is strong selection against mutations that cause obesity, since chubby animals are more likely to be taken by predators. The biggest animals will provide the biggest meals, making them targets, and their high weight will hamper their ability to run away. We know from bite marks on bones that our smaller Australopithecine ancestors were frequently a tasty meal for big cats, dogs, bears, crocodiles and birds of prey.[18] Up to 50,000 years ago Neanderthals were eaten by hyenas in Italy.[19] Modern humans, however, have wiped out the large predators that used to hunt us. We do not tolerate the existence of any animal that kills us and so have driven numerous big predators to extinction, using our talents for teamwork, language and hunting. Turning the tables on our predators meant the demise of species such as sabre-toothed cats, giant cheetahs and dog-like bears, especially when modern humans reached new lands like the Americas, Australia and the Pacific Islands. Once animals that might hunt us were wiped out, it was less of a handicap to be overweight. Thus humans with mutations that led to obesity could survive, or indeed prosper, instead of being eaten.[15]

Studies from twins and families show that there is some genetic basis to obesity. The most common way in which DNA varies is called a single nucleotide polymorphism (or SNP, pronounced 'snip'), where one base of the DNA sequence (A, T, G or C) is swapped for another. Hundreds of SNPs and genes seem to affect the likelihood of being obese, each making a small but just about measurable contribution.[20] Various suggestions have been made as to why SNPs that promote obesity have spread, in addition to being thrifty genes, generally based on the idea that a particular gene can have multiple effects. For example, the generation of new fat cells may be beneficial for the development of babies, particularly their brains, and help them fight off infection.[21] While being good for babies, these fat cells can lead to obesity in later life. Many genes and SNPs work in this way – they have multiple effects, some good and some bad. This means that we must be very careful in considering whether a particular SNP is beneficial or not. Just because it increases the likelihood of one disease does not mean it is bad overall. We might not even be aware of some of its good effects.

Obesity has numerous negative effects on health. A BMI of 40–44 takes 6.5 years off your life on average; extreme obesity, with a BMI of 55–60, takes off 13.5 years. Obesity increases death rates from heart disease, cancer, diabetes, kidney failure, chronic lower respiratory disease, influenza and pneumonia.[22] Overall, it is about as bad for you as smoking.

The most frequent cause of death in total, by a considerable margin, is coronary heart disease, which can lead to a heart attack. Oxygen-rich blood leaves the heart by the aorta, the largest artery in the body. From the aorta, the coronary arteries branch off and loop back to the heart muscles. Over time, fatty material forms plaques, which build up inside the walls of the coronary arteries. These plaques make the arteries harden and narrow, restricting blood flow, so that they struggle to deliver enough oxygen to your heart. Narrow arteries are at risk of a blood clot forming a blockage; if this happens, blood flow to the heart can suddenly be cut off, causing heart failure. The brain can then die within ten minutes, as it no longer receives the oxygen-rich blood that it needs. Stroke is the second biggest killer and is another disease of blood vessels – this time when they are blocked in the brain, resulting in the death of brain cells downstream of the blockage. Both are more likely in obese people.

Fat tissue in an overweight person needs oxygen and nutrients supplied by blood. The heart therefore needs to work harder to pump blood through these additional blood vessels, increasing blood pressure and heart rate. Arteries under higher pressure are more likely to burst, killing tissues downstream of the artery. Carrying extra weight also puts more stress on joints, particularly knees and hips, which take much of the higher load. Osteoarthritis can follow, where the protective cartilage on the ends of your bones breaks down, causing pain, swelling and stiffness. The joints grow extra bone matter and become inflamed. Joint-replacement surgery may eventually be needed. Overweight men are more likely to get prostate or colon cancer; overweight women are more likely to get cancer of the breast, colon, gallbladder and uterus, among others. Fat cells emit chemical signals affecting other cells in the body. They increase levels of insulin, produce oestrogen, which induces cell division in the breast and womb in post-menopausal women, and stimulate inflammation. All these processes promote cell growth and division, key processes in cancer cells.[23]

Obese people have an increased risk of sleep apnoea, which causes breathing to stop for brief periods, so they frequently wake, missing out on a good night's sleep. The additional weight of the chest wall squeezes the lungs, causing restricted breathing and respiratory problems. Obesity puts the kidneys under great strain, causing the gradual loss of kidney function over years.[24] This can manifest as water retention, giving swollen feet or hands, shortness of breath, blood in urine, fatigue, insomnia, nausea, muscle cramps and other symptoms. People who are obese in middle age are more likely to have dementia later in life.[25] Why this is the case is not yet clear, but it does seem that if you look after your heart, you are also looking after your brain.

Diabetes involves resistance to insulin, the hormone that regulates blood sugar, so that blood sugar becomes elevated. The major cause of type 2 diabetes is obesity. Type 2 diabetes typically begins in adulthood, but we are now starting to see significant numbers of cases in children. Even moderate obesity substantially increases the risk of diabetes. In 2016 the WHO reported that 422 million people had diabetes, a staggering fourfold increase since 1980. It is growing fastest in low- and middle-income countries, in parallel with their rising obesity. It killed 1.6 million people in 2016, with many more affected indirectly by higher chances of heart attack, stroke, blindness, kidney failure and the amputation of lower limbs.

Obesity is bad for mental health as well as physical. Most modern cultures view being thin as desirable and attractive. Overweight people can therefore suffer by being seen as lazy, lacking willpower to lose weight. Disapproval can be overt, or manifest as bias, discrimination or ridicule.

One way of looking at the obesity epidemic is that it is a result of our natural instincts, behaviours and bodies being unsuited to the modern world. A maladaptation is a feature of an organism that is harmful, even though it is written in its DNA.[26] Evolution takes time, as it needs many generations for the harmful effects of a gene to be reflected in a decrease in the number of people carrying that gene. Hence, if we suddenly change our environment, we may be stuck with a set of behaviours that are not well suited to the new way of living. Thrifty genes would be examples of these.

Our love of sweet foods provides an obvious mismatch between what we want and what is good for us. Before we started farming, our ancestors rarely encountered foods rich in simple sugars. They could either find them in honey, which is not easy to get from thousands of bees intent on defending their winter food supply, or from fruits. Desiring sweetness made us eat fruit so that we could get vitamin C.[27] We therefore may have evolved a craving for sugar to avoid scurvy. Over the last few thousand years, we developed bigger and sweeter fruits (for example, compare apples in the shops to their wild crab-apple ancestors), began cultivating and trading sugar cane, sugar beet and maple syrup, and started beekeeping. Our desire for sugar is now a maladaptation, since we are still driven to eat sweet things despite already having all the vitamin C we need. Obesity, diabetes and tooth decay thus follow.

Loving sugar too much is not the only way in which we are maladapted to the ways we live today. Ancient humans who lived in hot, humid areas often did not have enough salt in their diet. They therefore evolved genes to favour salt retention. Now these adaptations have turned into a maladaptation, increasing hypertension in modern populations eating salty food.[28] Disrupting our natural circadian rhythms with night-time light[29] or poor sleeping habits[30] also result in obesity.

Maladaptations to the modern world don't end just with diet. A whole host of health problems have been attributed to us having bodies better suited to being hunter-gatherers. For example, reading, sitting and wearing shoes lead to short-sightedness, back pain and bunions, respectively.[31] Lack of exercise causes hypertension. We may have increased our life expectancies to eighty, but often at the cost of many years of chronic ill health.

One strategy to increase life expectancy and avoid these pitfalls of the modern world is to look at the people who live the longest and find out how these role models do it.

The general increase in life expectancy has its most dramatic effect at the extremes, with the numbers living to be 100 climbing from 3,041 in the UK in 1983 to 13,781 in 2013; 0.1 per cent of them live to be supercentenarians at 110 years. Numerous studies have been carried out on what makes these people special, such as the Boston University New England Centenarian Study. This started in 1995, focused solely on eight towns near Boston, Massachusetts, with a population of 460,000 people in total, which contained about fifty centenarians. It has now grown to be the largest study of centenarians in the world, enrolling approximately 1,600 centenarians, 500 of their children (in their seventies and eighties) and 300 younger controls. More than a hundred of them are supercentenarians.[32]

A second centenarian study is on the island of Okinawa, which lies about 500 miles south of the major Japanese island of Kyushu. While part of Japan, the Okinawan people are genetically distinct and speak languages incomprehensible to standard Japanese speakers. Okinawa has the world's greatest life expectancy and highest prevalence of centenarians in the world – 50 per cent more than Japan and three times than the USA.[33] Even more remarkably, the Okinawan centenarians were born when life expectancy on the island was little more than forty. They survived infectious diseases, natural disasters and one of the most brutal battles of the War in the Pacific in 1945. Today death rates from heart disease are currently three times lower than in the USA and the death rate from Alzheimer's is an amazing ten times lower. The goal of the Okinawa Centenarian Study, taking genetic and lifestyle factors into account, is to find out why.[34]

Studying the oldest people has shown the following: there are about five times as many centenarian females as males, and the excess of females increases still further with age. In January 2020 the twenty oldest people in the world were all females. Many were Japanese. Few were obese or smoked at any point in their lives. Even though Alzheimer's is strongly linked to age, the very old usually escape dementia and have healthy brains. Cardiovascular disease and diabetes are also delayed. Women were often able to have children at a late age, consistent with slower ageing throughout life. Centenarians tend to have high levels of vitamins A and E, active red blood cells and a strong immune system. They are good at repairing the mutations that continually arise in their DNA, as DNA damage is a key feature of the ageing process.[35] The supercentenarians are astonishingly free from the major diseases of ageing (stroke, Parkinson's, cardiovascular disease, cancer and diabetes), often finally dying from organ failure.

You will not be surprised to find out that Okinawans eat a healthy diet, traditionally sweet potatoes, soy, green vegetables, roots, bitter melon, fruit, and a little seafood and lean meat. Their preferred drink is jasmine tea. Overall, their diet is high in complex carbohydrates and low in calories, with moderate protein content, and little meat, refined grains, sugar and dairy products. In addition to an optimal ratio of protein to carbohydrates, the Okinawans, like the Japanese, practise *hara hachi bun me*, which means eating a meal until you are only 80 per cent full, something rarely done in the West. Obesity is thus rare. Prior to the 1960s, when rice became a major part of the diet, Okinawans consumed 10–15 per cent fewer calories than would normally be recommended.[36] The idea that long-term restriction of calories consumed leads to longer life has been validated in many animal studies.[37] A simple, though challenging, way to live longer could therefore be to eat a little less every day.

Additional help for dieters can come from anti-obesity drugs that suppress appetite or reduce fat absorption.[38, 39] Unpleasant side effects are common, though. While promising research on drugs to beat obesity is continuing,[40] simply consuming fewer calories and burning more through exercise remains the best strategy that we have.

PART IV

A LETHAL INHERITANCE

All things are hidden, obscure and debatable if the cause of the phenomena is unknown, but everything is clear if its cause be known.

Louis Pasteur, *Germ Theory and Its Applications to Medicine and Surgery,* 1878[1]

14

Woody Guthrie and the Blonde
Angel of Venezuela

That children resemble their parents, and that medical conditions can be passed on down the generations, has been known for thousands of years. An easy-to-see example of this is polydactyly – being born with extra fingers or toes. In 1752, Pierre Louis Moreau de Maupertuis, president of the Berlin Academy of Science, reported on the Ruhe family of Berlin, which showed the trait in three generations and eighteen individuals. Polydactyly could be inherited from either the father or mother.[1] Inheriting other, more damaging, mutations can cause disease.

Genetic disease has been around for billions of years, ever since life started, since errors in copying DNA are inevitable. Here we shall look at four types of genetic disease: dominant, where the relevant mutation need only be inherited from one parent; recessive, where it must be inherited from both; sex-linked, where typically men can show a disease, while women are symptom-free carriers; and polygenic, where a huge number of variations in DNA change the likelihood of getting a disease. We shall see how long and careful study of selected conditions led to breakthroughs in understanding how genetic disease happens.

To date, managing the symptoms of genetic disease is all that we can ever do, as permanent cures that would spare people and their descendants would require altering our DNA. Since our DNA is present in every one of the trillions of cells that make up our bodies, tackling this root cause has always seemed to be an impossibility.

Recently, however, outstanding breakthroughs in molecular biology have brought the dream of curing genetic disease once and for all within reach, potentially benefiting not just a patient, but all their descendants. Before we see how this might be done, let us find out how a folk singer, an American family and a South American village led to the discovery of the location of a disease gene within our DNA for the first time.

Woodrow Wilson Guthrie was born on 14 July 1912, in Okemah, Oklahoma. In 1920 oil was discovered nearby, and the town was briefly transformed into a boom town. A few years later, the oil suddenly ran out and the local economy crashed. Woody therefore travelled south to Texas in 1931, where he married Mary Jennings, had three children and started performing music in bands. In the 1930s, the economic downturn of the Depression was made even worse in the US Midwest by the Dust Bowl. The conversion of grassland into cropland, followed by years of drought, led to massive dust storms where the fragile topsoil was blown away, ruining thousands of farms. Woody was one of the poverty-stricken 'Okies' who left the devastated prairies to seek work out west. Leaving his family behind, Woody hitch-hiked, rode freight trains and walked along Route 66 in search of the promised land of California. In exchange for bed and board, Woody painted signs and entertained in saloons, playing his guitar and singing.

These grim conditions for working-class people inspired the political views that strongly influenced his music. Woody Guthrie wrote and performed hundreds of folk songs, often with a left-wing political message, played on an acoustic guitar painted with the slogan 'This machine kills Fascists'. Many of his songs, such as those on his 1940 concept album *Dust Bowl Ballads*, are about his experiences travelling with homeless and poverty-stricken ex-farmers, learning their traditional folk and blues songs.

In Los Angeles Woody found a job on radio, singing traditional songs as well as his own compositions, which were especially popular with fellow Okies. He used his radio appearances to advocate social justice, denouncing corrupt politicians, lawyers and businessmen, and to praise union organisers who were fighting for the rights of migrant workers. In 1940 he moved to New York, where he continued his activism, and began recording music and writing songs professionally. He married for a second time, to Marjorie Mazia, wrote hundreds more songs and served in the Merchant Marine and army in the Second World War. After the war, he returned to Marjorie and it finally seemed that Woody had achieved stability, peace and success. It was not to last.

In the late 1940s Woody's behaviour became increasingly disturbed. He stumbled on stage and forgot his lyrics. At home he showed bursts of anger and other personality changes, frightening Marjorie. He was arrested in 1949, thought to be drunk, as he staggered around and slurred his speech. It took three years in a variety of institutions before he was finally correctly diagnosed with Huntington's disease. Doctors tried to hide this from him, but Woody guessed that he had the same condition as his mother Nora, telling a friend that Nora died at forty-one from that 'old three-way disease of chorea, consisting of St Vitus dance, epilepsy and mild insanity'. In 1927, Nora Guthrie had set her husband Charley on fire with a kerosene lamp while he slept on the sofa. She was admitted to the state psychiatric facility in Norman, Oklahoma and died there two years later.

Woody described his condition as follows:

> Face seems to twist out of shape. Can't control it. Arms dangle all around. Can't control them. Wrists feel weak and my hands wave around in odd ways. I can't stop. All these docs keep asking me about how my mother died of Huntington's Chorea. They never tell me if its pass-onable or not. So I never know. I believe every doctor ought to speak plainer so us patients can begin to try to guess partly what's wrong with us. If it's not alcohol which has me, I wonder what it's going to be.[2]

Woody was unable to look after his family and left Marjorie, though she later returned to care for him. A benefit concert for his family in 1956 reunited many of his musician friends, ending with his most famous song, 'This Land is Your Land'.[3] Folk music was becoming a huge phenomenon in the USA and Woody was recognised as one of its greatest performers and inspirations. The young Robert Zimmerman, later to change his name to Bob Dylan, met his idol Woody in 1961 in hospital. 'Song for Woody' is included on the first album on which Dylan revealed his genius, released a year later. Woody Guthrie died on 3 October 1967 at the age of fifty-five, leaving nearly 3,000 song lyrics, two novels, artworks, and numerous published and unpublished manuscripts, poems, prose, plays, letters and news articles. Despite only modest success during his lifetime, he is now widely seen as one of America's great songwriters, inspiring musicians such as Bruce Springsteen, Joe Strummer, Billy Bragg and Jerry Garcia. In addition to his music, Woody's life and death made a substantial contribution to understanding Huntington's disease.

Huntington's disease (in Woody Guthrie's time known as Huntington's chorea) is a classic example of a dominant genetic disease, caused by a mutated form of the huntingtin gene, which encodes the sequence of the huntingtin protein. The disease typically first shows symptoms between the ages of thirty and fifty, as jerky, random and uncontrollable movements called chorea. Rigidity, writhing motions, abnormal postures and facial expressions, and difficulties chewing, swallowing and speaking then follow. Despite these physical manifestations, the body's muscles are unaffected directly – rather, it is the brain's ability to control the body that is going wrong (as with motor neurone and Parkinson's disease).

Psychiatric and personality changes include anxiety and depression, aggression, addictive behaviour and becoming generally unpleasant, making the disease highly distressing to those who have Huntington's and their families. Suicidal thoughts are common, with 10 per cent taking their own lives. Cognition is adversely affected, particularly executive functions that control behaviour, so that patients might blurt out what they are really thinking, rather than more wisely keeping their mouths shut. Various problems are apparent in both short- and long-term memory, which progresses to dementia. The disease is inevitably fatal, with a life expectancy of fifteen to twenty years from diagnosis. The huntingtin protein is not only found in the brain. Its presence in other tissues can cause muscular and testicular wasting, heart failure, osteoporosis, weight loss and glucose intolerance. Institutionalisation of the patient is usually necessary.

Huntington's disease was first recorded in the Middle Ages, though its inherited, dominant nature was not clearly explained until the mid-nineteenth century. People with the disease were sometimes treated as witches and burned to death. The gene may have come to Massachusetts with the Pilgrim Fathers on the *Mayflower*.[4] American physician George Huntington accurately described its pattern of inheritance, writing in 1872:

> Of its hereditary nature. When either or both the parents have shown manifestations of the disease … one or more of the offspring almost invariably suffer from the disease … But if by any chance these children go through life without it, the thread is broken and the grandchildren and great-grandchildren of the original shakers may rest assured that they are free from the disease.[5]

This is correct – you can only inherit the disease if one of your parents has it. On a road journey he described seeing, 'two women, mother and daughter, both tall, thin, almost cadaverous, both bowing, twisting, grimacing'.

Why does Huntington's disease show this pattern of inheritance? DNA is a gigantic molecule, present in the nucleus of cells, consisting of a sequence of bases, like letters in the alphabet. Bases are found in four different versions called C, T, G and A. The DNA of a simple organism, such as the *E. coli* bacterium that is happily living in your intestine right now, has DNA containing about 5 million bases. More complex organisms, such as the Norway spruce (used as Christmas trees), have 20 billion. Humans, lying somewhere between bacteria and Christmas trees in complexity, have 3 billion.

The function of DNA is to tell cells which other molecules to make, most importantly proteins. Typically, a gene is a region of DNA that encodes a particular protein. Proteins are chains of small molecules called amino acids, chemically joined into a long string. The DNA sequence is read in blocks of three and translated into a protein sequence. For example, we might have a gene whose sequence starts ATGCTATCC. The first triplet to be read is ATG, which encodes the amino acid methionine. Next is CTA, meaning leucine, then TCC for serine, and so on. The protein therefore starts methionine-leucine-serine, continuing for perhaps a few hundred more amino acids, before another triplet (TAA, TAG or TGA) acts as a stop sign, signalling that the end of the protein has been reached. Other parts of DNA show where a protein-coding region starts and control whether the gene is switched on to make protein.

Human DNA is organised into forty-six separate pieces called chromosomes. Twenty-two of the chromosomes, known as autosomal, and unimaginatively called chromosomes 1 to 22, are duplicated so that most cells have two copies of each. In total, we have about 20,000 different genes in our chromosomes that encode proteins. It is proteins that perform most of the functions in a cell, such as making chemical reactions happen (enzymes), transporting molecules (like red haemoglobin, which carries oxygen), acting as antibodies, or forming hair, skin, bone and tendons (made from the collagen protein).

Human sperm and eggs normally contain just one copy of each autosomal chromosome. A fertilised egg will therefore contain forty-four pairs of the autosomal chromosomes, with one copy from the father and one from the mother. The remaining two chromosomes are called X and Y; it is these that determine sex. The egg provides an X chromosome and the sperm either an X or a Y. If the fertilised egg gets the X from the sperm, its sex chromosomes will be XX and the offspring will be female. Conversely, acquiring the Y gives XY sex chromosomes and a male child. The image below shows the chromosomes of a male and female, neatly showing how they are all in pairs, apart from the sex chromosomes in a male.

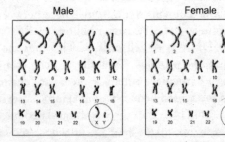

Human chromosomes. Male (left) and female (right) differ by the XY chromosomes in males and XX in females. In each pair, we get one chromosome from our mothers and one from our fathers.

The huge number of variations in DNA make us all different, with hundreds of millions of possible variations known, giving rise to our endless variety.[6] Many of these differences are SNPs, where the DNA sequence differs at a single position. If we pick a pair of unrelated people at random, they will have variations in their DNA at about 5 million sites – most of these are SNPs.[7] Even identical twins, formed when a fertilised egg splits to give two babies, have a handful of differences, made by random mutations in the process of development from egg to baby.

Most damaging mutations to a gene will result in its protein product not working properly. Disease will then only be manifest when someone is unlucky enough to inherit two faulty copies, one from each parent. The mutated gene is harmless when present as just one copy. This is a recessive genetic disease. In contrast, a mutation can occasionally mean that the altered protein is toxic. When this happens, the individual will get the disease when they have just one copy of the mutated genes. This kind of mutation is said to be dominant, since the toxic form overrides the presence of the normal, functional gene. A child of someone with a dominant gene will have a 50 per cent chance of acquiring it, since it is random which version they will get from the affected parent. This is what happens with Huntington's.

Unknown to George Huntington, a German-speaking monk called Gregor Mendel from Brno, in what is now the Czech Republic, had independently discovered recessive and dominant genes with his classic work on breeding tens of thousands of pea plants, published in 1865 and 1866.[8] A monastery might seem an odd place to carry out cutting-edge research, but Mendel's abbot, Cyrill Napp, had a keen interest in science and even built Mendel a greenhouse, solely for his genetic studies.[9] Mendel found that organisms contain heredity units, which we now call genes, which determine what is inherited. Genes exist in different forms, such as a gene for white or purple pea flowers, and are found in pairs. If the pea has two different forms of a gene, then one will be dominant, showing its effect, and the other recessive, where its effect is masked by the dominant gene. The effects of recessive genes are only seen when both recessive gene copies are present. With our flower-colour example, purple is dominant and white recessive, so we see white flowers when the peas have two white genes, purple when the peas have two purple genes, and purple when the peas have one white and one purple gene. Just like humans, each daughter pea plant inherits one gene from each parent.

When Mendel published his conclusions from peas, he had no idea of a physical mechanism that could explain them. Chromosomes were first described in the mid-nineteenth century after observing them in the nuclei of cells, but their role as the carriers of genes was not proposed until the early twentieth century, by German and American biologists Theodor Boveri and Walter Sutton.[10] Boveri was using sea-urchin eggs to study embryonic development, as their large, transparent eggs allowed easy viewing. Boveri saw that all the sea-urchin chromosomes had to be present for the egg to develop successfully into an adult. Sutton found that in grasshoppers, chromosomes occurred in pairs, and proposed that one came from each parent. In order for this to work, the sperm and egg must each contain just a single copy of each chromosome. How these single-copy cells are formed, by a process called meiosis, was first seen in 1876, again in sea-urchin eggs.[11] In the first stage of meiosis, the chromosomes are all copied, so that we have a big cell containing four copies of each chromosome. This cell then divides twice, giving four daughter cells, each with one copy. It is these daughter cells that will develop into eggs or sperm. During fertilisation, eggs and sperm join, giving the fertilised egg two copies of each chromosome, one from each parent. As genes are located on chromosomes, we have a beautiful physical explanation of why Mendel's laws of heredity are true.

Meiosis is the critical process that allows sexual reproduction, since its product, daughter cells, destined to become sperm, eggs or pollen, have only half the DNA needed to make a viable organism. An animal must therefore find a partner to provide the missing half of DNA. Sexual reproduction evolved about 1.2 billion years ago in a single-celled organism, the ancestor of all plants, fungi and animals. How sexual reproduction benefits a species, and why we don't simply produce cloned offspring with the same DNA as ourselves, as bacteria do, remains a contentious issue among biologists.

When Mendel's work became widely known in about 1900, Huntington's disease was one of the first diseases to be recognised as being caused by a dominant gene. The disease could be tracked in families across generations to show the dominant pattern of inheritance. Nothing more was known about the nature of the gene at that time. We did not know what kind of molecule it encoded, its normal function or on which chromosome it could be found. It was not until the 1960s that an American family took up this challenge.

Milton Wexler was born 1908 in San Francisco, then moved with his family to New York.[12] He first studied law at New York University, but switched to science, earning a PhD in psychology from Columbia University. After navy service in the Second World War, he moved to Topeka, Kansas, where he specialised in research and treatment of schizophrenia. Wexler married Leonore Sabin and they had two daughters, Nancy and Alice.

In 1950 Leonore's three older brothers (Paul, Seymour and Jesse) were all diagnosed with Huntington's. The three brothers had inherited it from their father, Abraham Sabin, who had died from Huntington's in 1926, at the age of forty-seven. Wexler moved to Los Angeles in 1951 to set up a more lucrative private practice, treating writers, artists and Hollywood stars, providing a good income to fund medical care for his three brothers-in-law. Shortly after, his wife Leonore's personality began to alter. She developed depression, moodiness and erratic behaviour. Neither Wexler nor his wife or children realised that these were signs of the onset of Huntington's disease, since they mistakenly believed that it could only affect men. Milton attributed her moods to stress from the early deaths of her parents and brothers. Leonore's personality changes made her increasingly difficult to live with, and the Wexlers divorced in 1962. With hindsight, Wexler realised that the early symptoms of Huntington's had destroyed their marriage.

In 1967, after getting out of her car at 9 a.m. while on jury service, Leonore Wexler was apprehended by a policeman, who screamed, 'How can you be drunk so early in the morning? Shame on you!' Leonore was not drunk. Just as with Woody Guthrie, the Huntington's was causing Leonore to stagger around, jerk and stumble, as her brain was losing its ability to control her body. Leonore called her ex-husband in a panic and went to his office. Milton brought in a neurologist colleague, who listened to her story and history of symptoms. He unhesitatingly diagnosed Leonore with Huntington's disease, meaning that all four of Abraham Sabin's children were affected. What was even worse was that Milton and Leonore now knew that their daughters could also have inherited the deadly gene.

Alice and Nancy were twenty-five and twenty-two at that time. That afternoon, Milton told them of the neurologist's verdict and explained that they each had a fifty-fifty chance of getting the disease and that there was no way to tell unless the symptoms started in about twenty years. Every time they might stumble, have trouble pronouncing a word or notice their bodies behaving strangely in any way, they would be wondering whether this was the start of Huntington's. Nancy and Alice decided there and then that they would not have children themselves. If they had the Huntington's gene, any children would see their mothers suffer and die at a young age and be in the same position of wondering whether the same would happen to them.

Milton was shocked into taking action, determined not to give up hope, but to fight the disease. He knew that Woody Guthrie had recently died from the same condition, so contacted his widow, Marjorie, who had already created an organisation to campaign for research. Milton set up his own branch in California. Later the same year, he started the Hereditary Disease Foundation, dedicated to funding research on Huntington's, a disease that had been largely ignored by researchers until then. Milton set up a board of experienced scientific advisors and a team of bright young scientists, happy to work in an area where they would essentially be starting from scratch. He raised funds from the US Congress and from a folk concert at the Hollywood Bowl, with many of Woody Guthrie's admirers performing. He organised parties where his scientists mixed with Milton's movie-star friends, and workshops where research ideas could be debated.

In 1970 Leonore tried to take her own life. She was found by her housekeeper, after taking a huge overdose of sleeping pills, lying on her bed with pictures of her daughters. Leonore was furious at her life being saved. This was the final event that pushed her daughter Nancy into being fully committed to Huntington's work. She worked closely with affected families and completed a PhD on the psychological effects of the disease on Huntington's families.

In 1972, the Hereditary Disease Foundation found the ideal group of people to study. At a workshop in Ohio, a Venezuelan doctor called Ramón Ávila Girón showed a film made at a village by the shores of Lake Maracaibo in northern Venezuela. In the film dozens of people could be seen, all with the characteristic movements of Huntington's. Ávila Girón explained that they were all from the same family. Many villages by the lake were affected. In some, over half the people would develop the disease. Local people would avoid marrying anyone from these villages, knowing what was likely to happen to any children. Nancy and her colleagues were used to working with families with just a handful of affected individuals. In contrast, thousands of people with Huntington's were living in villages by Lake Maracaibo, all of whom appeared to be descended from just one common ancestor. If it was possible to find a stretch of DNA that was always present in those with the disease and absent in others, then the gene that caused Huntington's had to be within that region. Nancy and her team visited the villages and collected family tree and medical information, as well as blood samples. She became known as the 'Angel Catira' – the Blonde Angel.

Thanks to the Hereditary Disease Foundation and the successful lobbying of Congress, the US-Venezuela Huntington's Disease Collaborative Research Project was started in 1979, with the primary aim of finding the responsible gene. Over 18,000 people in two isolated Venezuelan villages, Barranquitas and Lagunetas, were studied, most of whom were from one extended family. The disease had originated with María Concepción, who had lived in the area 200 years earlier and had ten children. María's father was probably an unknown European sailor who also had Huntington's disease.

More than a hundred scientists worked on the project for ten years, before finally pinning the gene down to a location on chromosome 4. How did they do it? Nothing this ambitious had been attempted before, so new techniques had to be invented. Key to the success was using linkage analysis. Linkage analysis relies on the fact that pieces of DNA that are close to one another on a chromosome are likely to be inherited together during meiosis. Scientists can use this knowledge to work out which genes are where on a chromosome.

The work was difficult and tedious. It was also a triumph, not only succeeding in finding the first dominant gene using linkage methods, but also in developing methods later used for sequencing the human genome. It was found that Huntington's was closely linked to a marker on chromosome 4 called G8.[13] In other words, people who inherited a G8 marker also inherited the Huntington's gene, and this must be because G8 and the Huntington's gene are close together on chromosome 4. Other techniques allowed the team to home in more closely to the precise location on the tip of chromosome 4 and a gene known as IT15 (standing for 'interesting transcript 15'), which turned out to be the Huntington's gene. When it was sequenced, the exact nature of the Huntington's mutation was revealed.[12]

As we have seen, most mutations are SNPs, where a single base in the DNA is replaced by another base (for example, G for A or C for T). The mutation that causes Huntington's is very different. Within the Huntington's gene there are repeats of the triplet CAG over and over again. Normal healthy people have six to thirty-five CAG repeats, but someone with Huntington's will have more. The Huntington's gene encodes a protein called huntingtin. The exact function of the huntingtin protein is not clear, but we know it is essential, as mice that lack the protein die. It could be involved with cells communicating with each other or transporting materials. It is most abundant in nerve cells and in the brain, as we might expect from the disease symptoms.[14] A CAG encodes the amino acid glutamine, so the repeating CAG pattern will mean that huntingtin has a string of glutamines all in a row within the protein.

Fewer than thirty-six glutamines is harmless, with huntingtin functioning normally. However, when the chain is longer than thirty-six, enzymes can cut the huntingtin, producing fragments of polyglutamine protein. These fragments stick to one another, forming clumps within nerve cells. It is unclear at present whether it is the clumps that damage nerve cells or whether cells have trouble in processing the mutant huntingtin, leading to its build-up within cells, causing damage. In any event, we know that the longer the CAG repeats, the deadlier the protein, with Huntington's disease appearing at a younger age as the length of CAG grows. If thirty-six to thirty-nine are present, the individual might be fortunate enough to avoid the disease; if longer than forty, Huntington's is inevitable.[15]

What is especially distressing about diseases caused by CAG expansions is the phenomenon of anticipation. During DNA replication, the polymerase enzyme that copies the DNA can sometimes jump, resulting in the addition of an extra CAG. Adding two or three CAG sequences per generation is typical. This means that if a child inherits the Huntington's gene, it will produce huntingtin with a longer polyglutamine sequence than their affected mother or father, making a more toxic protein. The child will then start to show symptoms at a younger age than their parent. This means that people with thirty-something CAG repeats may have a child with Huntington's, even if they do not have the condition themselves, since the addition of a few extra CAGs could tip the protein beyond the threshold where it becomes deadly. Very long CAGs cause juvenile Huntington's disease, with onset under the age of twenty.[16]

The discovery of the gene enabled the development of a test for the condition. If a young person has a parent diagnosed with Huntington's, they can take the test to see if they will get it too. In practice, most people choose not to know until they are considering having children. There is still no cure for Huntington's disease. Recent work that aimed to inhibit the production of huntingtin[17] has not been successful,[18] though promoting the destruction of proteins with CAG repeats[19] is also under investigation. Approaches like these could be the first step towards a real cure. Time will tell.

Alice and Nancy Wexler both decided not to get their huntingtin sequenced. They had already decided not to have children when their mother was diagnosed with the disease, well before the test was available. Eventually, Nancy began to show the symptoms of Huntington's herself, with an unsteady gait, slurred speech and uncontrollable movements. Nancy kept her situation private for a long time before Alice persuaded her to go public. Living with Huntington's has not stopped Nancy's work, pushing forward research, publicising the condition, and continuing to live a productive, fulfilling and enjoyable life well into her seventies.[20]

15

Daughters of the King

In 1990, a boy with severe physical symptoms and intellectual disabilities was admitted to the office of paediatric neurologist Dr Theodore Tarby in Phoenix, Arizona. As the boy's condition was entirely new to him, Tarby sent urine samples to the University of Colorado, which specialised in rare genetic diseases. There, DNA sequencing revealed that the boy had an extremely rare disease called fumarase deficiency. Fumarase is an enzyme essential for generating energy in cells, so mutations here are likely to be catastrophic. A lack of fumarase causes severe epileptic seizures, an inability to walk or even sit upright, severe speech impediments, failure to grow at a normal rate, and terrible physical deformities.[1] Much of the brain is missing. Further investigation revealed that there were numerous other children with the same condition, including the boy's sister, all from the same small community. It was no wonder that Tarby had never seen fumarase deficiency before – until the 1990s there were only thirteen known cases in the whole world. By 2006, however, Tarby discovered more than twenty other children living with the condition, all in the same town.[2]

The community in question is the Fundamentalist Church of Jesus Christ of Latter-Day Saints (FLDS) in Colorado City, Arizona, and the adjacent town of Hildale, Utah, which straddle the state border. About half of the 8,000 people living there belong to two of the founding families, the Barlows and the Jessops, who settled in the remote area in the 1930s. The FLDS members practise polygamy, arrange marriages between relatives, marry young and encourage women to have as many children as they can.

Having multiple wives follows the practices and teachings of Joseph Smith and Brigham Young, the first leaders of the Latter-Day Saints (LDS), otherwise known as the Mormons. Following the death of Smith in Illinois in 1844, Young led the new Church west to found Salt Lake City in Utah. In 1890, following pressure from the federal government and a revelation from Jesus Christ, Church President Wilford Woodruff announced his manifesto, which ended polygamy. This allowed Utah to become a state of the USA six years later, when a ban on polygamy was included in the state's constitution. While this change was accepted by the majority of LDS adherents, some strongly disagreed, since this was a clear break with Church tradition. Those who rejected Woodruff's reforms broke away to start FLDS churches and new communities where they could follow their own beliefs. One of these was Colorado City/Hildale.

The Colorado churches founder Joseph Smith Jessop and his first wife, Martha Moore Yeates, had fourteen children. One of their daughters married John Yeates Barlow, another of the community's founders and religious leaders. By the time Joseph Smith Jessop died in 1953, he already had 112 grandchildren, most descended from him and Barlow. Marriages were arranged to preserve pure bloodlines, so they were always between cousins: sisters would marry the same first cousin; uncles married nieces; pairs of brothers married cousin pairs of sisters. Unwanted male teenagers, known as 'lost boys', were expelled, because if a select few men had numerous wives, then there was no place for those with no partner. After several generations, fumarase deficiency appeared, when children inherited the faulty fumarase gene from closely related parents. Now thousands of FLDS members are carrying the deficient fumarase gene. Fumarase deficiency is not their only genetic problem. Many are born with cleft lips, club feet, heart-valve abnormalities and hydrocephalus.[2, 3]

When Tarby explained at a town meeting that the community had to stop intermarriages between Barlows and Jessops, he got a hostile reception.[2] Keeping their bloodlines pure was more important than reducing the risk of disease, and any sick children were a test from God. Male Church members needed at least three wives in order to get into heaven, and the more wives a man has, the better.[4] Church leader Warren Jeffs personally has about eighty. In 2011 Jeffs received a life-plus-twenty-year sentence for aggravated sexual assault. He then instigated a sex ban for the whole community from prison.[5] Many members have since left the Church. The struggling Colorado City/Hildale community is now undergoing rapid change after years of control and abuse.[6]

Carrying a faulty gene rarely matters, as our partners will almost certainly have two functional copies. Our children are therefore bound to inherit a copy of the functional gene from them, even if we are a carrier of a deficient gene. The situation is not so reassuring, however, if parents are related; then both parents may have inherited a faulty gene from a common ancestor, as with the fumarase gene in the FLDS community. The closer the relationship between a couple, the more likely a genetic disease is to appear in their children. Relatives having children are playing genetic roulette with their offspring.

Brothers and sisters marrying is therefore illegal in nearly all human cultures for excellent reasons. Laws against the practice are probably not even necessary, as finding one's sibling sexually attractive is very rare. Disgust is a rational response, evolved to prevent such unhealthy relationships. Nevertheless, brother-sister marriages have been practised at times, as in ancient Egypt. At present, about one in 3,600 people in the UK are the products of extreme inbreeding, such as their parents being brother and sister, or father and daughter.[7]

While brother-sister marriages are rare, children by first cousins, who share two grandparents, are common in many cultures.[8] In many parts of South Asia, North Africa and the Middle East, the marriage of a daughter will often be a great burden to a family, since she will require a substantial and expensive dowry. Marrying a daughter to your sibling's son will keep the dowry wealth in the family and make it easier to stay in contact with her after the marriage. Attitudes to cousin marriages vary enormously around the world. It is illegal in China, Korea, the Philippines and about half the states of the USA. While legal in Europe, there is stigma against the practice, due to (justified) suspicion of health risks in children and the incest taboo.

Cousin marriages are especially frequent in the Middle East. For example, more than 70 per cent of marriages in Saudi Arabia are to first or second cousins, substantially increasing the chances of a recessive genetic disease occurring in their children. Such practices have been common for thousands of years, magnifying the problem through generations. As a result, Arabs now have the highest rate of genetic disease in the world. Aware of these risks, countries like Qatar sensibly offer genetic screening to prospective married couples, to see if both are carrying genetic conditions.[9] It wouldn't be a bad idea to roll this out everywhere. SNPs that are known to be linked to genetic disease can be rapidly and cheaply identified. Despite this increasing awareness and screening, cousin marriages are, if anything, increasing in frequency.

A 2015 study investigated the effects of inbreeding on health in 354,224 individuals from 102 groups around the world.[10] The people with the highest genetic similarity to each other were within the Amish and Hutterite religious communities in the USA, who had small original populations and married within their own groups for hundreds of years. The most genetically diverse groups were in Africa. Sixteen measures of public health were studied, looking at height, intelligence, blood pressure, cholesterol levels, lung volume, body mass index and haemoglobin levels. Changes in genetic variation significantly adversely affected four of these traits: height, lung function, educational attainment, and g (a measure of general cognitive ability). Converting the numbers showed that the effect of parents being first cousins was on average equivalent to losing ten months of education and 1.2 cm from height. Such effects would be magnified with repeated generations of cousin marriage. There were no apparent effects on blood pressure, cholesterol or heart function.

Marriage between distant cousins can often occur between couples who don't realise that they are related. This is more likely when the husband and wife are both from a community descended from a small number of people. The FLDS community provides an extreme example of this. These bottleneck effects, which give high genetic similarity due to a small founder population, are also present in French Canadians. The city of Quebec was founded in 1608 and over the next 150 years the colony of New France slowly expanded. In 1663 about 2,500 people lived in New France, with 719 unmarried males and only 45 unmarried females. Most of the available professions in New France, such as soldier, fur trapper and priest, were exclusively for men, so they were the ones who emigrated from Europe, giving a severe population imbalance. Single women were very reluctant to travel to this new world, so the colony was heading for extinction, or assimilation with Native Americans or the British colonists to the south.

In order to increase the population, so maintaining the French colony and culture, Jean Talon, the chief administrator of New France, proposed to King Louis XIV that he could sponsor passage of at least 500 young women across the Atlantic. The king agreed, and eventually 800 were recruited. They were mostly between the ages of twelve and twenty-five, of sound morals (as certified by a priest), in good physical condition, making them suitable for work in agriculture, and generally commoners of humble birth. These *filles du roi*, Daughters of the King, were provided with the cost of a one-way ticket to Canada, dowries and chests containing personal accessories (a comb; two hoods; a belt; a pair of hose; a pair of shoes; a pair of gloves; a bonnet; shoelaces; four sets of laces; and sewing supplies), making them a prime catch for any lonely and frustrated Québécois.

The programme worked. By 1670 most of the girls who had arrived the previous year were already married and pregnant, following some speed dating, where the girls would interview their potential husbands, chaperoned by nuns, and choose between them. If none were acceptable, they could get on a boat to the next city up the St Lawrence River. By the next year, a total of nearly 700 children had been born to the *filles du roi*. The population of New France doubled in just nine years, as having ten or more children was not unusual; most of the current 5 million French Canadians have *filles du roi* in their ancestry. Angelina Jolie, Hillary Clinton and Madonna are three of their descendants.

The Seven Years' War, fought from 1756 to 1763 between Britain, Prussia, Portugal and other German states against France, the Holy Roman Empire, Austria, Russia, Spain and Sweden, brought French emigration to New France to a sudden stop. A complex set of territorial swaps at the war's end led to New France being ceded to Britain, in exchange for the much more productive Caribbean sugar islands of Martinique and Guadeloupe. Immigration to Canada was subsequently primarily from the British Isles, particularly Scotland and Ireland; or from American loyalists who wanted to stay in the British Empire after the loss of the thirteen colonies in the War of Independence. French Canadians thus show a strong founder effect and low genetic variation, with a large current population descended from the small number of *filles du roi*. This manifests in dozens of genetic diseases.[11, 12]

Population bottlenecks can arise when the population of a group crashes to a very small number, which subsequently expands again. Sharp population reductions can happen due to epidemics, natural disasters or warfare, particularly genocide. Before Europeans reached the Americas following Columbus in 1492, all Native Americans were descended from a small number of people who travelled around the coast from eastern Russia, across to Alaska and Canada, and then eventually all the way down to the tip of South America. This happened during the last Ice Age, about 14,000 years ago, when sea levels were lower, and land extended all the way from Russia to Alaska. When these intrepid travellers moved south, away from the bitter cold of a Canadian Ice Age, they found a rich land teeming with large animals ready to be hunted. Their population expanded enormously. Perhaps 50 million people lived in the Americas before Columbus, with the highest population density in Central America, home of the Aztec and Maya civilisations. Studying genetic data from present-day Native Americans shows that these 50 million were descended from less than a thousand founders.[13] Presumably this ancestral population was at its lowest during the crossing from Siberia to Alaska through the worst conditions of the epic journey.

As a result of this bottleneck, Native Americans show low genetic diversity, despite the great geographical distances from Canada to Chile. Almost all are blood group O, for example. SNPs that are distinct for Native Americans seem to have first arisen when their ancestors were living in Siberia. One factor that may have contributed to the horrific death rate of Native Americans from European diseases was this lack of genetic diversity. A diverse population has a large variation in susceptibility to a new disease, so there are always a fair number lucky enough to be resistant. In the case of the Native Americans, however, if one person was hit hard by a particular strain of infectious disease, then almost everyone else would be as well.

The arrival of Europeans may have had an even larger effect on dogs. Dogs first arrived in the Americas 10,000 years ago, also from Siberia, and flourished thereafter. If the DNA left by these ancient animals is compared to modern American dogs, they show almost no traces of DNA from these original inhabitants. The first American dogs may have been annihilated by diseases carried by European dogs.[14]

It is quite plausible that many of us are carriers of recessive lethal diseases, though this is not normally a problem unless we have children with cousins. We are unaware that one of our gene copies is non-functional, as its presence is masked by the normal gene, thus avoiding any disease. A recent study of the Hutterite community in South Dakota was able to estimate how likely someone is to be a carrier.[15] The Hutterian Brethren originated in Austria in the 1520s. After their numbers dropped to 400, they emigrated to North America, founding three communal farms in the 1870s, and speaking their own German dialect. The colonies thrived, giving three major subdivisions, with most marriages since 1910 taking place among individuals within the same group. The current population is 45,000. The Hutterites have kept extensive genealogical and medical records and suffer from thirty-five recessive disorders, including cystic fibrosis, again as a result of founder effects and inbreeding. Hutterites have a communal lifestyle, sharing all their possessions and minimising environmental differences, making them an excellent group for the study of genetic disease.

The analysis used data from thirteen generations, including 1,642 living Hutterites in South Dakota and 3,657 of their ancestors, all of whom can be traced back to sixty-four founders. Modern DNA sequencing technology allowed testing to see if someone was carrying a disease-linked variant. Each Hutterite founder carried on average 0.6 lethal recessive mutations. Assuming that the Hutterites are a good representation of the rest of humanity, about half of us are, therefore, carriers of lethal genetic disease.

Until recently, there was nothing that could be done to prevent children being born with recessive genetic diseases, though screening programmes or, more simply, not having children with cousins would decrease the risk, especially if a particular disease is known to be present on both sides of the family. As we shall see, a more exciting (though scarier) prospect is to alter human DNA, removing genetic disease for ever.

More boys are born than girls, with a natural excess of 3 per cent more male births than female worldwide.[16] This difference decreases with age, so that it is close to equal numbers for young adults. Men are more likely to be victims of violence, whether warfare, suicide or homicide, and more likely to die in accidents. Far more young teenage men die in accidental deaths than girls, when teenagers start riding motorbikes, driving dangerously and taking up risky jobs, sports and other activities. These behaviours tend to even up the numbers of young men and women. After the age of fifty, there are more women than men, as men die younger. Boys and young men also have higher death rates than girls, as they have a higher risk of genetic disease.

It is the presence of a Y chromosome that makes someone biologically male. Female is the default, so in the absence of the genes on the Y chromosome that makes someone male, we will get a female. As we saw with recessive genetic diseases, we normally have a spare copy of every gene, as chromosomes are in pairs. This is not the case for males, however, since they have just one X and one Y. Humans have about 20,000 genes in total that encode proteins, but the Y chromosome has by far the fewest with only around 70. The key gene for making someone male is called sex-determining region Y (*SRY*). If *SRY* is present on the Y chromosome, it switches on a number of other genes, leading to gonads developing into testes, rather than ovaries. The testes will then start making the male sex hormone testosterone. Male and female foetuses, which had started out developing identically, now follow separate paths.

Genetic diseases that are far more common in boys than girls are caused by dysfunctional genes on the X chromosome, as boys have only one X, so no spare copy. Diseases caused by mutations on the X chromosome are one reason why women have a longer life expectancy than men. For example, Duchenne muscular dystrophy is a severe muscle-wasting disease caused by mutations in the dystrophin gene present within the X chromosome. Dystrophin is a huge protein that binds to muscle fibres. If it is not functioning correctly or missing altogether, muscles will weaken and die. Muscle weakness is apparent as soon as a baby starts to walk; a wheelchair is needed from around the age of ten, paralysis below the neck is typical by twenty-one, and life expectancy is just twenty-six years. Girls carrying the mutated dystrophin gene are unaffected, since they have a functional gene on their other X chromosome. Boys are not so fortunate. Many other conditions are sex-linked in this way, such as red/green colour blindness. A classic example is haemophilia in European royalty.

Queen Victoria was famously a carrier of haemophilia. She had a single base change (from an A to a G) in her gene for blood coagulation factor IX, an essential protein for blood clotting. It was this tiny variation that changed history. The mutation makes the factor IX much shorter than it should be and hence non-functional.[17] The factor IX gene is on the X chromosome, so females, such as Victoria, will not be affected, since they have a normal version of the gene on their other X chromosome. If males have the mutation they cannot escape the condition. As they have only a single X, they are incapable of making factor IX and have a hugely impaired ability to make blood clots. Haemophiliacs will bruise easily and bleed for a long time after a cut. The brain is particularly susceptible to bleeding, causing permanent damage, seizures and loss of consciousness. The condition is typically first noticed when a newborn baby does not stop bleeding after the umbilical cord is cut.

Haemophilia was unknown in any of Victoria's ancestors, so it appears that the mutation started with her. More specifically, it probably came from a sperm from her father Prince Edward, Duke of Kent, who was fifty-one when she was born. Older fathers are more likely to have acquired mutations in their sperm, as the sperm cells will have had a longer time to accumulate mistakes. The first instance of haemophilia in the British royal family was in Prince Leopold, the fourth son and eighth child of Queen Victoria and Prince Albert. Leopold was born in 1853 and diagnosed five years later. When he was thirty, he slipped and fell, hitting his head, causing a cerebral haemorrhage that would not stop. He died in the early hours of the next morning. Leopold was the first of ten of Victoria's male descendants to have haemophilia, and the only one to have children. When Leopold had a daughter, Alice, she was inevitably a carrier, as she could only inherit a mutated factor IX gene from her father. Alice passed the condition on to her son Rupert and probably her youngest son Maurice, as well. Rupert died from injuries in a car crash at the age of forty, while Maurice died at five months. Luckily, Victoria's oldest children, Vicky and Bertie, avoided the haemophilia gene. Vicky married the German Emperor Frederick III and was the mother to Kaiser Wilhelm II; Bertie became King Edward VII of the UK. The German and British royal families thus escaped the curse of haemophilia.

The chart below shows known haemophiliacs and carriers in Victoria's descendants.

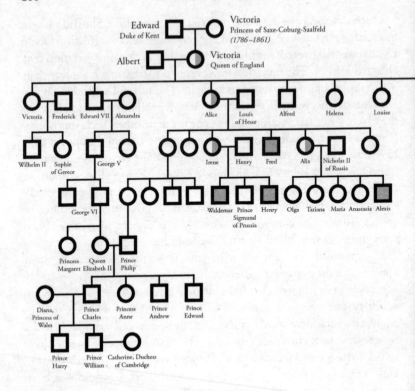

Haemophilia in descendants of Queen Victoria. The disease was transmitted into three royal families: those of Russia via Alice of Hesse and Alexandra; Spain via Beatrice and Victoria Eugenie; and Saxe-Coburg and Gotha and Saxony via Leopold. Some additional females may also have been carriers.

Victoria's children married into numerous royal families in Europe, resulting in ten haemophiliacs in total – the last was Gonzalo, born in 1914. Today, it seems that none of Victoria's descendants are carrying the gene, though there is a chance that it is still present in the Spanish royal family, in an all-female line descended from Beatrice.[18] DNA sequencing would tell.

Tsar Nicholas II of Russia, his wife Alexandra, his son and heir Alexis, and their four daughters were all murdered in 1918 during

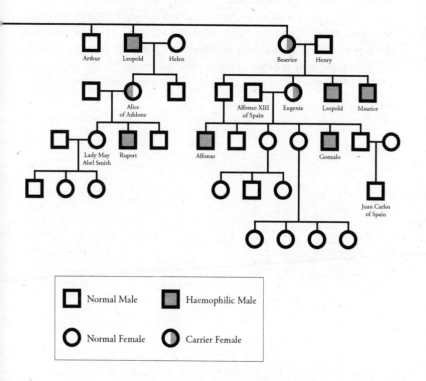

the civil war that followed the Russian Revolution. In 2009 their remains were conclusively identified within a mass grave discovered in 2007. Comparing the DNA in two burned skeletons to descendants of Victoria who were living at the time (such as Prince Philip, Queen Elizabeth II's husband, who is included in the chart) and a bloodstained shirt of the tsar confirmed that the skeletons were those of Prince Alexis and one of his sisters.[19] The DNA was well enough preserved to be able to sequence genes on the X chromosome known to be associated with haemophilia.

As expected for a carrier, both normal and mutant genes (one with A and one with G) were detected in the two X chromosomes from Alexandra. The DNA from Alexei's single X chromosome contained the mutant gene (with G). One of Alexei's sisters (either Maria or Anastasia, from the age of the bones) was shown to also be a carrier, like her mother.[17] If she had lived, she might well have passed the defective gene into another royal family.

16

The Brain of Auguste D

On 25 November 1901 a fifty-one-year-old woman was admitted to the Hospital for the Mentally Ill and Epileptics in Frankfurt am Main, Germany, where she was examined by senior physician Alois Alzheimer. Her name was recorded as Auguste D. Alzheimer moved to the Royal Psychiatric Clinic, Munich in 1903, though he continued to follow the course of Auguste D's condition until her death in 1906. Auguste's symptoms had started with a deep, irrational jealousy of her husband, followed by poor memory and understanding, difficulties with language, erratic behaviour, hallucinations and paranoia. Complete dementia followed and less than five years after her first symptoms, she was dead.

Alzheimer performed a post-mortem, including a detailed study of her brain. What he found was nothing like any other brain that he had seen before. Firstly, it was unnaturally small, clearly having lost much tissue. In the centre of many brain cells he saw some dense bodies, standing out due to their unusual thickness and 'peculiar impregnability', while outside the cells he saw larger deposits in the brain cortex.[1] Alzheimer was describing tangles and plaques, defining characteristics of Alzheimer's disease, and still used to diagnose the disease in a post-mortem. Remarkably, even though Alzheimer's is so prevalent now, Alzheimer himself reported on only a single patient with the condition, and it was believed at the time (1910) to be a new disease.[2]

How can we go from a situation where there was only a handful of cases of Alzheimer's disease to one where it is one of the leading causes of death, in just a hundred years? Given the age of Auguste D and other patients, Alzheimer's disease was first regarded as a type of so-called 'presenile dementia'. Dementia was seen as something that naturally happens to the brain in old age, while with Auguste D, the condition had set in prematurely. Senile dementia was often considered to be a normal part of ageing, and hence neglected, though there was much confusion on the issue. One of the problems was a lack of studies, as so few patients apparently had the condition.[2] Mental illness in general was neglected by conventional medicine at the time.

As life expectancy grew during the twentieth century, senile dementia became more and more prevalent, finally sparking increasing interest in the condition. The revolution came in 1976, when Robert Katzman of Albert Einstein College of Medicine, New York, pointed out that 'neither the clinician, the neuropathologist, nor the electron microscopist can distinguish between the two disorders, except by the age of the patient', and hence 'Alzheimer disease and senile dementia are a single process and should therefore be considered a single disease'.[3] Reclassifying senile dementia as Alzheimer's disease, and realising that senile dementia is not a normal part of ageing, immediately expanded enormously the number of cases of Alzheimer's disease. It was now apparent that Alzheimer's disease should be made a public health and research priority.[4]

Even though Alzheimer and others had identified his disease and found its key symptoms and brain features, no one knew what the plaques and tangles that Alzheimer had seen actually were. It wasn't until 1984 that George Glenner and Caine Wong, at the University of California, San Diego, discovered that the characteristic brain plaques are made of a small protein called amyloid-β.[5] Amyloid-β is a fragment of a long protein called APP. It is made by enzymes called β- and γ-secretase, which cut the APP chain in two places, releasing the amyloid-β; γ-secretase is a complex of several proteins, including two called PSEN1 and PSEN2. Amyloid-β is produced without any problems throughout most people's lives, but for poorly understood reasons, in the elderly it can start to stick together into a toxic form, ultimately forming large plaques surrounded by dead or dying brain cells.

Genetics also points to the importance of APP, PSEN1 and PSEN2: in about 5 per cent of cases, Alzheimer's symptoms appear before the age of sixty-five. This early-onset disease is caused by dominant mutations in *APP*, *PSEN1* or *PSEN2* genes, which lead to enhanced production of amyloid-β, changing γ-secretase activity, or altering the amyloid-β so that it is more toxic. Most mutations that cause early-onset Alzheimer's are in *PSEN1*, with nearly 200 currently known. The book and film *Still Alice* tell the true story of Alice Howland, a professor of linguistics at Columbia University in New York, who was diagnosed with early-onset Alzheimer's disease at the age of fifty due to a dominant *PSEN1* mutation. Of Alice's three children, two decide to take a genetic test to see if they are carrying the mutation and hence will develop the disease – one turns out to be positive and one negative. Alice's third child did not want to know.

Just like Huntington's disease and Parkinson's disease, Alzheimer's disease is a disease of protein aggregation, where proteins that were previously behaving themselves start to stick together, becoming toxic. Which disease symptoms arise depends on where the aggregates form and hence which types of cell they damage. Loss of cells in the brain that control muscles results in Parkinson's disease, for example. Alzheimer's disease starts with damage to the part of the brain responsible for short-term memory (the hippocampus); it then spreads to adjacent areas that give personality, emotion and language. If mutations turn a protein toxic, as with early-onset Alzheimer's and Huntington's, then the mutation is dominant.

The ways in which changes in DNA cause disease that we have looked at so far work in straightforward manners: they are either dominant (like Huntington's), recessive (like cystic fibrosis) or sex-linked, where the mutant gene is on the X chromosome, so (like haemophilia) it only manifests in men. The effects of most sequence changes in DNA are much more complicated than this, however. Firstly, some people may not get a disease, even if they are carrying a mutation that can cause it. For example, hundreds of mutations in the *BRCA1* gene have been shown to increase the risk of breast or ovarian cancer.[6] We can now screen for *BRCA1* mutations so that those with mutations that give high risk for the development of breast cancer could have a preventative mastectomy. However, *BRCA1* mutations differ from the CAG expansions in huntingtin in that the likelihood of getting breast cancer by the age of seventy if you have a *BRCA1* mutation is only about 60 per cent, whereas with mutant huntingtin it is 100 per cent. Many carriers thus never get breast cancer. This phenomenon is called incomplete penetrance, where not everyone with a disease-causing mutation actually gets the disease. Many mutations work in this way.

In diseases such as Huntington's, haemophilia and cystic fibrosis, the disease is straightforwardly caused by a mutation in a single gene. Most medical conditions, however, are multifactorial, where variation in many genes shifts the probability of getting a disease, on top of lifestyle and environmental factors. Thus conditions such as heart disease, schizophrenia, cancer and type 2 diabetes tend to run in families but disentangling exactly how multiple SNPs are linked to each condition is not easy. Getting the same health problems as your parents is by no means guaranteed.

Alzheimer's disease provides examples of both simple and multifactorial genetics. As we saw, about 5 per cent of cases of Alzheimer's are early onset, first diagnosed in people less than sixty or sixty-five, like the case of Auguste D. Early-onset Alzheimer's is caused by dominant mutations in *PSEN1*, *PSEN2* or *APP*. The great majority of cases of Alzheimer's are late-onset, however, starting over the age of sixty-five, with the likelihood of having the disease steadily increasing with age. Patients with late-onset Alzheimer's have the normal *APP*, *PSEN1* or *PSEN2* genes. There are genetic links to many other genes associated with late-onset Alzheimer's disease. There are no SNPs that give a 100 per cent chance of getting the disease in these genes – rather, there are many SNPs that change the probability of getting it. For example, a mutation in the gene called *CLU* causes a 16 per cent higher chance of developing late-onset Alzheimer's; MRI scans showed that white matter in the brain, which carries nerve impulses between neurons, is affected by changes in *CLU*,[7] explaining its link to Alzheimer's disease.

The most important SNPs for late-onset Alzheimer's are in a gene called *APOE* on chromosome 19, with the variant called ε4 being especially problematic. Having both your *APOE* genes as ε4 increases your chances of having Alzheimer's substantially and it is likely to start at a younger age.[8] While the effect of *APOE* ε4 is strong, it is still not absolute; most people with an ε4 variant do not get Alzheimer's disease. Late-onset Alzheimer's disease is thus polygenic, affected by variations in many genes.

If the *APOE* ε4 variant is so harmful in leading to Alzheimer's, then why is it so common? Shouldn't natural selection have removed it from our DNA? One argument is that genetic variants that only affect the elderly will not affect reproductive fitness and carriers will already have had children before the harmful effects of *APOE* ε4 are apparent. Things are not quite so simple, though. People with *APOE* ε4 are more likely to be carers for their parents or grandparents, since their relatives are also more likely to be *APOE* ε4 carriers. Having *APOE* ε4 therefore can lower fitness at a younger age, as being a carer can be so burdensome. Alternatively, *APOE* ε4 might have some advantageous effects that counteract its promotion of Alzheimer's. Studies have looked at how *APOE* SNPs correlate with cardiovascular responses, reproduction, foetal development, effects of head injury, and brain structure and function. Overall, while ε4 clearly decreases fitness in old age, it may well be beneficial to a foetus, infant or youth.[9] The ε4 variant thus persists.

If we look at the most important twenty or so SNPs found to alter the likelihood of Alzheimer's disease, we can make a fairly good prediction of whether someone will get it and, if so, at what age. Would you want to know, given that Alzheimer's is a miserable terminal illness with no cure? If you are at high risk, you might choose to alter your lifestyle by looking after your heart through exercise and a better diet, and staying mentally and socially active from middle age, measures known to reduce the risk. James Watson, co-discoverer of the double helix structure of DNA, was one of the first people to have their entire DNA genome sequenced in 2009, when he was seventy-nine. When the results were published, he requested that his *APOE* status was kept secret. He wanted to know everything else. He had seen one of his grandmothers develop Alzheimer's disease and did not want the worry of expecting it himself.[10] It is bad enough knowing that you have to die at some point in the future; it would be even worse to have the date.

Most diseases follow a complex polygenic pattern, with variations in many genes modifying the risk of getting a disease, rather than a single change determining it absolutely. Only about 6,000 diseases are known that are caused by mutations in single genes, like huntingtin. Most affect tiny numbers of people in single families. Testing whether someone is carrying a particular SNP linked to disease is now commonplace, especially if a relative is known to have disease. A more exciting prospect is not just to sequence small parts of our DNA, but to sequence all of it. This is the next revolution in healthcare. Thanks to vast improvements in DNA-sequencing technology, genomic data is now being generated at an amazing rate. It is now possible to sequence a human genome for about $1,000 and in less than twenty-four hours.[11]

Concerned parents recently took their five-week-old baby boy to the emergency room in the Rady Children's Hospital in San Diego, after he had been crying inconsolably for two hours. The parents were especially worried as ten years earlier, they had had a child with similar symptoms who progressed to severe epileptic seizures and death. X-ray imaging showed that damage was taking place in the baby's brain. Even though rapid action was essential, the doctors knew that at least 1,500 different diseases fitted the baby's symptoms and didn't have enough information to be able to tell exactly what was wrong. Many of the possible diseases were genetic. In addition, the parents were first cousins. The team therefore decided to try to make a diagnosis by sequencing the baby's DNA. Seventeen hours after admission, they sent a blood sample from the boy to the Rady Genomic Institute so that his DNA could be sequenced. While they waited, the baby began to have seizures.

Just sixteen hours after the baby's blood had been collected, the results from the DNA sequencing were back. A mutation had been found that caused a condition called thiamine metabolism dysfunction syndrome 2, a recessive genetic disease where a protein that transports vitamin B_1 is dysfunctional. Now the doctors knew exactly what to do. To compensate for the lack of transporter function, the baby was given a solution containing three simple chemicals, including vitamin B_1. After one more brief episode, the seizures stopped. Six hours after receiving his first dose of the solution, the baby stopped crying and was happily feeding. His parents took him home the next day. Six months later, he was thriving.[12]

Without the diagnosis from the sequencing, the doctors could only try one anti-seizure medication after another, desperately hoping they would hit upon one that worked before it was too late. Further sequencing later confirmed that both parents were carriers of thiamine metabolism dysfunction syndrome 2. It seems likely that their first child had died from the same condition, when doctors were helpless to prevent it. Rapid whole-genome sequencing for suspected genetic disease is the future of medicine, especially for newborns.[13]

DNA sequencing is so cheap, fast and information-rich that it is likely to become routine for everyone to have their genome fully sequenced. Cancer arises from mutations, so tumour cells can be sequenced to find out exactly what made that set of cells cancerous. Treatments can then be targeted to that type of cancer. This is an example of personalised medicine, where treatments are tailored for a specific patient and condition, rather than recommending the same treatment for every person diagnosed with a specific disease. DNA sequencing can even happen before birth, sequencing a sample of foetal DNA. Doctors will then know in advance if a baby will be born with a potentially life-threatening genetic condition, so can be ready to treat a newborn baby, if necessary. Combining DNA with computers trained with powerful machine-learning software shows whether a baby will be affected by all sorts of health conditions throughout its life. The genetics for nearly all diseases are polygenic, with many sequence variants changing the odds of getting that disease. If we know our risks, we can change our lifestyles and instigate early screening. For example, if our DNA means that we are at high risk of breast cancer, then mammograms can be carried out more frequently and from a younger age. Disease diagnosis can be improved using DNA information on top of a patient's symptoms.

We are already using DNA sequencing data to screen embryos for genetic diseases. If you suspect that you might be a carrier for a genetic disease, it is possible to get pre-implantation genetic screening. In vitro fertilisation (IVF) is first required to give a set of embryos at the blastocyst stage of just eight cells. A single cell is taken for screening and only the embryos that are free of the disease-causing mutations are placed into the womb. In the UK the service is available to couples who have already had children with serious genetic problems or if a genetic disease is known to be in their families. In July 2021 it was possible to test for over 600 conditions in this way.[14] The sequencing tests can show not only whether the embryo will get the disease, but also whether it is a carrier, with a single copy of the problematic gene, rather than two. Potentially, we might therefore choose to implant embryos that are not only free from disease but are not carriers either. The widespread use of programmes like these could eventually eliminate numerous genetic diseases. Whether you think this is ethical depends on your views on IVF, and the value and rights of an embryo.

Screening is fine as far as it goes, but instead of just observing DNA sequences, how about making changes to improve them? We could give people the gene variants that are common in centenarians, for instance, presumably improving their chances of a long life. In 2012 a remarkable paper was published that showed that it might be possible to eliminate Alzheimer's disease for ever by genetic engineering.

The 400,000 people of Iceland are one of the best studied population groups on Earth, due to the country's isolation and excellent genealogical records, often stretching back to the country's settlement 1,000 years ago. A group of mostly Scandinavian geneticists generated sequences of the *APP* gene in 370,000 Icelanders and compared these sequences to patient records. The team found a rare SNP, called A673T, present in about 1 per cent of Icelanders, that made getting Alzheimer's disease five times less likely than the usual sequence.[15] There seems to be no downside to having the A673T SNP. People with it are more likely to live to be eighty-five and they keep their mental faculties intact. This was the first time that a SNP had been found that prevents Alzheimer's, prompting a search for it in other population groups around the world. Not surprisingly, it showed up in other Scandinavian populations, but was very rare elsewhere with only 1 in 5,000 people in North America having it.[16] It seems to be something unique to people with ancestors among a small group of Vikings.

If this work holds up, and those with the A673T SNP really do avoid Alzheimer's disease at no cost, then maybe this is something that we should add to a human genome. This is a step beyond screening embryos for disease-causing genes: here we are considering editing the human DNA so that an embryo has a SNP that neither parent has. Technology to modify DNA in precisely the right place and in the right way is a hot area of research right now. The most famous method for DNA editing is called CRISPR/Cas9, but plenty of improved or alternative methods are being developed. If it can be perfected, we will be able to alter human DNA as we see fit. If we edit an embryo so that it has A673T, then it should grow into an adult that never gets Alzheimer's. Not only that, but the change would get passed on to their children, as some embryo cells would develop into egg or sperm cells that will also carry the altered DNA. Admittedly, trying this would be a somewhat long-term experiment, as we would have to wait eighty years to find out whether it had worked.

Experiments of this nature open the door to the world of trying to 'improve' or 'enhance' humans by changing their DNA. Geneticists have always looked for mutations that cause disease, but there is likely to be a vast number that protect from disease instead, as with A673T. Indeed, a second mutation that appears to protect from dementia and increase lifespan has now been found.[17] People with the normal APP sequence do not have a disease, so introducing the A673T SNP is not curing an illness. In that sense it is fundamentally different from taking out CAG repeats in the huntingtin gene that we know are certain to cause Huntington's. If you think that it is right to introduce A673T to prevent Alzheimer's or edit DNA to stop Huntington's, then why stop there? High blood pressure is the most important risk factor, so how about changing SNPs in an embryo to prevent hypertension? We know that SNPs that affect blood pressure exist.[18] Perhaps we could optimise our DNA to minimise risks from cancer, diabetes, stroke, heart disease and HIV. If we changed the CYP2A6 enzyme,[19] we could even create people who were resistant to the addictive effects of nicotine.

A host of practical and ethical issues have to be addressed before we start modifying DNA in this way. Firstly, our technologies for this purpose are not yet reliable enough. We might introduce unwanted mutations in addition to the one we want, only affect a subset of the cells and cause cancer, among other potential problems.[20] Using in vitro fertilisation is also likely to be necessary, which has a high failure rate. Even if we can accurately alter DNA just how we wish, we don't understand exactly what the changes would do. Few cases are as clear-cut as the CAG repeats that cause Huntington's disease every time. The hundreds of genes that appear to affect blood pressure will affect numerous other biological processes as well. It isn't possible to change propensity to get hypertension without affecting anything else. Genes interact with each other in fantastically complex ways that change with age, environment and location in the body. Changing the probability of having a heart attack in middle age might well have all sorts of unforeseen consequences in other times and places. In addition, as we are altering embryonic cells that will eventually develop into new sperm and egg cells, mistakes would get passed on to future generations, compounding any errors.

If the technology ever becomes reliable (and it isn't at the time of writing, despite a few reckless scientists pressing ahead anyway[21]), then we could go ahead with curing genetic diseases where there is a simple and direct relationship between having a mutation in a single gene and having the disease. This would include haemophilia, where Queen Victoria's SNP in the factor IX gene is all you need to get the disease, sickle-cell disease,[22] cystic fibrosis, fumarase deficiency and Huntington's. For Alzheimer's disease, we could correct the mutations in *APP*, *PSEN1* and *PSEN2* genes that are known to cause early onset of the disease, as these dominant mutations appear to have no benefit and undoubtedly cause great harm. In total, we know of nearly 3,000 so-called single-gene disorders, where a mutation in just the one gene is known to cause disease.[23] These are the first candidates for editing DNA to eliminate genetic disease. One might also go further and argue that it would be unethical not to repair single-gene disorders if you could safely do it. If it is a moral duty to take care of an unborn baby – by taking folate to prevent spina bifida, for example – then it should also be a moral duty to edit an embryo's DNA to prevent a short, miserable life with a horrific genetic disorder. Would you like to explain to your child suffering from muscular dystrophy that it was possible to prevent their disease by editing their DNA before they were born, but you chose not to? Having said all that, there is still little need for this editing, when we can screen embryos for their SNPs and choose which to implant.

In contrast, the likelihood of getting late-onset Alzheimer's disease is affected by dozens of gene variations. These SNPs have multiple effects that we don't fully understand, many of which could even be beneficial. Until we have a much better understanding of what is going on, we should leave these alone. Most health conditions work like this, with a huge number of SNPs in dozens, if not hundreds, of genes, all of which have small effects. The same holds for traits like height[24] and intelligence,[25] not just disease. In addition, it doesn't make much sense to alter our DNA to cope with lifestyle diseases, when our lifestyles are sure to change. Who knows whether we will still be struggling to cope with the effects of a glut of tempting but sugary food in fifty years? DNA editing is the wrong solution for nearly all diseases, particularly if solutions are already here.

17

Death Before Birth

In 1866 the British doctor John Langdon Down published a remarkably unpleasant paper, called *Observations on an Ethnic Classification of Idiots*.[1] The German anthropologist Johann Friedrich Blumenbach had previously proposed classifying people into five races: the Caucasian race was white, the Mongolian yellow, the Malay brown, the Ethiopian black and the American red. Down used Blumenbach's system to classify the occupants of the asylum where he worked, by photographing his guests, measuring them and assigning them into races. He proposed that disease could break down racial barriers, making the facial features of the offspring of Caucasians resemble those of another race. It was obvious to Down that having a baby born into a race other than Caucasian would make them inferior. Most of his report was on what he called 'the great Mongolian family', describing what we would now call Down syndrome. These were the most numerously represented in his asylum. In his words, 'A very large number of congenital idiots are typical Mongols. So marked is this that, when placed side by side, it is difficult to believe the specimens compared are not children of the same parents.' Down did accept that humans of different races were all members of the same species, a controversial viewpoint at the time.

In the Western world 'mongolism' remained an accepted term for Down syndrome for a hundred years. Nevertheless, Chinese and Japanese researchers in particular found the association between 'Mongol' and 'idiot' ridiculous and insulting. A delegation from the Mongolian People's Republic to the World Health Organization in 1965 naturally agreed.[2] In addition, it was known by 1961 that 'mongolism' had absolutely nothing to do with East Asia or a so-called 'race'. In 1961 a group of geneticists therefore wrote an open letter to the prestigious medical journal *The Lancet*, proposing banning the offensive term 'mongolism'.[3] After consulting Norman Down, John Down's grandson, the World Health Organization officially confirmed the switch in name to Down's syndrome in 1965 (later altered to Down syndrome).

To understand the true cause of Down syndrome, we need to look into the process of fertilisation. Here, one lucky sperm fuses with an egg within a fallopian tube, triggering several key processes: firstly, the surface of the egg rapidly hardens, making a barrier to any sperm that arrived just too late. It is clearly essential that only one sperm enters the egg, as only a single set of twenty-three male chromosomes are needed to work with the twenty-three female chromosomes in the egg. Remarkably, the barrier forms as little as ten seconds after the first sperm has penetrated the egg. Egg and sperm surfaces fuse and the paternal DNA is unpacked.

This highly complex process often goes wrong, giving an embryo with a chromosomal abnormality.[4] Humans should have forty-six chromosomes, forty-four of which are autosomal and two of which are the sex chromosome (XX or XY). As part of the fertilisation process, the chromosomes from the mother and father need to replicate, meet and assemble, so that the fertilised egg is ready to divide in two. Mistakes are frequent and can give embryos an incorrect number of chromosomes. A sperm may be missing one chromosome entirely, so that the embryo ends up with just a single copy, rather than two. Alternatively, a sperm or egg before fertilisation may have acquired two copies of a chromosome rather than one, so that the egg ends up with an extra copy. Any errors at this point will be passed on to every human cell in the body, as they are all descended from the fertilised egg.

Consider what happens if only one autosomal chromosome is present. Firstly, the embryo is at high risk of genetic disease. As with X-linked diseases in males, like haemophilia, the embryo will lack a spare copy of hundreds, if not thousands, of genes. There will therefore be no escape from the effects of any detrimental mutation in that single chromosome. Secondly, the amount of protein produced by each gene could be decreased if the protein is being made from one gene instead of two. Missing any autosomal chromosome is totally lethal at early stages of pregnancy.

What can sometimes be tolerated is having part of a chromosome missing. Children born with cri du chat (cry of the cat) syndrome have a low birth weight, respiratory difficulties and a malformed larynx causing a characteristic cat-like cry in babies. People with cri du chat syndrome have distinctive features, such as a small head and chin, an unusually round face, a small bridge of the nose and folds of skin over their eyes. Skeletal problems, heart defects, poor muscle tone and hearing or vision difficulties are common. Children are slow to learn to walk and talk, show behavioural issues such as hyperactivity or aggression, and have severe mental disability. About one in 30,000 newborns have the condition.[5]

French geneticist Jérôme Lejeune discovered the cause of cri du chat syndrome in 1963; he is also the person who discovered the genetic abnormality that causes Down syndrome. Cri du chat is caused by a deletion on chromosome 5. An alternative name for the condition is therefore 5p- (5p minus).[6] The size of the deletion varies from person to person, making all children with cri du chat unique, but there is one critical region that will cause cri du chat if it is missing. Within this region, it is the absence of a gene called CTNND2 that is responsible for causing severe intellectual disability.[7, 8] The CTNND2 gene encodes a protein called delta-catenin, which plays a crucial role in the function of brain cells and the early development of the nervous system. A missing CTNND2 gene has a dominant effect, causing intellectual disability. Eighty-five per cent of the time the deletion that causes cri du chat syndrome occurs by chance, usually during sperm development. Occasionally, however, the syndrome is inherited from a parent, where parts of the parental chromosome have been swapped around or broken off and reattached back to front. The parent will then be fine, as they still have all the right genes, but the chromosomes that they pass on to their children are now prone to breakage.

The most frequent chromosomal problem is to have an extra copy of a chromosome, normally acquired from an abnormal sperm cell. It is much deadlier to have an extra autosomal chromosome rather than an extra X or Y, with only three conditions capable of reaching birth.

Patau syndrome is caused by an extra chromosome 13. Most foetuses with Patau syndrome miscarry or are aborted; otherwise, 90 per cent die in their first year due to major problems with the brain and nervous system, bones, muscles, kidneys and genitals. An extra chromosome 18 causes Edward syndrome, with kidney and heart defects, small heads and severe intellectual difficulties. Again, most are miscarried or terminated, and babies are unlikely to live a year.

The most common condition with an extra autosomal chromosome is Down syndrome, where cells have three copies of chromosome 21, as Jérôme Lejeune found. The chromosome with the smallest number of protein-coding genes is Y with about 70; next is chromosome 21 with about 230, which is presumably why extra copies of Y or 21 are tolerated better than others. More rarely, some children with Down syndrome have a mixture of cells, some with the extra chromosome 21 and some with the usual 46; these tend to have weaker symptoms. Occasionally, the total number of chromosomes in the cells remains 46, but a full or partial copy of chromosome 21 attaches to another chromosome, usually chromosome 14. The presence of the extra genes causes some characteristics of Down syndrome. For example, the *APP* gene that is linked to Alzheimer's disease is found on chromosome 21. People with Down syndrome will therefore have an extra copy of *APP*, giving them more amyloid-β, and early-onset Alzheimer's disease, on top of their other health problems.

Down syndrome is well known to cause distinctive facial features, slow growth and intellectual disability. The average IQ of a young adult is 50, equivalent to a nine-year-old, though there are wide variations, so that many can live independently. Children with Down syndrome are often described as having sweet and loving personalities. About one in 300 pregnancies have the condition, though the probability is highly age dependent, increasing from less than 0.1 per cent in twenty-year-old mothers to 10 per cent in those aged forty-nine. Women lose fertility at this age, perhaps because the risk of chromosomal problems becomes so high. However, 80 per cent of children with Down syndrome are born to women under thirty-five years of age, who often have no idea they were carrying a baby with Down syndrome until it is born.

When Lejeune discovered the cause of Down syndrome in the late 1950s, he hoped that his work would contribute to a cure. Instead, to his horror, it led to more abortions, as his work brought about the development of a test that can see whether a mother is carrying a child with Down syndrome. In the UK women are offered a screening test for Down, Edward and Patau syndromes between ten and fourteen weeks of pregnancy. Ultrasound measures the size of a pocket of fluid at the back of the baby's neck which, together with hormone levels, gives a risk estimate. Women at high risk can have their amniotic fluid or placental tissue sampled. Foetal cells are grown in a culture medium, fixed and stained so that their chromosomes can be examined. If chromosomal abnormalities are detected, most mothers choose to have their pregnancies terminated. To this day, nothing can be done to cure chromosomal abnormalities. After his discovery, Lejeune became a prominent advocate of humane care for people with Down syndrome, led a French anti-abortion movement called 'Let Them Live' and worked as an advisor to Pope John Paul II.

In about 2 per cent of conceptions the foetus has a complete extra set of chromosomes, giving them sixty-nine instead of forty-six. These triploid foetuses rarely survive to birth, with most spontaneously miscarried as an embryo. The few infants that do survive to term have multiple severe birth defects, including growth retardation, and heart and neural tube defects, and die within a few days. Triploidy occurs when either the egg or the sperm has a complete set of forty-six chromosomes, from a failure of sperm development, or if two sperm enter the egg at the same time. As we saw, once a sperm has successfully penetrated an egg, it needs to rapidly create a barrier to any others; if this is too slow, two sperm can enter, so that the egg has a double set of chromosomes from the father. More rarely, tetraploidy can take place, when the embryo has four copies of each chromosome; early miscarriage is then highly likely.

The only chromosomes that can be deleted entirely are X and Y. This should be no surprise – after all, most men seem to manage perfectly well with only one X chromosome and women have no Y chromosome at all. Whether the baby turns out to be male or female depends on whether they have the Y chromosome, or more specifically, functional genes on the Y that will turn a developing embryo male, such as *SRY*, which initiates testes development. Many genetic conditions that are caused by alterations in the sex chromosomes are tolerated after birth.

People with Turner syndrome have forty-five chromosomes, instead of the usual forty-six, with only one X in every cell. Naturally, they are all female. The X chromosome that is present is usually from the mother, so the sperm had only the twenty-two autosomal chromosomes and no sex chromosome at all. Even though life expectancy is reduced by only thirteen years and adults can live normal lives, 99 per cent of Turner syndrome conceptions end in miscarriage or stillbirth (10 per cent of miscarriages in total). Women with Turner syndrome don't produce enough of the female sex hormones oestrogen and progesterone, though this can be treated with hormone replacement therapy to ensure that puberty takes place. Diagnosis is therefore crucial so that treatment can be given. Women with Turner syndrome often have problems with their hearts, kidneys, thyroid glands and bones, as well as tendencies to be obese and have diabetes. While they are good with language, sometimes they struggle to understand social relationships and mathematics, and are poor at spatial reasoning. Most women with Turner syndrome cannot conceive, but a small number have enough ovarian tissue in their teens to become pregnant with fertility treatment.[9]

One in a thousand females are born with triple X syndrome. Their symptoms are mild, so triple X syndrome is usually not diagnosed, though the women tend to be tall and may have some learning difficulties. Many other combinations of sex chromosomes have been found, such as XXY, XYY, XXXY, XXYY and XXXXX, with a range of symptoms. The mildest is XYY syndrome, present in one in 1,000 boys. It has few or no symptoms, so men with the condition usually have no idea. XYY men are even fertile.

After fertilisation, the human embryo undergoes multiple cell divisions, starting its way to the trillions of cells in an adult human. First produced is a ball of cells, called a blastocyst. Once the embryo reaches the blastocyst stage, approximately six days after fertilisation, it begins to implant into the wall of the uterus, where it will develop into a placenta and foetus. This requires a healthy embryo and extensive alterations to a receptive uterus, giving plenty of scope for failure. In fact, more than 50 per cent of fertilised eggs fail this implantation process.

If you think that human life starts at fertilisation, then the leading cause of death has never been cancer, heart disease or infectious disease, but rather failed implantation. This has always been the case and probably always will be so. If you believe that an embryo gains an immortal soul at conception, then about half of the souls in the afterlife are of nothing more than blastocysts.

Occasionally a blastocyst collapses and splits in half for unknown reasons. Each half will have the same genetic material but will form separate foetuses. These are identical twins. Alternatively, non-identical twins can form when two fertilised eggs implant in the uterus at the same time. Non-identical twin births are more common than identical, making one in forty-five people a twin. One in eight pregnancies start as twins, however, with one of the foetuses usually dying early and being reabsorbed, known as a 'vanishing twin'. Many of us therefore started development as a twin, though we are rarely aware of this.

Miscarriage is the death of an embryo or foetus before it is viable. After twenty-three weeks of pregnancy, the loss of a foetus is called a stillbirth. Bleeding from the vagina is the main symptom, often with pain. The mother may also simply feel that she isn't pregnant any more. Some mothers have no signs at all that their baby has died and only discover their loss when they attend a routine antenatal appointment and have an ultrasound scan. Medical treatment following a miscarriage is not usually needed, though emotional support and sympathetic counselling can help. Women often feel grief, anxiety, depression and a sense of guilt, even though this is almost always undeserved. I can assure you from personal experience that fathers find it upsetting too.

The frequency of miscarriage is very hard to know, as many take place before the mother is even aware that she is pregnant. As we have seen, unknown to the mother, perhaps 50 per cent of fertilised eggs fail to implant in the uterus. The death of an embryo shortly after implantation is nearly as frequent, particularly with twins. Once a woman knows that she is pregnant, the miscarriage rate is roughly 10 per cent to 20 per cent.

The risk of miscarriage decreases substantially once the foetus is about twelve weeks old. By this stage, many major organs will be in their initial forms and have started to function. If an essential organ does not work or fails to develop properly, then the embryo will be lost. For example, the heart should be beating by three or four weeks, pumping essential nutrients around the tiny embryo. With no heart, the embryo will miscarry at this very early stage.

The specific reason why a miscarriage has happened is rarely known. Nearly always the miscarriage could not have been prevented, as is the case with chromosomal disorders. In addition to chromosomal disorders, a number of conditions are common causes of miscarriage.

The thyroid gland in the neck produces hormones, such as oestrogen, to control metabolism and growth. An overactive thyroid will produce too many hormones that can interfere with oestrogen's ability to make the uterus favourable for implantation. Similarly, an underactive thyroid can lead to stillbirth. Fortunately, this is easily treated with synthetic thyroid hormone.

Diabetics lack the hormone insulin or develop a resistance to it, even though it is still made by the pancreas. Insulin signals to the body that blood glucose levels are high, so if insulin is absent, the body will send glucose into the bloodstream, even if it is not needed. Poorly controlled blood sugar levels can cause many complications in pregnancy, such as heart and neural tube defects, miscarriage and premature birth. Careful monitoring of blood sugar levels, nutrition and medication will help.

As you might guess, drugs, alcohol and smoking all increase the risk of early miscarriage and stillbirth. Most women do not realise that they are pregnant until a couple of weeks after their missed period. By this time the foetal spinal cord is formed and the heart is beating, so the damage could already be done.

Rarely, miscarriage can be caused by physical problems in the mother, such as uterine abnormalities or a weak cervix, which cannot hold the pregnancy. These tend to be late in pregnancy.

The immune system has evolved to attack things that it recognises as foreign, such as infections by bacteria or viruses. This immediately creates a potential problem when an embryo forms, as it could appear foreign to the mother's body. When functioning correctly, the immune system can recognise a pregnancy as a desirable condition. The embryo will suppress the mother's immune system and initiate processes where the mother's immune system is directed to protect the embryo from attack. If her immune system is defective, due to an autoimmune disorder, these processes may not occur. Then her immune system can attack the embryo, causing recurrent miscarriage.

An autoimmune disorder – such as multiple sclerosis, type 1 diabetes or Crohn's disease – is a condition where the body's immune system attacks and destroys its own healthy tissue. Lupus is an autoimmune disease that can result in an increased miscarriage rate, due to additional antibodies that these women carry. While it is not possible to control whether you have these antibodies, they can be detected, and treatments then given to reduce the risk of miscarriage.

Eating healthily, avoiding harms like smoking and alcohol, and managing conditions like diabetes can thus lower the risk of miscarriage. Beyond screening in embryos, there is little that can be done about chromosomal abnormalities, however. The conditions are not inherited, so a parent cannot be a carrier, apart from rare cases like cri du chat, where a chromosome prone to breakage might be present with no symptoms. Once a baby is born with a chromosomal abnormality, the condition is present in many, if not all, of their cells and cannot be repaired. All we can do is manage symptoms to help the child live the best life that they can. Not all diseases have a cure within sight.

PART V

BAD BEHAVIOUR

The old law of an eye for an eye leaves everybody blind.

Martin Luther King, *Stride Toward Freedom:*
The Montgomery Story, 1958[1]

18

Thou Shalt Not Kill

So far we have looked at reasons for dying that are little more than bad luck, like catching an infection or inheriting some kind of genetic condition. Now, however, we shall change tack, to consider causes of death that arise from our own choices.

We are the most dangerous animal on the planet. We often harm ourselves or others – we kill each other, legally in wars and illegally by homicide, cause accidents, abuse drugs, eat the wrong food and even take our own lives. All are a central part of the human condition. Since we are large predators, no cause of death is more basic or more ancient than murder.

Ten thousand years ago a group of nomads made a temporary camp by a lagoon near Lake Turkana in Kenya. This fertile region was home to elephants, giraffes and zebras, and was a popular spot for bands of humans. One such band was not there to hunt big game, however. Instead they were there to hunt people. They launched an attack on the campers, killing dozens of them. Many of the corpses of their victims seem to have been left as they had died, to be covered by silt and the waters of the lagoon, with their corpses rotting to skeletons. Over thousands of years the lagoon dried up and turned into a desert. Finally, wind eroded the surface, exposing the bones once more.

In 2012 professional fossil hunter Pedro Ebeya discovered fragments of human bones at the site. Pedro was part of the In-Africa project, a five-year research programme to investigate the origins of our species, *Homo sapiens*, in East Africa.[1] The team found the remains of twenty-seven people, including twelve complete skeletons. Ten of the twelve skeletons showed damage from weapons, suggesting that they had died at the hands of other people. Skeletal features included an arrowhead still embedded in a skull, neck damage, and seven head injuries from being struck. There were also two cases of broken hand bones, possibly from the victim trying to ward off blows. The two people with no evidence of bone damage from weapons may have had their hands tied to die. One of these was a pregnant young woman.[2] The attackers had used bows and arrows, clubs, axes with wooden shafts and sharp stone blades – weapons designed to be used on people, rather than for hunting animals.[3] The type of stone used in the axe heads was not found near the lagoon, suggesting that the attackers had travelled a long way for the purpose of killing. Dating of the human remains showed that the massacre was one of the earliest known cases of conflict between groups of people.[4]

Humans are hunters, yet compared to other predators of the same size, our weapons are weak. We have useless claws, small teeth, weak jaws and poor arm strength compared to our chimp cousins. We are excellent at throwing, though, able to kill at a distance, with stones, spears, slings and bows. Where we really find success in hunting is through teamwork. Even so, hunting very often fails and when it is successful in making a large kill, there can be too much for any small group to eat by itself. It therefore pays to share the spoils, in the form of feasts for neighbours, so that they will feed you in return in the future. Risks are also shared to even out the dangers of hunting. Human behaviour thus evolved to be cooperative, as working together is vital for successful hunting. Communication in the form of speech may have started as simple commands used in hunting ('Stop! Shhh! Now!').

In 2012 American anthropologist Christopher Boehm analysed the culture of fifty modern-day hunter-gatherer groups.[4] All used social rules that worked like laws to prevent selfishness, bullying, theft, or unduly favouring close relatives or friends. Punishments were public humiliation, telling-off, ridicule, shaming, shunning, expulsion from the group or even death. Exile would often be a death sentence in effect, since humans living alone in a dangerous environment stand little chance of long-term survival. Cooperative behaviours have been selected for thousands of generations, so that a sense of justice and fairness is part of what makes us human. Indeed, we punish ourselves severely for bad behaviour by feeling shame and guilt. These emotions can be so powerful that they can even drive us to suicide.

What was remarkable about the hunter-gatherer lifestyle is how likely it was to end in a violent death.[5] In a survey of twenty-seven non-state societies in the modern world by Max Roser, on the Our World in Data website,[6] the percentage of deaths from violence varies from 4 per cent to 56 per cent; around 25 per cent is typical. Top is the Waorani people from the Amazon rainforest in Ecuador, who had a policy of killing all outsiders until the last few decades. The most peaceful are the Anbara people of Northern Australia, where 'only' 4 per cent suffer deaths from violence. Perhaps this situation reflects something special about modern-day hunter-gatherers who might need violence to survive? An alternative approach is to use archaeological evidence. Within twenty-six archaeological records of groups over the last 14,000 years, violent death rates vary from 0 per cent to 60 per cent, with an average of 16 per cent, comparable to modern non-state societies. Skeletons frequently show evidence of violent deaths in the Palaeolithic period, such as arrowheads embedded in bones and fatal head injuries from weapons. Studies of present-day mobile forager bands suggest that most incidences of lethal aggression seem to have been one-on-one events, rather than fights between groups like the Lake Turkana massacre.[7] Even so, anthropological studies of traditional non-state societies, like those in highland New Guinea, confirm that small-scale conflicts are frequent and often end in mass slaughter of the defeated group.[8] Fertile young women stand the best chance of being allowed to live.

Nomadic hunter-gatherers lived in bands of perhaps a few hundred people at most. People within these societies would see each other every day and know each other very well. Social rules to enforce good behaviour worked well in groups this small, as everyone knew everyone else; however, they could break down when the size of the group grew too large. By 3000 BCE the Sumerian city of Uruk was the largest in the world, with a population of about 40,000. Punishments such as public rebukes and ostracism might work in a band of a hundred people, but in a city this size they would be less effective, as the target could simply move to a new group of friends and colleagues within the same community. A new system was needed.

One of our finest inventions is writing, turning language into images that we make, store and share. Writing was independently devised at least three times – in the Middle East, China and Central America. The oldest writing comes from the Middle East, as with many other inventions. Writing was invented by accountants to facilitate trade, and later extended to inscriptions, religious writings, poems, stories and recording deeds of kings. Shortly afterwards the first codes of law were written down. The earliest legal code that we know about is named after the Sumerian king Ur-Nammu and dates to about 2100 BCE. A more comprehensive legal code is the Code of King Hammurabi of Babylon, also in Iraq. It was found in 1901 carved onto a huge block of stone, clearly meant for public display. It was written in the name of Hammurabi in the Akkadian language and is now on show in the Louvre in Paris. At the top, the king is shown receiving the law from the god Shamash. Underneath is the entire legal code, carved in stone on a 2.25-metre-tall slab using the Akkadian script.

The code contained 282 laws in total.[9] This was sufficient to administer an entire empire. (In contrast, the USA adds about 40,000 new laws per year and no one is really sure how many laws there are in total.[10]) All of Hammurabi's laws are written in the form: IF <u>you do this bad thing</u> THEN <u>this is how you will be punished</u>.

The laws cover family law, commerce and administration, and have the full backing of the Babylonian gods. Laws often varied depending on your sex or which class of Babylonian society you belonged to. For example, a doctor who cured a severe wound could charge ten silver shekels to a gentleman, five to a freedman and only two shekels to a slave. Similarly, a doctor who killed a rich patient would have his hands cut off, while if a slave was killed there would only be a fine. Most punishments were fines, though the death penalty was frequently used too. There was no imprisonment. Here are examples of some of the laws:

If anyone bring an accusation of any crime before the elders, and does not prove what he has charged, he shall, if it be a capital offence charged, be put to death. [Do not bear false witness.]

If anyone is committing a robbery and is caught, then he shall be put to death. [Do not steal.]

If anyone open his ditches to water his crop, but is careless, and the water flood the field of his neighbour, then he shall pay his neighbour corn for his loss. [There were many laws for farmers. Irrigation of fields from the Tigris and Euphrates rivers was of critical importance in Babylon, as there was very little rain. Compensation from a farmer is in the form of crops, rather than money, presumably because that would be easier for a farmer.]

If anyone be guilty of incest with his mother after his father, both shall be burned. [A sexual law.]

If a man put out the eye of another man, his eye shall be put out. [An eye for an eye.]

If he put out the eye of a man's slave, or break the bone of a man's slave, he shall pay one half of its value. [Slaves are worth less than free men.]

There were no religious laws, even though Hammurabi's laws carried Divine approval. It seems that Hammurabi was unconcerned about which gods his citizens did or did not worship, in contrast to the Old Testament of the Bible, much of which was also written and compiled by the rivers of Babylon 1,000 years later. God is much more central in the legal books of the Bible, with 'You shall have no other gods before me' in the Ten Commandments (Exodus 20:3). Encouraging the worship of other gods carries the death penalty: 'If your very own brother, or your son or daughter, or the wife you love, or your closest friend secretly entices you, saying, "Let us go and worship other gods" ... do not yield to them or listen to them. Show them no pity. Do not spare them or shield them ... Stone them to death' (Deuteronomy 13: 6–10). Here the state is seeking to control what people thought, not just what they did.

Reading the Code of Hammurabi, what is striking is how little human nature has changed. Even 4,000 years later, we can generally agree with Hammurabi on what deeds count as a crime. The glaring exception is the legality of slavery. These law codes were a big advance on the arbitrary systems of justice previously used, in terms of transparency and fairness. The laws were carved on huge durable stones to be set up for all to see and read (assuming they were literate). The consequences of bad behaviour were thus plain, to act as a deterrent. Gods were frequently invoked to add weight to the laws. People were innocent until proven guilty. Everyone in each social class had the same punishment for the same crime. Previously, an intimidating, related or rich criminal might get more lenient treatment compared to someone who was disliked or weak. As it says at the top of the code, Hammurabi's purpose was to 'bring about the rule of righteousness in the land, to destroy the wicked and the evil-doers; so that the strong should not harm the weak ... and enlighten the land, to further the well-being of humanity',[10] which are still laudable aims.

States can be defined as organised political communities under a government with authority over a set area. They first appeared in Sumeria about 5,000 years ago, as walled cities, ruling over their surrounding land. In contrast, stateless societies do not have power concentrated in one or a few individuals, such as a king or a group of nobles. Stateless societies are not necessarily nomadic, as they can be self-governing villages. They lack job specialisation into monarchs, soldiers, administrators, priests and tax collectors, and hence lack the products of taxes and centralised power, like pyramids, palaces and temples. Since states can leave long-lasting records in the form of well-built cities and writing, our view of the past is dominated by them. Nevertheless, for nearly all of history, most people lived in stateless societies. Four thousand years ago states only occupied tiny areas within a sea of stateless so-called barbarians. States have only dominated most of the planet since about 1600, when Europeans established control over most of the Americas.

In 1651 Thomas Hobbes published *Leviathan*,[11] one the most influential books ever written on politics. In it he argued that it was desirable for people to give up their freedom to act as they choose in order to avoid an anarchic state of war of all against all, with continual fear and danger of violent death. War can, and should, be avoided by handing over the right of governing to a sovereign. This sovereign would establish laws and do whatever is necessary to preserve peace and society, avoiding the catastrophe of civil war, which for Hobbes was the worst possible situation. Hobbes was writing during the English Civil War. This was a complicated struggle primarily over the governance of England, though with a large dose of Catholic versus Protestant violence, as usual in the seventeenth century in Europe. It was fought throughout the British Isles, with Ireland treated especially brutally. In terms of percentage of total population that were killed, this war was the worst in British history. Hobbes thus witnessed the appalling effects of loss of government.

Comparing hunter-gatherer societies with states based on agriculture shows that Hobbes had a point. The first rulers might appropriate wealth for themselves, and remove freedom and power from the masses, but they did tend to make the world a less violent place. Consider what might happen when two groups of hunters meet in the Palaeolithic period. If they are related, they would have better reasons to cooperate, so lengthy discussions on possible family connections might come first. What if they are unrelated strangers, though? Should they fight or depart in peace? Fighting is obviously a dangerous business that could easily result in injury or death. It does have potential rewards, however: the winners would be able to seize the loser's possessions, including territory and women, not just goods. If one band felt they were substantially bigger and stronger, an easy win would surely be tempting. Secondly, now that the two groups have discovered each other, it might be safer to eliminate the other one completely if they can. If not, the beaten survivors might be back later with many more fighters. The safest option could be to attack them now. Ideally, all will be killed, so that none can flee to plot their revenge. Finally, a successful warrior could earn a tremendous boost to his reputation and status within their band. Hot-headed and downtrodden young men would be keen to demonstrate their mettle to their peers. Killers might be able to display their newly earned high status in clothing or tattoos, permanently cementing their position. Murdering strangers could be rewarded rather than punished – after all, there were no laws against it.

In contrast, in states with codes of law, an individual seeking out their own justice, such as revenge killings, is not tolerated. As German sociologist Max Weber pointed out in 1919, states award themselves a monopoly on the legitimate use of violence.[12] Indeed, Weber went further and defined a state as an organisation that is able to hold the exclusive right to use and authorise physical force against people within its territory. Revenge is forbidden, as it is the state that decides on guilt and punishments. Good rulers, such as Hammurabi, promise the people that criminals will be punished fairly. Consequences of misbehaviour are literally spelled out in advance, so that ignorance is no excuse. However weak an individual is, they can have confidence that the state will administer justice on their behalf. Similarly, a criminal will fear that the entire system will be against him, not just a victim's family. There is no point in slaughtering all the relatives of their victim to avoid their revenge, as it is the state that will be punishing the criminal, not just the victim's family. Might is no longer right. In addition, gods often give their backing to the law, adding authority and the risk of punishment from deities who see all.

The downside of states taking over the right to determine the use of violence is loss of freedom, even if that freedom is being able to kill with impunity. We do not have the right to reject the rule of law or seek personal revenge if we live in a state. We are born into legal systems and cannot refuse to accept values and laws that we disagree with, even if tyrannical rulers abuse their position to exploit and oppress the people. The benefit of state-based rule is a great decrease in crime, particularly murder. This is the social contract,[13] much discussed by moral and political philosophers. As such, codes of law are one of our greatest inventions.

As well as laws, states created professional armies to enhance their power.[14] Rather than all the men of the village going out to fight when necessary, this job was now left to highly trained soldiers, equipped with armour, sophisticated weaponry and horses. Even if a city was conquered, there wasn't much reason to kill the farmers. Peasants were an asset, as they produced food. As they were hopeless at fighting compared to professional soldiers, they couldn't take revenge even if they wanted to. By 2,000 years ago, this had led to peace within a vast area inside the Chinese and Roman empires, with the borders protected by walls and armies. Cities inside the walls could be hundreds of miles from any potential enemy. The chances of being killed in battle thus fell greatly as states grew larger.

The most violent state of all time, as far as we know, is the Aztec state in Mexico, which lasted from about 1345 until 1521. The Aztecs engaged in extensive warfare with the aim of conquering neighbouring states and exacting tribute from them. Taking captives was a second vital goal: prisoners who were to be sacrificed to the gods. All Aztec boys started warrior training from the age of fifteen and could be drafted into the army, even if they had other jobs. Warfare was so important to their culture that the Aztecs fought so-called Flower Wars that were arranged in advance with neighbouring states, rather as we might arrange sporting fixtures. The two sides agreed before battle on the sizes of the two armies to keep the fight fair. They fought to give individual warriors the opportunity of gaining prestige by taking captives. Football matches are a preferable recent substitute.

Captives were sacrificed by having their hearts cut out on the top of pyramids. This occurred on a staggering scale: the Spanish chroniclers who invaded Mexico in 1519 reported that skull racks could be found at Aztec temples, where thousands of skulls were skewered through their temples on poles. There had been speculation on whether the Spanish accounts were exaggerated to justify their conquest and destruction of the Aztec civilisation. In 2017, however, the remains of a twelve-metre-wide skull rack, just as described by the Spanish, was found in Mexico City.[15] It was located at the base of the Templo Mayor – a pyramid with two temples on top, dedicated to the war god, Huitzilopochtli, and the rain god, Tlaloc. On either side of the rack were two five-metre-tall towers, built from skulls taken from the rack when they began to fall to pieces. The Spanish were horrified by the Aztec religion, particularly after witnessing some of their fellow soldiers having their hearts cut out while still alive at the top of the temple after being taken prisoner. After their conquest and destruction of the city in 1521, the Templo Mayor was torn down. The site was paved over and became part of Mexico City.

Even though 5 per cent of the citizens of the Aztec Empire met a violent end, this is still low compared to hunter-gatherers. In the USA and Europe from 1900 to 1960 the violent death rate was only 1 per cent, despite two world wars. At present, homicide rates are highest in Latin America, the Caribbean and Southern Africa. El Salvador, Honduras and Venezuela topped the list in 2016, with murder rates fifteen times higher than the USA, which is itself fifty-five times higher than Japan.[16] If a state is weak, other groups, like criminal gangs, are able to use violence as they see fit. Central America is home to extensive organised crime, where gangs fight each other and the state, engaging in robbery, kidnapping, extortion and the drug trade. Availability of firearms and high drug and alcohol use are additional risk factors, especially for young men. Poverty and crime form a vicious circle where crime drives away legitimate businesses, creating more poverty and unemployment. Perhaps we are seeing a switch to new forms of organised-crime-based conflict, as in El Salvador, away from just those between states.[17]

The next section and its links contains information about suicide which may be upsetting to some people.

For young people aged sixteen to forty or so, the number one cause of death is suicide. The next time you look in the mirror, consider that the person you are looking at is by far the most likely to kill you – you are more dangerous to yourself than every other person on the planet combined. Humans are the only species known to use violence against themselves, using weapons to take their own lives.

Guyana, Lesotho and Swaziland apparently have the most suicides per person, though statistics on suicide are not trustworthy, as many countries do not collect accurate data.[18] In 2021, the World Health Organization estimated that only about eighty countries recorded good-quality data on suicide.[19] Suicide has high stigma or can even be illegal, so many deaths recorded as accidents, such as driving a car straight into a tree under good road conditions, are actually deliberate. The high rankings for Guyana, Lesotho and Swaziland, therefore, at least partly reflect that suicides are more likely to be recorded there. Suicide is a global phenomenon, with 77 per cent of suicides occurring in low- and middle-income countries in 2019. It is the fourth leading cause of death for fifteen- to nineteen-year-olds.[20] On top of this, for every death by suicide there are about twenty attempts.

The Golden Gate Bridge, which connects San Francisco to Marin County to the north, opened in 1937. If you jump from the bridge, it takes four seconds to make the fall, plenty of time to think about it; you then hit the water at 75 mph. If you survive the impact, you will have extreme pain from broken feet, legs and back. These injuries prevent swimming in the freezing bay, so you drown. Nevertheless, some survivors are occasionally picked up by a boat, albeit often with permanent disabilities. When interviewed afterwards, many say that they regretted their decision the moment they jumped. They most certainly were not at peace with their choice. Similarly, of 515 people who went to the bridge with the intention of jumping, but were prevented by California Highway Patrol officers, only about 10 per cent went on to die by suicide at a later date.[20] The decision to take one's life is therefore nearly always a temporary one. People who manage to get through their anguish are later glad that they did.

Suicide has a complex set of causes, manifest in intense emotional pain. Many suicidal people are struggling to cope with a psychiatric condition, especially depression or bipolar disorder. Depression is particularly insidious, as it is invisible and can last for decades. People who attempt suicide are more likely to have a lower social status, be in a sexual minority and have no children. Humans are highly social animals, caring intensely about how other people see them. A deep sense of shame can propel someone into a suicidal state. Irresponsible reporting of suicides by the press or social media, such as describing methods used by someone that a vulnerable person identifies with, can lead to imitation.

Some cultures are relatively accepting of suicide, while in others it is even criminal. Major religions condemn suicide, saying that life is a gift from God, not to be thrown away or it will condemn you to hell or generate very bad karma for your next rebirth. But for those of us without religious beliefs, why is suicide wrong? Surely you have the right to do what you want with your body? One can take a utilitarian perspective on this issue. While taking your own life might end your own (temporary) torment, it will cause deep, long-term suffering for all those people who love and care for us, making the net effect of a suicide highly negative in terms of the total amount of pain caused. Unfortunately, a common delusion when in a suicidal state is that you are not cared for, you are a burden and that your passing would be some kind of relief to other people. It is also hard to imagine that things will get better. These false beliefs help lower the barriers to self-harming. Spending time with vulnerable people and reminding them that they are loved therefore reduces the risk of suicide. Any human contact that is not unkind can help.

In 1935 a young Church of England curate called Chad Varah conducted his first funeral. A thirteen-year-old girl had taken her life, believing that she had contracted a venereal disease and was sure to die a shameful and painful death. In reality she was not ill at all – she had just had her first period. This tragic and pointless suicide transformed Varah's life. He vowed at her graveside to dedicate his life to overcoming the shame, isolation and ignorance that led to the girl's death. He would do this with a combination of education about sexual matters and emotional support for those with suicidal thoughts.

As well as his priestly duties, Chad authored stories for the children's comics *Girl* and *Eagle*, helping create Dan Dare, the Space Age hero with a stiff upper lip. He also provided sex education, making his youth-club talks highly popular, particularly with young couples thinking of marriage. In 1952 he wrote an article on sex for the widely read *Picture Post*. While conservatives were predictably outraged by the subject matter, Varah was more struck by 235 letters he received afterwards from people who needed someone to talk to – someone with whom to share their fears, worries and secrets. A few of the writers even admitted to having suicidal thoughts. At that time, three suicides a day were reported in London. Varah realised that there was a great need for desperate people to have someone to talk to.

In 1953 Chad moved to a new parish of St Stephen in the City of London, working with his secretary, Vivien Prosser. Unusually for the time, his new church was equipped with the height of modern technology in the form of a telephone. This gave him the opportunity to start a new service, a '999 for the suicidal'. He used his contacts in newspapers, found through his comics, to publicise the new service. The *Daily Mirror* came up with the phrase 'Telephone Good Samaritan', named after the Bible story, in which a member of a despised religious minority called the Samaritans helps a stranger in dire need. Chad and Vivien were soon inundated with people who needed support on the phone or a face-to-face talk. Many also volunteered to help. Some volunteers would sit with people while they waited for an appointment to speak with Chad. Often the visitors did not wait, but instead poured out their troubles to the volunteers before leaving, removing any need to see Chad. He soon realised that 'the volunteers were doing the clients more good than I was'.

After only a few months, Chad handed over the task of supporting callers solely to the volunteers. From this simple beginning, with two people and one phone, the Samaritans now has 20,000 volunteers and 201 branches across the UK and Republic of Ireland, answering a call every six seconds, night and day. The Samaritans meet a need for those in emotional distress. A caller can speak with someone who will not criticise or judge, but will listen confidentially, ask open questions and show empathy and understanding, whatever they have done. The

Samaritans spread abroad as Befrienders Worldwide, operating in more than thirty countries. The Samaritans and similar organisations save many lives by providing hope, support or simply someone who will listen in a safe environment.

Chad continued as director of the London branch from 1953 to 1974, and Samaritans president from 1974 to 1986. He did consultancy work for the sex-education magazine *Forum*, and became patron of the Terence Higgins Trust, the UK's largest HIV and AIDS charity. While in his eighties, he founded Men Against Genital Mutilation of Girls, which met with immigrants from East Africa, persuading them not to continue with this cruel practice. The Rev. Dr Edward Chad Varah CH, CBE, died in 2007, aged ninety-five. With the Samaritans' complete anonymity and inability to track a caller, it is hard to estimate how many lives his work has saved. Undoubtedly, it is many thousands.[21, 22, 23]

19

Alcohol and Addiction

In 1948 the village of Slyozi in western Russia was beginning to prosper again; the German invaders had been driven out four years before, after three years of occupation. Most of its one hundred inhabitants were working in the nearby collective farm, though some also kept their own bees, chickens, cows and pigs. Fifty years later, however, the village was almost dead. Most buildings were empty and rotting, and its population had dwindled to just four, with Tamara the youngest at seventy-nine. The last male inhabitant of Slyozi had died the previous year.

This scene of villages populated entirely by old ladies or completely abandoned is commonplace throughout Russia. In 2010 nearly 40,000 villages in Russia had fewer than ten inhabitants, almost all of them old women.[1] The young move to cities for work and better opportunities, leaving their mothers and grandmothers in the villages, and their fathers and grandfathers in the graveyards. This situation is reflected in the astonishingly large difference in life expectancy between men and women in Russia – ten years. Women can expect to live to seventy-eight, not great for Europe, but about average for the world. However, for men it is only sixty-eight.

Various social factors contribute to why the men have gone: poor healthcare, dangerous jobs, smoking and unemployment, for instance. But the number one reason is alcohol. Many Russian men drink on average a bottle of vodka per day, leading to frequent deaths before the age of sixty.[2]

The Russian women know very well why they have lost their men. Zinaida Ivanovna, aged seventy-nine, lived in the neighbouring village of Velye. She said, 'Drink is a huge problem around here. It's a nightmare. The men here drink their pensions as soon as they get them. They sell whatever they have to get more booze. They drink anything – moonshine and even window-cleaning fluids.'[3]

How did Russia arrive at this state? What explains our complex relationship with our favourite drug? To answer these questions, we must go back thousands of years to when our nomadic ancestors first encountered alcohol.

We don't know when humans first started consuming alcoholic drinks or even what they were made from. We do have a good idea of where wine originated, however.[4] The wild Eurasian grape, ancestor of the modern wine grape, still grows in eastern Turkey, Armenia and Georgia. We can imagine what happened: early nomadic humans moving into a fertile valley found wild vines full of fruit along the sunny slopes above the river. The people had far too many grapes to eat all at once, so ripe fruit were put into wooden containers, carved out by their stone axes. Many of the overripe grapes burst or were crushed, releasing their juice to be left at the bottom of the container. Now something interesting starts to happen to the forgotten fruit: the juice bubbles and froths, releasing dense carbon dioxide, which forms a layer above the liquid, excluding oxygen. The grape juice is undergoing fermentation, being transformed into wine.

A few weeks later the red murky liquid is discovered at the bottom of the container. Someone brave takes a sip. They like it. Not only is the taste better than grape juice, but it produces a pleasant, calm feeling. Sadly, this accidental invention made only a small amount of wine, but it is enough to encourage further experimentation when the group returns to the valley next year. Now copious quantities of grapes are deliberately left in containers, giving many litres of product to be shared around.

This is the first time humans have access to alcoholic drinks in large amounts. It therefore doesn't take too much for the effects of drunkenness to set in. People are happy and sociable. They chat more, sing and dance around the fire. As they keep drinking, bad behaviour sets in. Some get aggressive, while others lose inhibitions. Some vomit and others pass out. The next morning, the group encounters the hangover. Happily, their vows to never drink again are soon forgotten and the partying goes on. A few weeks later any remaining wine has oxidised from contact with air into vinegar. Vinegar is good with some food in small quantities, but you wouldn't want to down a bottle of it. The group will therefore have to wait until next year before making a new batch.

With time and much trial and error, the winemaking process is further improved: a tight-fitting lid to the container helps slow its conversion to vinegar. A brown sludge can be found at the bottom of the wine. If some of this is added to a new batch of grape juice, then wine production is quicker and more reliable. Grapes are now deliberately crushed to release the juice – trampling with bare feet is the traditional method for this. Other varieties of grape can be used or blended.

While the story above is conjecture, we do have solid evidence for wine production in the first towns, near to the areas where vines grow wild. Godin Tepe is an ancient site in western Iran excavated by a Canadian expedition from 1965 to 1973. Clay jars recovered from Godin Tepe have residues of tartaric acid, a chemical produced in fermentation, and anthocyanin pigments, which give red wine its colour. The jars appear to be designed to make wine, with small holes suitable for allowing carbon dioxide to escape, while excluding too much air. (A tightly sealed fermenting container runs the risk of exploding as the pressure builds up.) These jars are 5,000 years old.[5] Even older traces of wine have been found on pottery fragments from Sicily[6] and Armenia.[7]

Winemaking became an important part of the earliest civilisations of the Middle East, close to the Caucasus, before becoming the most popular manufactured drink in the Greek and Roman worlds.[8] As with many other inventions, wine was probably independently discovered by the Chinese. Grape seeds from Jiahu in Henan province in China are about 8,000 years old. Pottery from the same site showed traces of tartaric acid and other chemicals found in wine.[9]

Beer-making goes back to the dawn of civilisation and could be 13,000 years old.[10, 11] Wheat and barley grains were some of the first crops to be cultivated. Wet grain can ferment into an alcoholic mush after being colonised by yeast spores from the air. Yeast turns sugar into carbon dioxide and alcohol, to generate energy so that it can grow. Some of our oldest writing from Sumeria is a hymn to Ninkasi, goddess of beer, which doubles as a recipe. It includes lyrics like:

> Ninkasi, you are the one who soaks the malt in a jar.
> Ninkasi, you are the one who spreads the cooked mash on large reed mats.
> You are the one who holds with both hands the great sweet wort Brewing [it] with honey [and] wine.[12]

It was probably sung by the female brewers, though the tune is lost. Early beer was drunk through a straw to avoid the sediment. Beer-making spread from Sumeria to Egypt, Greece and Rome. It became particularly popular in northern Europe, where it was too cold to grow grapes. The Romans looked down on beer as a drink of barbarians, with the historian Tacitus writing, 'To drink, the Teutons have a horrible brew fermented from barley or wheat, a brew which has only a very far removed similarity to wine.'[12] Tacitus may be showing some prejudice here, as he also claimed that Germany had the worst climate in the world[13] and the Germans were a race of liars.[14]

Beer was valued not just for its taste and ability to intoxicate, but also because it was a safer drink than water. Polluted water can be rife with disease-causing microorganisms that can be killed by alcohol and the brewing process. Most popular in the Middle Ages was small beer. This murky brew could be made in only a few days and was flavoured with all sorts of substances, including tree bark, herbs and eggs. Everyone drank it, including children. This did not mean that the entire population was drunk all the time, as the alcohol content was only 1 per cent. Beer of about 4 per cent alcohol content, like modern brews, was rarer and more expensive. The other major yeast product is bread. Bread therefore also contains some alcohol, though most evaporates during cooking.

Modern beer consumption reflects its roots, with highest consumption per head in northern and Central Europe.[15] The Czechs come top. Around the world, a fondness for beer is indicative of influence from these regions. Namibia, a former German colony, is second in the world, for example. Wine consumption is highest in southern Europe and other countries that are producers, like Australia, Uruguay and Argentina. Uruguay and Argentina were settled mostly by Spanish and Italians, who brought winemaking skills with them. Number one is the Vatican City, which has an all-male, all-adult population that tends to eat together and share wine.[16] Spirits are preferred in Eastern Europe and East Asia.[17]

If fermentation is pushed to its limits, by feeding the yeast with lots of sugar, eventually it will make too much ethanol and the yeast dies. This happens at about 14 per cent ethanol content, depending on the variety of yeast. This gives the upper limit of wine strength.

There is a way to make much stronger drinks, however: distillation. Ethanol boils at 78° C, compared to 100° C for water. This means that if a mixture of ethanol and water (for example, wine) is boiled, the ethanol will boil off as a gas first. If this gas is cooled so it turns back to liquid and is collected, it will have a much higher ethanol content than the starting mixture.

Distillation was used thousands of years ago in China and the Middle East to make medicines, perfumes and drinking water from sea water, as well as alcoholic drinks. A significant improvement in the process came with the invention of a coiled cooling pipe. This allowed the gas to cool down more effectively than previous distillation equipment, which used a straight pipe, so that more of the gas was condensed back to liquid. Ibn Sina, the Persian all-round genius of the eleventh century, described the method in one of his many books. He distilled oil from rose petals to make rose essence, used as a medicine for heart conditions.

Spirits could now be made by distilling the fermented products of all sorts of plants. Most important for Russia was the invention of vodka in either Poland or Russia about a thousand years ago. (The Poles and Russians are still arguing over who takes the credit.) The word vodka comes from the Russian word *voda*, meaning water. The idea of distillation came to Eastern Europe from the Middle East via the Turks. As Eastern Europe is too cold to grow grapes, other plants had to be used. The first record of the production of vodka comes from ninth-century Russia, and a distillery was first mentioned in 1174. The Polish claim of the discovery of vodka goes back to the eighth century, but this may have been brandy, distilled from wine. In the fifteenth century Russian monasteries began making vodka from grain.

A major reason for the popularity of vodka in the Russian Empire was that it was heavily promoted by the tsars as a source of income. In 1540 Tsar Ivan the Terrible brought in high taxes on vodka and set up a network of taverns that had exclusive rights to sell vodka. Private manufacturing in a home distillery was banned, unless you were in the nobility. By the seventeenth century vodka was well established as the national drink of Russia, regularly served at the royal court and used during celebrations. All these measures gave vodka prestige, encouraging its consumption. Vodka taxes became so lucrative that they reached 40 per cent of the entire annual revenue of the state. In 1863 the government monopoly on vodka production was ended by Tsar Alexander II. Common people could then produce and sell their own drinks, leading to lower prices, exports outside Russia and even more consumption. Vodka was now deeply embedded in Russian culture.[18]

During the Soviet era, the government's attitude to alcohol varied between prohibition and promotion. Following the Russian Revolution in 1917, Lenin tried to ban vodka, with predictable lack of success. In his view, only sober workers of the world could unite. In contrast, Stalin was a keen drinker and late-night meetings with his Politburo friends would inevitably end up as huge vodka-drinking sessions.[19] Stalin went back to the tsar's method of using vodka taxes to fund the state. By the 1970s these were back to one-third of government income and alcohol consumption had risen to 15.2 litres per person per year. Allowing mass drunkenness may have helped preserve the communist regime, by reducing political dissent. The Russian historian and dissident Zhores Medvedev argued in 1996 that: 'This "opium for the masses" [vodka] perhaps explains how Russian state property could be redistributed and state enterprises transferred into private ownership so rapidly without invoking any serious social unrest.'[20]

In 1985 Mikhail Gorbachev, the great reformer and inadvertent ender of the Soviet Union, decided to take on the massive problems caused by alcohol. By this time alcoholism had become the third most common killer in the Soviet Union, after heart disease and cancer. Gorbachev's war on alcohol included a large-scale media campaign, higher prices for wine, beer and vodka, and restrictions on sales. People who were found drunk at work, on trains or in public could be prosecuted. Even scenes of alcohol consumption were cut from movies. Many wineries were destroyed.

Gorbachev's plan worked in that wives started seeing their husbands more when they were sober (raising the birth rate), life expectancy increased, and work productivity improved. However, many switched to illegal home production instead and some poisoned themselves with alternatives like antifreeze. Tax income fell as spending on alcohol at state outlets dropped. Gorbachev had hoped that this loss of income would be offset by increases in productivity from now sober workers without hangovers, but this did not happen. His anti-alcohol campaign was one reason for Gorbachev's deep unpopularity in Russia.

Following the fall of the Soviet Union, Boris Yeltsin became first President of the Russian Federation. A keen drinker himself, Yeltsin dropped the state's monopoly over alcohol that had been reintroduced under communism, leading to a big increase in supply. In 1993 alcohol consumption was back up to 14.5 litres of pure alcohol per person per year, making Russians some of the heaviest drinkers in the world. Also in the top ten for alcohol consumption are Belarus, Moldova, Lithuania and Ukraine.[21] All these countries used to be part of the Russian Empire and Soviet Union. Bottom of the list are Islamic countries, where alcohol is often illegal, if not strongly disapproved of.

It is logical to assume that our liking for alcoholic drinks only began in the last 10,000 years, when people in the Middle East and China began to make wine and beer. Recent DNA evidence, however, suggests that it goes back very much further.

Alcohol is a poison, so when we drink it, we need to break it down into something less toxic. The first step in this process is the oxidation of ethanol to acetaldehyde, catalysed by the alcohol dehydrogenase enzyme. Alcohol dehydrogenase is found at high levels in the liver, but also in the stomach, so it can start work on ethanol as quickly as possible. The ADH4 version of alcohol dehydrogenase catalyses the breakdown of many molecules, but in most species it has little affinity for ethanol. The exceptions are in humans and our great ape cousins, where ADH4 breaks down ethanol forty times faster than in other primates. About 10 million years ago our ancestors evolved this fast version of ADH4, suggesting that ethanol was then becoming a part of our diet. These early apes, the common ancestors of gorillas, chimps and us, were not brewing beer or making wine. Instead, they were eating overripe fruit that had fermented using natural yeasts to make ethanol. This would be consistent with large apes eating fruit that had fallen to the forest floor, rather than picking fruit from branches, as monkeys do.[22] Ethanol may therefore have been part of our diet for 10 million years, long before our species even existed. It dates to a time when our ancestors began to live more on the ground instead of in trees.

Humans have about twenty genes that make alcohol dehydrogenases to metabolise ethanol. These produce slightly different enzymes, due to changes in their DNA sequences, so that the effect of ethanol varies considerably from person to person. For example, one sequence variant that is common in East Asia leads to a bad reaction to alcohol, with a red face, headaches and nausea.[23] Alcoholism is less common in East Asian and Polynesian people than in Europeans, due to these genetic differences.[24]

What probably happened is that 10,000 years ago, when alcohol was rarely consumed, and certainly not in large quantities, all people were sensitive to alcohol. As it became a major part of our diet, mutations that made alcohol less toxic were selected. Human populations that have only recently encountered alcohol therefore tend to have less tolerance, as they have not had as much time for DNA changes that can deal with ethanol to accumulate.

The ethanol molecule has a wide range of effects, some beneficial and some harmful. Much of this research is from epidemiology. We study two groups of people, one consuming a high amount of alcohol, and one consuming little or none. We then see if the two groups have any differences in health and, if so, we may conclude that any variation is caused by alcohol.

This approach is fraught with problems. One is that the two groups might not be the same. For example, the reason why some people consume little alcohol is that they can't afford it. This group could then have all sorts of health problems associated with poverty that are not present in the richer, alcohol-buying group. Just because one group is sicker than the other doesn't necessarily mean that alcohol is the reason. Additional experiments are needed.

Working out the health effects of alcohol is therefore a tricky business. Nevertheless, we can draw some conclusions based on careful studies, ideally repeated by multiple research groups using different methods. Moderate drinking of alcohol does seem to have some benefits for health,[25, 26] including reduction in cardiovascular disease, stroke, stress levels, type 2 diabetes, gallstones and Alzheimer's disease.[27] A moderate level of drinking means about ten units of alcohol per week, spread over several days. That's about one bottle of wine a week. Red wine is probably better than beer, as it contains more antioxidants.

These studies compare moderate drinkers to people who never drink alcohol. But it's not necessarily bad to be a teetotaller. Even if your heart benefits from a little alcohol, your liver might prefer that you didn't drink any at all.

The blood-brain barrier normally serves to keep out toxic molecules from our most precious organ. Ethanol can easily cross it, however, causing its well-known effects on state of mind and behaviour. Low doses improve mood, increasing sociability and self-confidence. People become more reckless when drunk. For example, 40 per cent of people bitten by rattlesnakes are drunken men. Of those who decide to play with a rattlesnake deliberately, so only have themselves to blame, 93 per cent are drunk.[28] Higher amounts of alcohol cause violence, injuries, blurred vision, confusion, lethargy, lack of understanding, loss of balance and memory, impaired speech, nausea and vomiting. The risk of accidents, hypothermia and drowning is much higher. Very high amounts cause loss of consciousness, coma or even death from acute alcohol poisoning.

Heavy drinking over a lengthy period has many bad effects on your health: cardiovascular problems include weakening of heart muscle, irregular heartbeat, higher blood pressure and risk of stroke. Your liver does most of the work in breaking down alcohol, so loses function, potentially fatally. Scar tissue slowly builds up, a condition called cirrhosis, eventually leading to liver failure. The pancreas becomes inflamed and swollen. The brain is affected, changing mood and behaviour, making it harder to think clearly and move with coordination. In particular, drinking in adolescence has the strongest effects, as this alters the DNA in the part of the brain responsible for mood and emotion.[29] Alcohol causes cancer, particularly in the head, neck, throat, liver, breast, womb and colon. Birth defects are more common if the mother drinks heavily during pregnancy. Chronic drinkers are more likely to get infectious diseases like pneumonia and tuberculosis[30] and take their own lives. Finally, drinking too much can weaken the immune system, making your body an easier target for disease. Currently, 3 million deaths per year are now caused by alcohol, because of injuries, digestive diseases, cardiovascular diseases, diabetes, infectious disease, cancer, epilepsy and other disorders.[31]

In 2018, a highly comprehensive review was published that analysed 592 studies on the health effects of alcohol in 195 locations for both sexes and all ages from fifteen years. After weighing up all the positive and negative effects, it turns out that the optimal number of units per week to maximise the benefits of drinking alcohol is… zero.[32] Sorry about that.

The most insidious effect of alcohol is its addictive nature. An addiction is the persistent compulsive use of a substance or behaviour, even though the user knows it has damaging effects. Addictions start with activities that the user finds pleasurable, such as drug use (including alcohol), gambling, the internet or shopping. The enjoyment creates a mental high, leading to a strong urge to repeat the activity to recreate that feeling. Winning at gambling is a classic example of this.

Gabor Maté is a Canadian doctor who worked with drug addicts in Vancouver. His own addiction is to buying classical music, where he can spend thousands of dollars on CDs that he already owns and never listens to. It is quite astonishing, to non-addicts at least, how the brain can be hijacked. His irresistible compulsion once made him abandon delivering a baby to rush to the music store.[33] People vulnerable to addiction can latch on to more or less anything that gives pleasure, leading to catastrophic effects on health, wealth and relationships.

A widely accepted explanation for how the brain adapts and begins to crave something that gives pleasure, leading to addiction, centres on the role of the neurotransmitter dopamine. This model holds that whatever the addiction, it takes over the brain in the same way,[34] by releasing dopamine in the nucleus accumbens, a group of nerve cells involved with motivation, reward, pleasure and reinforcement learning. Near the nucleus accumbens is the hippocampus, which lays down memory, and the amygdala, which processes emotion. The hippocampus and amygdala store memories of a sense of satisfaction and pleasure. Repeated exposure to an addictive substance or behaviour stimulates the prefrontal cortex, which is responsible for planning and executing tasks; the pleasure of the addictive activity thus gets linked to desiring and seeking it.

There is plenty of evidence that dopamine is involved in drug addiction: animals that lack dopamine lose motivation to do anything, to the point that they will starve to death. They never learn to find food and shelter, or to avoid stimuli that cause pain. This is because bursts of dopamine release from neurons are needed for the formation of long-term memories that link a stimulus to a reward. The brain can adapt to habitual use of addictive drugs by reducing the levels of dopamine receptors in the brain. Cocaine, amphetamines, opiates, alcohol, caffeine, nicotine, cannabis, barbiturates and benzodiazepines all activate the dopamine system, though with varying intensities and mechanisms. Overeating and addiction to damaging behaviours like gambling may also work in similar ways.[35] Nevertheless, despite the popularity of the dopamine model, attributing all addiction to a craving for a single neurotransmitter must be an oversimplification.[36] Addiction is a complex behaviour that varies with both the identity of the drug and from individual to individual. Some stimulants can generate huge increases in dopamine with little effect on pleasure or addiction, while the release of opiates in the brain seems to be more important than dopamine for alcohol addiction.[37]

Injecting or smoking drugs is more addictive than swallowing them, as these give a quicker, stronger effect. Over time the brain adapts so that the addictive activity starts to lose its pleasurable effect and the same amount of a chemical will produce less reward and pleasure. Tolerance has developed. The addict will need a bigger and bigger hit to generate the same high. Thus, coffee fans prefer a stronger brew, gambling addicts feel the need to bet larger sums and drug addicts take increasing doses.

Now with full-blown addiction, the addict will often get little pleasure from their activity, though they continue to experience powerful cravings for it. The addict might say, 'I don't know why I am smoking. I don't even like it.' The brain wants the addictive substance or activity, but gets little joy in satisfying the craving, only relief from it. It remembers environmental cues associated with the desired substance, such as the situation where the addict indulged. These cues will trigger a conditional response and intense cravings: a gambling addict might be resisting temptation until they walk past their favourite betting shop, when they are compelled to enter and place another bet; an alcoholic might be sober for years until presented with a whisky bottle, when they are unable to resist.

In Gabor Maté's work with drug addicts, he got to know many of their life stories, described in his book on addiction, *In the Realm of Hungry Ghosts*. What every one of the addicts he worked with had in common was trauma in childhood – family violence, parental divorce, drug abuse or alcoholism in the family, death of a parent, or physical or sexual abuse. Every adverse childhood experience triples the risk of becoming a substance abuser.[33]

Drug addicts are therefore often self-medicating to relieve emotional pain caused by childhood trauma and stress. In addition, their brain development was damaged by their traumatic experiences.[38] Dopamine circuits, the amygdala and prefrontal cortex can be permanently affected, as shown by blood flow, electrical activity and seizures. These people have a higher sensitivity to stressful situations, so respond strongly to substances or activities that provide short-term stress relief, even if they cause long-term damage. Given this, we can see why punishing addicts is counterproductive, since the misery of punishment will only increase the desire for relief through drugs. Situations that humans find particularly stressful are those with uncertainty, loss of control, conflict and lack of emotionally supportive relationships.[39] All the traumatic situations listed above are likely to have these features. A child is especially vulnerable to insecurity, as they rely so much on parents for love and protection.

Now we can see why alcoholism is so prevalent in Russia: firstly, the tsars deliberately set out to hook its people on alcohol, to make money for themselves and the rest of the Russian nobility. This tax income was needed to fund the Russian army and to maintain their lavish lifestyle. Vodka was promoted via state taverns and by making it part of Russian culture. The policy worked in generating lots of income, but at a terrible social and medical cost.

Secondly, few peoples have suffered as much childhood trauma as those in Eastern Europe in the last century. Russia fought horrific wars with Japan (1904–5), the Central Powers (1914–17) and Germany (1941–45). The First World War came to a messy end with two revolutions in 1917, which turned into a civil war between numerous factions until 1923. The worst effect of the civil war was famine from 1921 to 1922, in which about 5 million died. The Bolshevik victory enabled the formation of the communist Soviet Union. Famines were a regular occurrence under the misgovernment of the Soviet Union, with especially bad ones in 1932–3, the Second World War and 1947. The Soviet Union suffered far more casualties in the Second World War than any other country, with about 20 million killed. Nearly half the Soviet population lived in fear under German occupation at some point. Stalin's reign of terror from 1924 to 1953 featured widespread police surveillance, suspicion of saboteurs, arbitrary executions and sentences to brutal prison camps. Millions were killed or persecuted. All these events left a vast number of children traumatised, losing parents to war, famine or the secret police. No wonder they later sought refuge in the bottle, as a temporary relief from their emotional pain.

In any country, alcoholics often make poor parents, neglecting their children or even being violent towards them. This creates another generation with trauma – meaning the misery goes on.

Illegal drugs, such as heroin, cannabis, cocaine, LSD and ecstasy, are widely believed to be highly addictive and extremely dangerous. I chose to write about alcohol, rather than these banned substances, for two reasons. Firstly, the number of users of alcohol is far greater, due to its cultural acceptance, legality, long history of use, and because alcoholic drinks taste great. The only drug that comes close for amount of use is tobacco.[40] Secondly, I cover alcohol because of its dangers. In 2010, a paper led by University of Bristol Professor David Nutt presented the results of a workshop by an independent scientific committee on drugs. Twenty drugs were scored on sixteen criteria: nine related to the harms that a drug produces in the individual and seven to the harms that the drugs cause to other people. Criteria were weighted to indicate their relative importance, resulting in an overall score out of 100.[41]

All twenty drugs are harmful, but as the illustration below shows, alcohol is the worst. It may only be fourth in terms of harm to self, after crack cocaine, heroin and methamphetamine, but it is the worst by a considerable margin in harm to others. Alcohol causes more injuries, accidents and violence than any other drug. Hospital emergency rooms on a Saturday night are full of the victims of alcohol. While cigarettes are undoubtedly dangerous, no one starts a fight or crashes a car because they have been consuming nicotine.

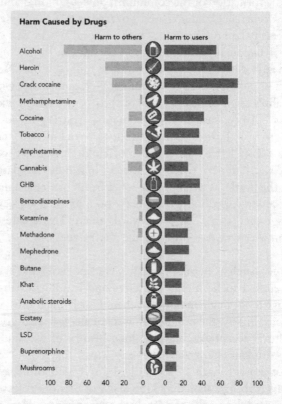

Drugs ordered by their overall harm scores, split into scores of harms to users and harm to others.[41, 42] GHB=γ hydroxybutyric acid. LSD=lysergic acid diethylamide.

Can you now see from this why tobacco and alcohol are legal, but magic mushrooms, cannabis and LSD are not? Me neither.

David Nutt had been chair of the British government's Advisory Council on the Misuse of Drugs. In October 2009 he was widely reported as saying that alcohol and tobacco were more harmful than many illegal drugs, including cannabis, LSD and ecstasy.[43] Home Secretary Alan Johnson did not want to know. The following day David Nutt was sacked.[44]

20

The Black, Stinking Fume

On 3 August 1492 Christopher Columbus set sail from Spain on the most important sea voyage of all time, with a crew of ninety men on three different ships. Columbus was an Italian from Genoa, though he was working for the Spanish monarchs Queen Isabella and King Ferdinand. At that time, Spain's rival Portugal was making substantial profits from trade with the Indies, sailing east around Africa and bringing back spices and other exotic goods. Columbus claimed that he could reach the Indies by a quicker route, travelling in the opposite direction around the globe, west across the Atlantic. He persuaded Ferdinand and Isabella to fund his voyage so that they could access the same wealth. None of them had any idea that the vast continents of North and South America lay in the way.

Just over two months after setting out, Columbus and his men made landfall in the Bahamas before going on to the larger islands of Cuba and Hispaniola. When he returned to Spain, his account of the discovery of the New World electrified Europe, initiating a colossal transformation in both the Americas and the Old World. The Columbian Exchange led to swaps of plants, animals, diseases, minerals, ideas and peoples across the Atlantic that affected us in multiple profound ways. Politics, power, religion, food, health and countless other things were never the same again.[1]

This contact was a catastrophe for the Native Americans. The Spanish returned in numbers in 1493, set on conquest and imposing their own culture, particularly Christianity. Worse still were dozens of deadly diseases brought from Europe, which killed perhaps 90 per cent of the inhabitants of the Americas. Unlike the Spanish, the Native

Americans had no resistance to measles, smallpox, typhus, cholera, influenza, diphtheria, scarlet fever, whooping cough and others, and often caught multiple infections at the same time.

In return, the Europeans were given syphilis. This was first recorded in 1495 in Naples, during an invasion by a French army that employed Spanish mercenaries who had served with Columbus. A date of 1495 suggests that the first Europeans to catch the disease brought it back to Europe on Columbus's first or second voyage. Syphilis seems to have been one of the most widespread diseases in Europe up to the twentieth century, though good data is lacking, due to its stigma from being acquired by sexual contact, particularly with prostitutes. Nowadays it can be treated with antibiotics, though there are still 6 million new cases per year,[2] causing ulcers, meningitis, stroke, dementia, blindness, heart problems, infertility and birth defects. A hundred thousand people currently die per year from syphilis worldwide.[3]

Deadly as syphilis was, its lethal effects pale in comparison to another gift from America. The friendly inhabitants of the Bahamas, who were the first to meet Columbus and his men, gave them presents, such as exotic fruits that they had never seen before. Also included were some dried leaves from a plant the natives called 'tabacos'. The puzzled Spanish tried eating the leaves, but found them to be inedible so threw them overboard. One month later, they realised what you are supposed to do with tobacco leaves. They saw native people in Cuba chewing them or rolling the herbs inside dried leaves, lighting one end and inhaling the smoke. Columbus recorded in his diary on 6 November 1492, seeing 'men and women with a half-burnt weed in their hands, being the herbs they are accustomed to smoke'. Some of his sailors tried smoking themselves, and found it pleasurable, though its addictive qualities were soon noticed. One of the sailors who took up smoking tobacco was Rodrigo de Jerez. Back in Spain, he scared people by blowing smoke out of his mouth and nose, a practice previously associated with demons. Jerez was accused of doing the work of Satan by the Inquisition, arrested and put in prison for seven years, where he had plenty of time to reflect that sticking to throwing the tobacco overboard would have been wiser.

The tobacco plant (*Nicotiana tabacum*) grows wild on the eastern slopes of the Andes in Bolivia and northern Argentina. It is one of over seventy naturally occurring *Nicotiana* plants.[4] Native Americans smoked it in pipes, used the leaves to dress wounds and chewed it as a painkiller for toothache. By 500 CE the Mayan people of Central America were cultivating tobacco plants, from where it spread as far as the Mississippi valley. Shamans also smoked a different tobacco species called *Nicotiana rustica*. This was far more powerful than the usual *Nicotiana tabacum*, with up to ten times the nicotine concentration, plus various psychoactive chemicals. Smoking *Nicotiana rustica* allowed the shamans to have spiritual experiences. It never really caught on in Europe, apart from in Russia, where it grew easily, so providing a high that was virtually free.

The voyage of Columbus triggered a huge wave of exploration, conquest and settlement by European countries in the Americas. The English were late arrivals. By the late sixteenth century, Canada and the Midwest of the USA had been claimed by France, Brazil was ruled by Portugal, and the Spanish ruled a huge expanse of territory encompassing most of South America, Mexico, Texas and California. English involvement in the Americas mostly involved acts of piracy, with their sea dogs attacking Spanish ships taking treasure across the Atlantic. Seizing plunder from the Spanish was easier than taking it directly from the Incas and Aztecs. As the skirmishing at sea intensified, the English concluded that it would be useful to establish permanent settlements in the New World that could act as bases for their ships. They might also be good places to send the ever-growing numbers of poor people who were not wanted in London and Bristol. How the poor felt about this plan was of little concern.

After failures in Newfoundland and at Roanoke in North Carolina in 1585 (where all the colonists died or abandoned the settlement), the next attempt to establish an English settlement in the Americas was in Virginia. Private investors set up the Virginia Company of London with the aim of colonising North America for a profit, as Queen Elizabeth I was wary of funding any more settlements herself after the Roanoke disaster. The Spanish had made a fortune from their colonies in gold and other treasure from Peru and Mexico, so the investors hoped that a British colony further north would do the same. In 1607 144 English men and boys founded the Jamestown colony, named after the new King James I of England.

The colonists were told that they were there to make money for investors – otherwise support from home would end. Many men therefore wasted time searching or harassing their native neighbours for non-existent gold, rather than trying to set up new farms. The first winter was harsh and malaria infected many colonists. After the first year, all but thirty-eight of the original 144 had died. Even worse was the winter of 1609–10, which the colonists called the Starving Time. Nevertheless, the Virginia Company persisted in sending further boatloads of colonists, including women, until it finally went bankrupt in 1624. Virginia then became a royal colony – an early example of a state bailout of a failing company.

Once it was accepted that Jamestown was never going to make a profit from gold, settlers tried other sources of income, such as glassblowing, silkworm cultivation and vineyards. Only one Virginia crop sold for a good price when exported back to England, however: tobacco. Smoking had already caught on in England, despite opposition from King James. In his *Counterblaste to Tobacco* of 1604, he wrote, 'Smoking is a custom loathsome to the eye, hateful to the nose, harmful to the brain, dangerous to the lungs, and in the black, stinking fume thereof nearest resembling the horrible Stygian smoke of the pit that is bottomless.' James managed to overcome these views in 1619 when he granted himself a monopoly on tobacco and a handy source of income from taxes.

Settler John Rolfe (and husband of Pocahontas) imported tobacco seeds to Jamestown from the West Indies and found they grew well. Within ten years copious quantities of leaf were being exported to England. Tobacco growing had profound effects on the British colonisation of North America. Firstly, it made the new settlements a financial success. In contrast to the settlers' earlier schemes, tobacco was a sustainable and growing industry, encouraging further emigration. Immigrants often worked as indentured servants. They were given a free ticket to Virginia in exchange for being obliged to work as a farm labourer for a fixed term of five years or so. At the end of this time they were free. Secondly, tobacco made big demands on the soil, draining it of nutrients, so that it had to be left to recover after three growing seasons. This was a big driver to settle new lands, expanding the colonies to the west. Finally, the indentured-servant system was not attractive enough to potential immigrants, even if they were promised land, so slaves began to be imported from West Africa instead. Slaves were not bound to the plantations for just five years – they could be used for life and made to work harder than free men from Britain. African slaves were also more resistant to malaria. It was therefore the demands of the tobacco industry that turned Virginia into a slave state and hence on the side of the Confederacy in the American Civil War, fought between northern free states and southern slave states 250 years later. The states of North Carolina, Kentucky, Georgia and Virginia in this region remain the largest centres of tobacco production in the USA.

Before the twentieth century, tobacco was primarily consumed in clay pipes, by chewing, in cigars or snorted as snuff. We now know that pipe and cigar smoking cause cancers of the lung, throat, colon and pancreas, as well as heart disease and lung disease.[5] Chewing tobacco causes mouth cancer, gum disease, cardiovascular disease and loss of teeth. Inhaling snuff causes nose, throat, pancreas and mouth cancer, heart attacks and stroke.[6] Bad as these are, smoking cigarettes is a lot worse.

Prior to 1880 cigarettes were made by hand, with workers rolling only a few per minute. This kept cigarettes rare and expensive. What made them plentiful and cheap was the mechanisation of cigarette production. In 1880 James Bonsack invented a machine that could roll 210 cigarettes a minute, fifty times the rate of handmade cigarettes. He was motivated by a prize from the industry of $75,000 for anyone who could build a reliable rolling device. The machine made a long cigarette that was chopped into sections by rotating shears. This not only slashed the cylinder, but also slashed the price of manufacturing, giving a superior, neatly rolled product.

Bonsack went into business with James Buchanan Duke, known as 'Buck'. Duke had started in the handmade cigarette business in 1880, with his Duke of Durham brand, based in Durham, North Carolina. Shortly afterwards, he heard about Bonsack's invention and realised its potential. Other companies had been reluctant to invest in Bonsack because the machine often broke down; they also thought that there was no market, as consumers preferred hand-rolled cigarettes. Duke was willing to take a chance on Bonsack, however. Working with a mechanic from the Bonsack Company,

Duke improved the machine's reliability and negotiated a deal so that he had a monopoly on its use.

Duke now potentially had a huge competitive advantage, with his unique ability to mass-produce cigarettes. The problem that Duke had was that there was little demand for cigarettes at the time. In 1890 cigarette sales were tiny compared to pipe tobacco, cigars and chewing tobacco. Duke therefore set out to change the way we used tobacco with a series of masterful marketing campaigns.

Machine-made cigarettes looked neat and were promoted as being more hygienic than cigars that were manufactured using human hands and saliva. Cigarettes could be smoked in restaurants where cigars and pipes might not be allowed. They were less fiddly to use and quicker, making them ideal for a coffee break. The word cigarette means 'little cigar', so it was assumed that they were safer. Indeed, they were often promoted as being beneficial for health, not just in advertising, but in pharmaceutical encyclopaedias until 1906. Doctors sometimes even prescribed cigarettes for coughs, colds and tuberculosis. These doctors were not idiots. The decades-long delay between smoking and any adverse health effects meant that it took a long time to understand the harm caused by cigarettes.

In 1902 Duke formed British American Tobacco, currently the fourth biggest tobacco company in the world, by merging his American Tobacco Company with his British rival, Imperial Tobacco.[7] Cigarettes were a spectacular success. Not only did they mostly replace other forms of tobacco consumption, but the total market grew as well. Cigarette usage jumped in the First World War (1917–18), Second World War (1941–45) and the Korean War (1950–53), where the US government ensured that soldiers received a plentiful supply in their rations to keep up morale. Tobacco companies even sent millions of free cigarettes to the soldiers, giving them loyal (addicted, to be more precise) customers when they came home.

The same patterns of growth operated in other countries. Although tobacco was first introduced to Britain in the sixteenth century, smoking only grew to become a major part of British culture from the late nineteenth century. By the mid-twentieth century, 80 per cent of men and 40 per cent of women were smoking. This works out at 3 kilograms of tobacco per adult per year.[8]

Buck Duke died in 1925, having created a huge new industry, hooking the world on cigarettes. Duke was not a bad man, seeking to make money from a product that he knew was lethal. He had no idea how dangerous cigarette smoking could be. Even at the time of his death, lung cancer was still rare. Duke donated more than $100 million to Trinity College in Durham, North Carolina, which was renamed Duke University after his family and became one of the world's foremost universities. If Duke had not taken on Bonsack's machine, then undoubtedly someone else would have begun mass production of cigarettes, as other prototypes were under development at the same time. What is more arguable is whether cigarettes would have taken such a hold without Duke's talents in marketing, advertising, psychology and pricing. Perhaps without Buck Duke, we would still be chewing tobacco and smoking cigars, and death rates from smoking would be a lot lower.

One problem that the tobacco industry faced is that whatever the brand, cigarettes were much the same product. They therefore used packaging and marketing to appeal to diverse groups of consumers. Advertising to differentiate brands was crucial.

As an illustration, let us look at how the R. J. Reynolds Tobacco Company (RJR) promoted its Camel cigarettes. Camels were first manufactured shortly before the First World War, as a 'mild' cigarette. They used the slogan 'I'd walk a mile for a Camel' for decades. RJR alleged health benefits from Camels using the slogan 'For digestion's sake – smoke Camels' and a dubious claim that it was the choice of doctors. RJR had given doctors a free pack of Camels immediately before asking them what their favourite brand of cigarettes was. The results from this survey led to RJR using the slogan 'More doctors smoke Camels than any other cigarette'.

In 1987, RJR changed tack, creating the cartoon character Joe Camel. Always controversial, Joe Camel was attacked by the American Medical Association for targeting children: a 1991 study found that 91 per cent of six-year-olds correctly associated Joe Camel with smoking.[9] Camels became the cigarette of choice for the junior smoker, with the share of the cigarette market among eighteen- to twenty-four-year-olds nearly doubling. In 1997, however, RJR lost a lawsuit, which forced it to pay $10 million for anti-smoking education for children in California.[10] In the face of further legal action and controversy, RJR withdrew the Joe Camel character.[11]

The addictive nature of smoking was quickly noted after its introduction to Europe. In 1623 Francis Bacon wrote: 'In our time the use of tobacco is growing greatly and conquers men with a certain secret pleasure, so that those who have once become accustomed thereto can later hardly be restrained therefrom.'[12] Bacon, of course, had no idea of how exactly tobacco does the conquering.

Smoking enhances mood, either directly or by relief of withdrawal symptoms. Inhalation of smoke carries nicotine into the lungs, where it is rapidly absorbed into the blood and transported to the brain within seconds. There it binds to receptor proteins that normally bind to acetylcholine, a neurotransmitter that brain cells use to signal to each other. Stimulation of these receptors releases a variety of other neurotransmitters in the brain. As is common with addiction, one of these is dopamine, which leads to pleasure and compulsion.[13]

Tolerance, craving and withdrawal develop with continual exposure to nicotine. Smokers typically use cigarettes so often that they keep their acetylcholine receptors permanently saturated with nicotine. The rewarding psychoactive effects that were present when they started smoking tend to be lost with repeated exposure. Instead of seeking these pleasurable rewards, smokers are therefore trying to avoid the withdrawal symptoms that would arise if their nicotine levels dropped, freeing their brain receptors. Nicotine withdrawal causes irritability, low mood, anxiety and stress, again via neurotransmitters, giving strong incentives to take up smoking again.

As usual with addictions, the effect is enhanced by conditioning effects of associating certain situations with smoking: smokers might routinely take a cigarette after a meal, with coffee, beer or smoker friends. These environments, the taste, smell and feel of smoke, or the physical handling of a cigarette all become associated with the pleasure of smoking. The short time between inhaling smoke and getting a hit of nicotine helps link the physical act of smoking with a good mood. Bad moods can also become conditioned cues for smoking when a smoker learns that smoking makes you feel better. Irritation from any source can then become a stimulant for smoking.[14]

People's responses to smoking are, in a large part, genetic. Nicotine dissolves in blood and circulates round the body. It is removed by being broken down in the liver by an enzyme called CYP2A6, which converts it to a much less potent chemical called cotinine.[15] Many different versions of CYP2A6 are present in humans, and they vary in their efficiency at converting nicotine to cotinine. People who break down nicotine rapidly are more likely become addicted to smoking, as they need to smoke more often to keep their nicotine levels up. They also find quitting harder. Conversely, those with versions of CYP2A6 that break down nicotine slowly tend to smoke fewer cigarettes, inhale less deeply, as they crave less nicotine, and are not as likely to suffer from severe withdrawal symptoms if they try to give up.

If you wanted to design a product that causes addiction, the cigarette would be hard to beat. How many other drugs compel their users to get a hit dozens of times every day, as chain-smokers do? All in all, cigarettes combine a number of features that make them especially addictive – far more than cigars: they are cheap, calorie-free, easy to use, and give a drug response in seconds that fades within hours. Smoking is an appetite suppressant, so people who give up may gain weight, further discouraging quitting. They are also legal. All this would not be such a problem if cigarettes were not quite so bad for you.

It was not at all obvious at first that smoking was harmful. Indeed, in the 1570s, the Spanish doctor Nicolás Monardes recommended tobacco as a cure for dozens of conditions including, astonishingly, cancer.[16] His book introduced the words 'tabacco' and 'nicotaine' and initiated a debate on the health benefits (or not) of smoking. For example, in 1659, Giles Everard's book, *Panacea; or the universal medicine, being a discovery of the wonderfull vertues of tobacco*,[17] was published in English. Everard claimed that tobacco could do away with the need for doctors, as 'It is no great friend to physicians, though it be a physical plant; for the very smoke of it is held to be a great antidote against all venome and pestilential diseases.' Others were not convinced, with critics calling tobacco 'hurtfull and dangerous to youth'[18] or saying 'this custome of taking the fume downe into the stomack and lungs is very pernicious. The lungs will consequently become unapt for motion, to the great offence of the heart, and ruine at length of the whole body.'[19] As early as 1868, a publication by John Lizars, operating surgeon to the Royal Infirmary of Edinburgh, was warning that smoking caused mouth cancer, saying, 'injury done to the constitution of the young may not immediately appear, but cannot fail ultimately to become a great national calamity'.[20] Even so, by 1900 lung cancer was still a rare disease. By the mid-nineteenth century, few doctors were claiming that tobacco was capable of curing diseases, though smoking other substances as a treatment for asthma lingered on. Medicated cigarettes designed for respiratory problems were promoted and used by doctors until well after the Second World War.[21]

The number of cases of lung cancer had increased twentyfold from 1905 to 1945 in the UK, though the reason why was a mystery. So-called 'smoker's cough' became commonplace, which progressed to shortness of breath from the slightest exercise, chest pain, weight loss and coughing up blood. Concerned about the rapid spread of lung cancer, the Medical Research Council (MRC) asked Austin Bradford Hill, an epidemiologist at the London School of Hygiene, to investigate. Bradford Hill made the inspired choice of recruiting Richard Doll to help, who had been working on the causes of stomach ulcers at the MRC. At first, Bradford Hill and Doll did not think that smoking was causing the lung cancer epidemic. While a few small-scale studies had pointed in this direction, their leading hypothesis was that the problem was caused by the growth in road traffic. Fumes from car engines or road tar could be damaging lungs. After all, road traffic had grown in parallel with the increasing incidence of lung cancer in the first half of the twentieth century.

In 1949 Doll and Bradford Hill visited 709 patients in London hospitals who were suspected of having lung cancer, giving them a questionnaire on family history, diet and previous diseases. Naturally, they asked whether they had worked on the roads and, fortunately, whether they smoked. The lung cancer patients were compared to a control group of 709 patients who were in hospital for a different reason. A link between smoking and being in the lung cancer group jumped out. They also found evidence that the risk was larger if you smoked more often. Growth in lung cancer paralleled growth in cigarette smoking, but with a twenty-year lag. It was this lengthy time span between taking up smoking and its lethal effects becoming apparent that made cigarettes so deadly. Smoking was a ticking time bomb, with millions of users already addicted and on the way to cancer.

Doll promptly gave up smoking, yet others took more convincing. Perhaps the results reflected something special about London? Doll and Bradford Hill therefore extended their work to 5,000 patient records from Cambridge, Bristol, Leeds and Newcastle. The results were the same.

In 1951 the MRC funded them to try a different strategy – sending a questionnaire to all 60,000 doctors in the UK to ask about their smoking habits:[22] 40,500 replied. Thereafter, the Registrar General of births, marriages and deaths sent Doll and Bradford Hill a copy of the death certificate for every doctor who had died. After three years, thirty-six doctors had died of lung cancer and every one had been a smoker. While this is an apparently striking result, one problem was the small size of the non-smoking control group – only 13 per cent of doctors did not smoke. It therefore took many years to acquire sufficient data on why non-smokers died. As the work continued, additional conclusions emerged: smokers died younger than non-smokers by about ten years, and quitting smoking, especially at a young age, increased life expectancy. Other groups confirmed and extended their findings: smoking causes cancer in numerous other tissues; smoking causes heart disease, stroke, bronchitis, emphysema, pneumonia, asthma, type 2 diabetes and impotence; passive smoking is also dangerous; smoking damages blood vessels; and smoking while pregnant can lead to miscarriage, stillbirth and premature birth.

Why does smoking cause cancer? Cancer occurs when cells start to grow when they shouldn't. Every human cell in our bodies is descended from just one cell – a fertilised egg, which divides and differentiates into all our tissues and organs. Some cell types will need to keep dividing: those in the bone marrow, skin and gut, for instance, to replace those that die. Others will need to divide after injury to repair damage. Cell growth is normally kept under tight control. When cells fail to respond normally to signals meant to halt their growth, they can develop into cancerous tissue. These failures arise because the DNA of the cells has acquired mutations that change the way in which proteins involved in regulating cell growth work. Oncogenes are genes that will stimulate cell growth if they are mutated. Tumour suppressor genes encode proteins meant to inhibit the growth of damaged cells; if tumour suppressor genes are mutated, then cells will grow when they shouldn't. One example of a tumour suppressor gene that is supposed to be activated if cells acquire too much DNA damage is $TP53$, which encodes a protein called p53. Normally, p53 blocks division of damaged cells and can even make the cell kill itself, thus ridding the body of a cell that might develop into a tumour.

Anything that can mutate DNA is therefore prone to cause cancer. Tobacco is spectacularly good at this, producing numerous mutagenic chemicals delivered straight to the lungs that can generate oncogenes and dysfunctional tumour suppressor genes. One such chemical is benzopyrene. This reacts with guanine bases in DNA, disrupting the DNA structure and introducing mutations. Benzopyrene is especially effective at mutating three critical guanines in the p53 gene, stopping p53 working as it should, thus turning lung cells cancerous.[23]

Benzopyrene is just one of dozens of substances present in tobacco smoke known to cause cancer. These are not just organic chemicals – smoke contains toxic metals, such as lead, arsenic and cadmium. Psychoactive compounds, in addition to nicotine, can also be generated at the high temperatures found in a burning cigarette, which may add to the addictive nature of smoking.

The effect of ending smoking on public health would be enormously beneficial, comparable to vaccination, sanitation or antibiotics. But how could this be achieved? No country has a complete ban on smoking, and rightly so: making the sale of cigarettes illegal would create a huge outbreak of crime. Millions of addicts would seek out dealers. Organised crime would soar, with gangs fighting for control of the multibillion trade. Prices would rise, so addicts would turn to petty crime to get quick cash for their next pack. Nicotine addiction is so strong that many smokers would never give up, even if their habit became criminal. We see all these consequences from drugs that are currently illegal. Prohibition in the USA from 1920 to 1933, when the production and sale of alcohol was banned, also led to organised crime taking over the business. Given the numbers of smokers and the powerfully addictive nature of nicotine, trying to ban smoking would be far worse than the results of banning heroin, cocaine or cannabis.

Governments trying to stop their citizens smoking is not just a recent phenomenon. The first public smoking ban was by Pope Urban VII, who forbade smoking in churches in 1590, under penalty of excommunication. A quick puff in the porch of a church while waiting for Mass to start could therefore put your immortal soul at risk of burning in the fires of hell for eternity. Papal laws against smoking lasted until 1724. Ottoman Sultan Murad IV made Pope Urban look like a wishy-washy liberal by banning all alcohol, coffee and tobacco from his empire in 1633, under penalty of death. He took care of offenders personally, investigating the taverns of Istanbul in disguise to catch smokers, then whipping off his civilian clothes to reveal his true identity (Surprise!) and chopping their heads off. You could do that sort of thing if you were a sultan. Fortunately for Turkish smokers and coffee-lovers, his successor and brother, Ibrahim the Mad, reversed the ban. Ibrahim had acquired his traumatised mental state after Murad had killed his other three brothers to prevent any chance of them leading a rebellion; Ibrahim grew up effectively imprisoned in the palace in Istanbul, terrified that he would be next. The Russian tsars also took on tobacco at the same time, but with more lenient punishments than the Turks. A first-time offender received a slit nose, a vicious beating, or a one-way trip to Siberia. Only a second offence carried the death penalty.

Many American states turned against smoking at the start of the twentieth century. In 1900 North Dakota, Washington, Iowa and Tennessee had all banned cigarettes, with eleven more joining them by 1920. Consumption of cigars soared as a result. Adolf Hitler loathed smoking and imposed high taxes, banned smoking in government buildings and funded scientific projects to look at the effects of smoking on health, also finding links to lung cancer. In 1945 Hitler's laws were scrapped, tainted by their sponsor. By 1950, while there might be an age limit for buying tobacco, its use had few restrictions anywhere.

Measures to move against smoking were steadily introduced after the publication of Bradford Hill and Doll's results from 1950.[24] The first task was to convince public health bodies that smoking posed a threat to health. In the UK, the government accepted that smoking caused lung cancer by 1954; Health Minister Iain Macleod told parliament that there was a 'real' link between the two, followed by a press conference the same day. Macleod's announcement to the press was rather undermined by him smoking during his own speech and his half-hearted words, saying, 'It is desirable that young people should be warned of the risks apparently attendant on excessive smoking,' and, 'The time has not yet come when the Ministry should offer public warnings on smoking.' Macleod grudgingly accepted the conclusions of Doll and Bradford Hill, but he wasn't going to do anything about it.[25]

Similar moves took place in the USA, with the Surgeon General Leroy Burney declaring in 1957 that the official position of the US Public Health Service was that 'the evidence pointed to a causal relationship between smoking and lung cancer'. The 1964 report, *Smoking and Health: Report of the Advisory Committee to the Surgeon General of the United States*, had the greatest impact, with widespread media coverage.[26] Millions quit – simply due to public education and cessation campaigns.

Political action against the tobacco industry followed: health warnings were first placed on cigarette packs in the USA in 1965 and in the UK in 1971, which grew steadily more explicit. TV advertising was banned in the UK in 1965 and in the USA in 1970; eventually all tobacco advertising and promotion was stopped. In numerous countries, smoking was restricted and then prohibited on planes, buses and trains. No-smoking areas, then outright bans, followed in workplaces, restaurants and other enclosed public places; in 2011 New York extended the prohibition to city parks and beaches. Smokers were forced to huddle outside pubs in the cold and rain. The legal age for smoking was raised, taxes increased and smuggling targeted. Social pressure against smoking intensified, with people supporting tougher legislation and insisting on their right not to be a passive smoker.

At first it was assumed that simply presenting information on the dangers of smoking would be enough to get people to stop, with smoking commonly being described as a 'habit' rather than an 'addiction'. The US Surgeon General only acknowledged the addictive nature of cigarettes in 1988. Nicotine patches became available in 1992, followed by vaping, which mimics more closely the act of smoking, helping addicts satisfy their psychological and chemical cravings. Quitting is also more likely to be successful with the help of a support group, as with other addictions.

Tobacco companies were attacked with lawsuits, with lung cancer victims claiming that the companies knew about the dangers of smoking but had deliberately hidden them from customers. Naturally, companies fought a long, hard, but losing campaign, seeking to deny the risks and addictive nature of smoking. With their traditional markets in decline, they turned to other countries for their profits, such as former communist countries that were once closed for trade, particularly China. Japan, South Korea and Taiwan were made to allow US companies to sell tobacco products in their countries after the American government threatened economic sanctions.[27] In 2015 the highest rate of smoking was in Indonesia.[28]

Anti-tobacco measures work, especially when used in combination. Cigarette consumption per person in the USA decreased from 1960, when the link to cancer was first acknowledged and publicised; a drop in lung cancer rates followed in parallel twenty years later. Numerous diseases caused by smoking, such as cancer, emphysema, heart disease and stroke, have all decreased substantially in the last few decades in the USA, UK and other countries that tackled the problem, noticeably increasing life expectancy. Indeed, cutting smoking rates has had the biggest effect on public health of any measure in recent years. Currently about 1.3 billion people worldwide are regular smokers (mostly men), with tobacco killing over 9 million per year.[29] It is on the rise in Africa and the Middle East, as tobacco companies turn their attention to new markets.

Whatever you might think of tobacco-company executives, they don't want to kill their customers. A long-cherished dream of the industry is therefore to develop a harmless cigarette. Nicotine should be retained to keep customers hooked and because nicotine in isolation has few direct health risks – its dangers only flow from its addictive nature. From the 1950s, industry scientists tried to find ways to reduce carcinogen delivery while maintaining the nicotine, through modifying cigarette design or by finding new strains of tobacco plant. One difficulty companies faced was that even if they were successful and then tried to market a new type of cigarette as 'safe', this would be an implicit admission that all their other cigarettes were 'unsafe' – something that they were resisting hard.[27] The high temperature generated by burning tobacco unavoidably generates carcinogens. The search for the harmless cigarette therefore ultimately led to modern alternative ways to deliver nicotine at low temperature, such as vaping. It is doubtful whether vaping is entirely harmless, and we are still waiting to find out its long-term effects, but it is surely better than inhaling cigarette smoke.

Will we ever totally eliminate smoking? In 2014 the British Medical Association voted for a simple, yet radical, plan to end smoking.[30] It was to make tobacco sales illegal for anyone born in the year 2000 or later. In this way, smoking would vanish entirely by the year 2100 or so. Laws that change by age are commonplace: children cannot drive, vote or avoid education, for example. Laws that depended on date of birth would be a new precedent, though. It is certainly odd to think that someone who is thirty-eight might be able to smoke, while someone who is thirty-seven cannot.

The proposal was ignored by the British government and so far, no country has tried to implement such unprecedented legislation. With the continual decline of smoking because of the policies discussed above, perhaps it is not necessary. Hopefully, we will eventually become a smoke-free world, and cigarettes will be stubbed out in the ashtray of history.

21

Unsafe at Any Speed

Until the last century, land transport meant walking or, if you were lucky, horse power. Of course, horse-based transport has now been largely replaced by motor vehicles. While cars are safer than horses in terms of deaths per mile travelled, the enormous growth in transport over the last hundred years has meant that motor vehicles have become major killers.

As with numerous inventions, the development of the car was a gradual process, with many people making substantial contributions. Most credit, however, can be given to Karl and Bertha Benz, who built the first three-wheeled, two-seater automobile, powered by an internal combustion engine of their own design, in Mannheim, Germany in 1885. Benz filed a remarkable array of patents, including those for a speed-regulation system, ignition using sparks with a battery, the spark plug, carburettor, clutch, gear shift and water radiator. All were in Karl's name, though some had been invented in partnership with his wife Bertha, who as a married woman was not allowed to be named on a German patent. In 1888, without telling Karl, the intrepid Bertha took her teenage boys on a long-distance test drive in their new creation to visit her mother in Pforzheim, pausing to invent the brake pad on the way. During the trip, Bertha used one of her hatpins to unclog a fuel pipe and a garter to insulate a wire. She stopped at a pharmacy in the small town of Weisloch to buy fuel. A memorial outside commemorates her achievement and the world's first petrol station. This 180-kilometre journey gave welcome publicity and helped make the Benz business a success.

While the first commercial car and engine manufacturers were in France and Germany, it was in the USA that motoring really took off. We will therefore concentrate on how the USA handled the grave dangers that follow from allowing people to drive one-ton metal boxes at high speed. At first, cars were expensive, luxury items, built in small numbers. Henry Ford changed this with his Model T Ford, first introduced in 1908. The Model T was simple to drive and cheap to buy; indeed, the price dropped every year. Ford installed the first conveyor-belt-based assembly line in his car factory in Highland Park, an enclave within Detroit, Michigan. Assembly-line production slashed manufacturing time for the Model T.[1] High pay rates and shorter working hours attracted the best workers and allowed them to recycle their wages back to the company by buying one of the cars that they were making. Good conditions and pay also helped compensate for the mind-numbing boredom of repeating identical tasks over and over on an assembly line. In 1913 Ford became the world's biggest car manufacturer and by 1918 half of the cars in the USA were the Model T. By 1927, the final year of production, 15 million Model Ts had been built – a record that stood until 1972.

In 1950 there were 25 million registered automobiles in the USA, the majority of which were made before the Second World War; by 1958 there were 67 million, meeting Henry Ford's goal that any man with a good job should be able to afford a car. By the end of the 1950s one in six working Americans was employed in the automobile industry. Now that they were available to the middle classes and not just the rich, cars became a central part of American culture, more so than in any other country. New types of businesses were created to support the 1950s car-based lifestyle, with shopping malls, drive-through restaurants and drive-in movie theatres. Cars took leading roles in music, TV shows, books and an uncountable number of movies that featured car chases. New interstate highways, begun in 1956, helped accelerate car usage, as the graph opposite shows.

While the number of miles travelled on the roads steadily grew over the last hundred years, the death rate over the same period shows a quite different pattern. The graph below shows the number of deaths in car accidents per 100 million miles driven from 1921 to 2017 in the USA. In 1921, the first year for which we have data, this value was 24.09; in 2017 it was only 1.16, an amazing twentyfold reduction in deaths per mile. How was this achieved?

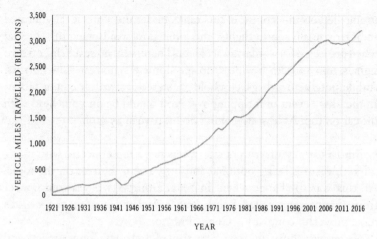

Billions of miles driven in the USA from 1921 to 2017.[2, 3]

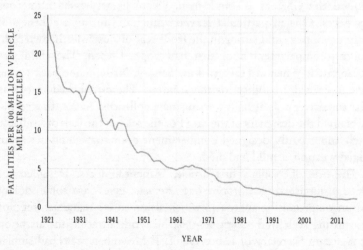

Motor vehicle deaths per 100 million vehicle miles travelled in the USA from 1921 to 2017.[2, 3]

While the Model T Ford was the first bestselling car, it was also highly dangerous. It featured ineffective rear-wheel brakes and no front brakes; a hand-crank starter that could break your arm when the engine caught; a cast-iron steering column pointing at your heart, ready to impale you in a collision; fuel tanks under the seats, ideally located to burn you alive; poor lights; and a flat glass windscreen to slice you when projected forward in an accident. There were no seat belts, no turn signals, no windscreen wipers, no speedometers, no rear-view mirrors, and definitely no airbags, cup holders, stereo system, air con or satnav. In the likely event of it tipping over, you would be on your head with the car on top. At least it couldn't do more than 45 mph.

For most car manufacturers safety was not a top concern, with many safety measures being optional and little research done on the topic. All this was to change when, in 1965, a thirty-two-year-old lawyer from Connecticut called Ralph Nader declared war on the world's most powerful company – General Motors (GM).

Nader was born in 1934, the son of Lebanese immigrants, and educated at Princeton and Harvard Law School. Nader had been interested in car safety (or the lack of it) since his time hitch-hiking around the USA as a young man, where he witnessed numerous accidents. One in particular stayed with him: during a collision at only 15 mph, a child sitting in the front seat of a car was thrown onto a glove-compartment door that had popped open. The child was decapitated. When at Harvard Law School, Nader came back to the case to consider liability for the accident. The established view was that the driver was at fault for causing a collision; Nader disagreed – he blamed the designers of the car.[4] For the sake of the lack of a reliable latch and a badly designed compartment door that could act as an edged weapon, a child had died.

The title of Nader's first article, 'American Cars: Designed for Death', published in *Harvard Law Review*, gives you some idea of his uncompromising approach, which slammed car manufacturers for prioritising style over safety. In 1964 his work attracted the attention of Assistant Secretary of Labor Daniel P. Moynihan, who had similar interests in car safety, having written an article of his own in 1959 titled 'Epidemic on the Highways'.[5] In 1965 Moynihan hired Nader as a part-time consultant at the Labor Department to write a report recommending increased federal regulation on highway safety. This had little effect.

Frustrated with his inability to make an impact, Nader quit his job to begin writing his devastating book, *Unsafe at Any Speed: The Designed-In Dangers of the American Automobile*.[6] Once he had an outline and a few chapters completed, he began to send them to potential publishers. The reception was generally frosty, as few foresaw many sales. One told Nader that the book would be 'of interest primarily to insurance agents'. Finally, he was approached by New York publisher Richard Grossman, who was impressed by an earlier article by Nader on car safety. Grossman wanted to publish the book, though doubted whether many copies would sell. As he said in 2007, 'The issue about marketing that book always was, even if every word in it is true and everything about it is as outrageous as he says, do people want to read about that?'[7]

'For over half a century,' Nader's book began, 'the automobile has brought death, injury, and the most inestimable sorrow and deprivation to millions of people.' Technologies existed that could make cars much safer, he argued, but car manufacturers would not use them, as they might eat into profits. *Unsafe at Any Speed* highlighted numerous features of cars that manufacturers knew were dangerous. These included:

1. Extensive use of chrome wipers, steering wheels, front bonnet, bumpers and dashboards that reflected sunlight into a driver's eyes.
2. Lights that were not visible from some directions, as they were buried in bumpers or obscured by other parts of the car body.
3. Tinted windscreens that made driving at night difficult.
4. Lack of standardisation of the arrangement of gears, particularly for automatics. When drivers bought a new car, they often put the car into 'drive' instead of 'reverse' or vice versa, as they were used to a different pattern.
5. No concern for driver error in dashboard design. One accident occurred when a driver shut off his headlights when trying to turn on the cigarette lighter. The knobs for both controls were identical and next to each other.
6. Poor manufacturing and lack of quality control. Nader reported the results of tests on thirty-two new cars bought in 1963. Every one had defects, including:

   rain leaks, a window running out of its channel, door handles that fell off, a broken distributor cap, a speedometer needle that fell back to zero and remained there, a broken seat adjuster, an ignition lock that wouldn't lock, a door that wouldn't latch, engines that leaked oil, directional signals that wouldn't cancel, a grossly inaccurate gas gauge, front wheels out of alignment, and headlights, as the late Mildred Brady of Consumers Union put it, 'that aimed at the ground or at the eyes of approaching motorists or at birds in trees'.

7. Sharp protuberances on the exterior that could harm passengers, like the tailfin on a 1959 Cadillac, which bore 'an uncanny resemblance to the tail of the Stegosaurus'. In 25 per cent of passenger fatalities in New York, the vehicles were moving at only 14 mph or less – hence the book's title. The victims' bodies were penetrated by ornaments, bumper rims, fins and other pointy bits. The shapes of bumpers could push the victim down where they would be run over, rather than deflecting them to the side.

8. Instrument panels with sharp, unyielding edges, no padding, and protruding knobs and controls.

9. Seatbelts only available as optional extras. GM's chief safety engineer, Howard Gandelot, argued that they were useless, saying:

> I find it difficult to believe that the seat belt can afford the driver any great amount of protection over and above that which is available to him through the medium of the safety-type steering wheel if he has his hands on the wheel and grips the rim sufficiently tight to take advantage of its energy absorption properties.[6]

He claimed there was 'little interest on the part of the motoring public in actual use of seat belts'.[6] In addition, seat belts restricted his ability to reach some of the vehicle controls, rumpled his suit, and gave him aches.

While each of these car problems could be corrected, Nader's primary target was the attitude of the auto manufacturers. They came up with a remarkable variety of reasons why they should not make cars safer: accidents were never due to poorly designed cars, but 'some nut at the wheel'.[6] If a mechanical problem was the cause of an accident, this was because the motorist had not maintained their car properly. Design decisions belonged to stylists and stylists were simply following customer demand. Non-glare finishes, to stop the sun shining in a driver's eyes, could not be introduced as they would incite a customer revolt. It was sometimes safer to be ejected from a vehicle in a collision than to remain inside. It was impossible to provide secure protection in an impact by any amount of design modification, or by any restraining device that the average driver would be willing to use.[6]

Nader claimed that a thriving industry of medical, police, administrative, legal, insurance, automotive repair and funeral services were earning a living from accidents, while casualty prevention earned little. Profit always came first, even if maximising profit meant the deaths and injuries of tens of thousands of people every year; in a nutshell, auto manufacturers were killing for money. 'But the true mark of a humane society must be what it does about prevention of accident injuries, not the cleaning up of them afterward.'

Auto-company executives were outraged by Nader's book, not least because many were named and shamed. They had several options in how to respond. They could:

- Ignore the book. Sales were not strong at first, so the bad publicity might just go away.
- Acknowledge that mistakes had been made, learn from them, and start to produce safer cars.
- Discredit the book on the grounds that it contained numerous errors, inaccuracies and exaggerations.
- Try to destroy the credibility of Ralph Nader. They could tap his phones, hire private investigators to look into his financial and private life, make menacing phone calls to friends and family, or perhaps try to hire prostitutes in an attempt to catch him in a compromising situation. Each of these approaches would help smear his reputation, damage his character and credibility, and serve as a warning to anyone else who might dare to mess with GM.

They chose the final option.

Shortly after publication, Nader was working as an unpaid consultant for Democratic Senator Abe Ribicoff. He told Ribicoff that he suspected that he was being followed. Ribicoff took Nader seriously, and convened an inquiry into the harassment, which took place in a US Senate committee room, in front of TV cameras and many reporters. GM CEO James Roche was called as a witness. Under oath, Roche was forced to admit that GM had hired a private detective agency to investigate Nader. An angry Ribicoff said, 'And so you [GM] hired detectives to try to get dirt on this young man to besmirch his character because of statements he made about your unsafe automobiles?' Ribicoff threw the GM report on the table, shouting, 'And you didn't find a damned thing!' Nader then appeared on news shows for all three national TV channels and the front page of newspapers across the country.[4]

As a result of this publicity, sales of *Unsafe at Any Speed* soared. Grossman and the rest of the publishers that Nader had sounded out had therefore been entirely wrong about his book's lack of commercial potential – thanks to generous help with promotion from GM, *Unsafe at Any Speed* become the bestselling non-fiction book of 1966 in the USA.

Nader sued GM for invasion of privacy, and two years later won $425,000, the largest out-of-court settlement in the history of privacy law. He used the proceeds to found the Center for the Study of Responsive Law,[8] which still campaigns on consumer issues.

Nader's book was timely in that it had an audience that was prepared to listen and politicians that were finally ready to take action. While car crashes didn't kill as many people as heart attacks, cancer and stroke in the 1960s, they were still the number one cause of death for Americans under forty-four.[9]

Another bright idea that took fifty years to implement fully was getting car owners to pass a driving test before being allowed on the road. New owners were frequently only shown how to drive by salesmen who were unlikely to say that they couldn't sell you the car as your driving wasn't good enough. Rhode Island was the first state to require a driving test before issuing a licence in 1908, the same year the Model T made its entrance. By 1930, twenty-four states required a licence to drive, though just fifteen had mandatory driving tests. In 1959 South Dakota became the last state to impose a driver's exam requirement, though the early tests were not especially challenging.

By 1960 numerous improvements to car design had been made, with windscreen wipers, rear-view mirrors, turning indicators, headrests to reduce whiplash injuries, collapsible steering columns, hydraulic brakes and padded dashboards, all as standard. Safety glass was first used in windscreens in 1927 to prevent them shattering on impact. In the 1930s GM began experimenting with crash tests to see what actually happened on impacts at various speeds; later, crash-test dummies were included. The benefits of better design of cars and roads, and driver training, are apparent in the steep decline in deaths on the road until 1960 (as the graph on p. 281 shows).

Many advances in car-safety technology were invented in the 1950s, including airbags, crumple zones to absorb the energy of a crash and disc brakes. Three-point seatbelts with a diagonal shoulder strap, as well as a lap belt, were invented by Volvo in 1959, but they were an optional extra at first and few owners paid up the extra money to have them installed. Nader was therefore not complaining that car designers needed to work on devising new safety features; rather, he was pointing out that while the technologies existed, companies were not using them.

The first congressional hearings on traffic safety were held in July 1956, though little was achieved in terms of legislation and regulation for the next ten years.[10] After *Unsafe at Any Speed*'s publication, and the exposure of GM's bad behaviour, however, Congress was not slow to appreciate that public opinion was now firmly on the side of the lone hero, Ralph Nader, fighting the evil giant General Motors.

The National Traffic and Motor Vehicle Safety Act[9] was passed by US Congress and signed by President Lyndon Johnson in 1966. It required car manufacturers to use safety standards to reduce the risk to the public from accidents caused by poor design, construction or operation of automobiles. A related Highway Safety Act, passed at the same time, legislated on highway design and set up the National Highway Safety Bureau to impose the new rules. A range of mandatory safety features for automobiles followed, including padded steering wheels and dashboards, seat belts, safety glass, rear 'back-up' lights and emergency flashers. Airbags, anti-lock brakes, electronic stability control, rear-view cameras and automatic braking followed. Making these compulsory meant that no manufacturer was at a competitive disadvantage. Similar measures took place in other countries around the same time.

The last fifty years have seen a continual improvement in car safety from manufacturers, driven by consumer demand, as well as legislation.

New inventions include inertia-reel seatbelts; intermittent wipers; traction control to maintain grip; head restraints; in-car electronics; computer-aided design and simulations; impact-protection systems, designed to spread the force of an impact; stronger steel and other materials; blind-spot information systems that use cameras and motion sensors to avoid collisions when parking; self-steering systems to keep a car in a line; side-impact airbags; and anti-skid and pedestrian-detection systems. Throughout the world new laws forced the use of seat belts, front and back, and made driving tests more rigorous.[11] Government agencies begin crash-testing all cars, publishing the results and giving safety scores for vehicles. Risks to pedestrians who might be hit were considered, as well as drivers and passengers. Self-driving cars that share information with each other and even check whether the driver is still awake, as well as pedestrian-detection systems, may be next.[12]

Nader's book was – not unreasonably – criticised for being inaccurate, unfair and full of errors. It contains a lot of engineering information that could be over the heads of its readers, targeted cars that were not even manufactured any more and hardly reads like a great piece of literature, often resembling something a prosecutor might read out in a trial. None of this matters. Nader's goal was to make manufacturers start taking safety seriously and stop making cars that they knew were dangerous. Self-regulation did not work, so this had to be done via legislation. In this, *Unsafe at Any Speed* was a huge success. New laws and government agencies inspired by Ralph Nader have prevented around 3.5 million deaths in the fifty years since it was published.[13]

Nader continued to work for consumer rights, founding other consumer-action groups, including Public Interest Research Groups, the Center for Auto Safety and the Clean Water Action Project. He ran for president four times, doing best in 2000 with 2.7 per cent of the vote. Despite these achievements, Nader is still loathed by many. In 2005, a panel of fifteen conservative scholars and public policy leaders voted *Unsafe at Any Speed* the twenty-second most harmful book of the nineteenth and twentieth centuries.[14] I doubt he minds.

Criminalisation of driving while drunk goes back to the start of motoring. On 10 September 1897 twenty-five-year-old Londoner George Smith achieved the dubious distinction of being the first person ever arrested for drink-driving, after smashing his taxi into a wall. In the USA the first laws against operating a motor vehicle while under the influence of alcohol were introduced in New York in 1910. There was no way of measuring intoxication at first, so it was up to each arresting officer to decide whether a suspect was too drunk to drive. While it was known that blood testing was a reliable way to quantify drunkenness, checking blood was not practical at the roadside. In 1927, however, it was shown that alcohol levels in the breath correlated closely with blood alcohol level, pointing to the value of a breathalyser, or 'drunkometer', as it was first known. Even though drunken driving was illegal and could now be straightforwardly detected using chemicals that reacted with alcohol in the breath, few people were convicted. If a case went to a jury, defendants were nearly always let off, as the general public rarely saw it as a crime that deserved the harsh punishment that would follow a conviction. Laws that people regard as unjust are unenforceable. Even in the 1960s, there was a debate about whether driving when drunk posed any danger at all.[15]

On 3 May 1980, in Fair Oaks, California, thirteen-year-old Cari Lightner was walking to a church carnival with a friend when she was hit from behind by a car driven by an intoxicated Clarence Busch. Cari was knocked out of her shoes, thrown 125 feet, and died in the street. Busch did not stop to help Cari, but went home, telling his wife 'not to look at the car' before passing out. When Busch killed Cari, he was out on bail from a hit-and-run crash when driving drunk two days earlier. He had had three previous drink-driving convictions in the past four years. None of this was sufficient to invalidate his California driver's licence.[16]

After police officers told Cari's mother, Candace (Candy), that the driver would probably receive little punishment for his latest crime, a furious and grief-stricken Candy founded Mothers Against Drunk Driving, or MADD, to campaign against drunk driving. Candy gave up her job and put her savings into the project. Her goal was to get tougher laws introduced, end tolerance and raise awareness of the 'only socially acceptable form of homicide', as she put it.[17] This was the turning point in changing the public's tolerance towards drink-driving.

Candy's work with MADD, California Governor Jerry Brown and President Ronald Reagan helped turn around attitudes towards driving under the influence of alcohol and other drugs in America.[17] As a result, the legal limit for alcohol in blood was lowered. The minimum legal age for alcohol consumption was raised and is now twenty-one in all US states. Drunk drivers are no longer let off but are convicted. They receive prison sentences or fines, lose their driver's licence and have to buy more expensive insurance. Ignition interlock devices can be compulsorily installed so that the car engine will not start without a successful breath test using a sensor attached to the dashboard. Despite public awareness, disapproval and stiff penalties, drink-driving remains a serious problem. In 2017, 10,874 people were killed by drunk drivers in the USA, about 20 per cent of total motor vehicle fatalities.[18]

While cars are now much safer per mile, thanks to all these changes and better medical care of crash victims, increasing usage has ensured roads are still major killers. The graph opposite shows the total number of deaths caused by motor vehicles in the USA since 1921. Worst was 1972, after which the reforms instituted by the US government began to make a real difference. The total number of miles driven since 1972 is 2.5 times higher, but the number of deaths has fallen. Emergency services have improved their handling of road-traffic accidents, in addition to better medical care.

While deaths on the road remain high in the USA, they could be a lot worse. Visitors to India and Africa have often commented on their relaxed attitude to the rules of the road. In 2016, the West African state of Liberia topped the table for road-traffic deaths, with a rate of 35.9 deaths per 100,000 people per year; bottom was San Marino with zero. San Marino's position is a statistical fluke, given its tiny size; next best were the Maldives and Micronesia, states composed of small islands where you can never drive far before reaching the ocean.[19] Western European countries score highly for road safety, with the USA mid-table. The most dangerous countries on the road are those that have only recently achieved enough wealth for car ownership to become widespread. A lengthy programme of driver education and attitude adjustment is required for these new drivers.

Twenty-somethings don't get dementia. Nor are they at risk of imminent death from heart disease, cancer, stroke, lung disease or diabetes. For those in their teens, twenties or thirties, injuries on the road remain the number one cause of death.

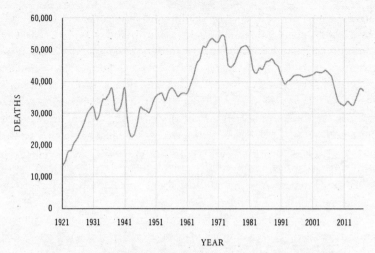

Total motor vehicle deaths in the USA from 1899 to 2017.[2, 3]

Conclusion: A Bright Future?

Nothing in life is to be feared, it is only to be understood.
Now is the time to understand more, so that we may
fear less.

Marie Curie, quoted in *Our Precarious Habitat*[1]

The reasons why we die have changed profoundly in the last 10,000 years. The oldest anatomically modern human, with a skeleton that matches modern people, is 200,000 years old.[2] For at least 95 per cent of this time, we lived as hunter-gatherers, with a healthy diet and active lifestyle. Many common infectious diseases, like measles, smallpox, plague and typhoid, were then almost unknown. The world was a dangerous place, however. Accidents were frequent, especially when hunting. Many people were killed by large animals – either our predators, or our prey fighting back – or other people. Abandoning a nomadic existence for living in permanent settlements, with crop planting and animal husbandry, gave us more food and less violence, but at great cost. Surviving on only a few plants as the main food source brought malnutrition and the risk of famine if harvests failed. Working in the fields was a miserable existence for most, with the joys of hunting and fighting reserved for the elite. In exchange rulers provided justice and security, protecting city dwellers from the barbarians (ideally). In the longer term, living in large settlements led to the accumulation of endemic infectious diseases, mostly caught from the animals or foul water that we now lived with. When we were nomads, catching a disease from an animal, such as plague from rodents, might well kill the entire band. However, that would be the end of it, as the pathogens would all die along with their victims. Populations were so low, and contact between groups of people so sporadic, that disease could not be maintained in groups of humans. In contrast, high densities of people and pathogens adapted to each other in cities, eventually leading to a host of illnesses that were routinely caught in childhood, like chickenpox, scarlet fever and rubella. Infectious disease was now the leading cause of death.

Defeating infectious disease resulted from some of the most brilliant and important ideas that we have ever had. Most of these ideas now seem so obvious that it is hard to believe that there was a time when they were not widely accepted. Firstly, collecting and analysing data. Before we began to systematically record information on death, starting with the Bills of Mortality in London about 1600, linking causes to disease was rarely more than speculation. In contrast, when John Graunt studied the data in the Bills of Mortality, he could conclude that living in the city was less healthy than the country because he had the numbers to prove it. Similarly, John Snow was only able to convince sceptical authorities that infected water caused cholera after he had painstakingly visited afflicted households in Soho and found that they had all been using the Broad Street pump.

The greatest revolution in thinking in medicine was germ theory – the idea that tiny organisms, invisible to the naked eye, were the primary cause of disease. Germ theory rationalised why we should drink clean water, wash bodies, clothes and living spaces, eat fresh food, perform operations in sterile conditions, and so on. Implementing cleanliness meant that hospitals became safe places to recover, rather than hothouses of infection. Beating famine and malnutrition with better food, in terms of both quantity and quality, also yields bodies better able to fight off disease. The identification of specific disease-causing organisms naturally led pioneers to search for ways to kill them or turn them into vaccines. Finding out whether a drug works requires a clinical trial. Groups must be compared that differ only in the potential cause or cure under investigation, like James Lind's pairs of sailors testing various foods against scurvy.

All these approaches use the scientific method, the best way for discovering reliable information about the natural world. An important, though sometimes overlooked, part of the way we do science is that credit for a discovery is only given when it is published. New inventions are next to useless if no one knows about them, as with the case of using forceps in a difficult childbirth, which was kept secret for a hundred years. Knowledge must be available to everyone, so it can be used, verified and built on. Science is the main reason why we now live in the healthiest and wealthiest period that we have ever had.

Beating violence, famine, malnutrition and infectious disease sent life expectancy soaring from the late nineteenth century, bringing in cancer, diabetes, stroke and heart failure as our main causes of death. While age is the most important risk factor for these non-communicable diseases, widespread obesity, smoking, alcohol and avoidance of exercise compound these problems. In addition, genetics has always had a profound influence on health.

Diseases like measles, childbed fever and cholera have straightforward solutions, such as vaccination, hand-washing and sanitation. In contrast, we have had to deploy a vast array of sophisticated measures, such as better diagnosis, prevention, surgery and drugs, to reduce the death rates from non-communicable diseases. Despite these challenges, again we have made remarkable progress. The graphs below show major causes of death in England (a typical industrialised country) from 2001 to 2019 for males and females. These are death rates, so they give the number of people that will die in each year from each cause in a representative sample of 100,000 people.

Age standardised rate, per 100,000 males

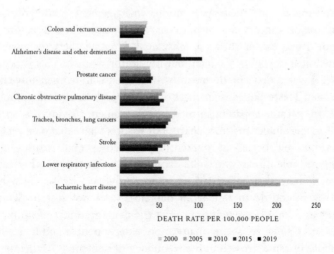

Main causes of death for males in England from 2001 to 2015.[3]

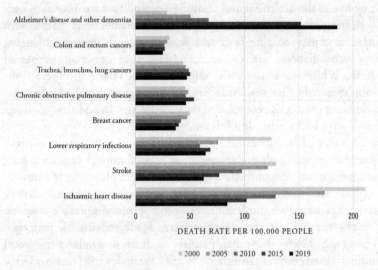

Age standardised rate, per 100,000 females

DEATH RATE PER 100.000 PEOPLE

■ 2000 ■ 2005 ■ 2010 ■ 2015 ■ 2019

Main causes of death for females in England from 2001 to 2015.[3]

Death rates from heart disease and stroke, which were the biggest killers in 2001, have now roughly halved, thanks to huge improvements in their prevention, management and treatment. Most major cancers are also in retreat, notably breast, colon and rectum. Lung cancer shows a substantial difference between men and women: it is declining for men, but not so for women. This is because smoking was at first a predominantly male habit, with women only taking it up later. The health consequences of starting and then quitting smoking therefore became apparent in men before women. Covid-19 is sure to make an appearance in future charts, but we don't have that data yet.

As we get better at preventing, detecting and treating non-communicable diseases, and life expectancy keeps rising, other causes of death take their place. Most importantly, we are seeing a huge increase in the death rate from dementia, and not just in Western countries. Countries passing through the demographic transition, like India and China, are seeing many more elderly people and hence have particularly rapid growth in the frequency of dementia. Alzheimer's is now the most expensive disease in the world. Not only is it common, but it often requires family members to give up work to look after their loved ones, who might later need years of care in a nursing home. In contrast, diseases that kill suddenly, like heart attacks or stroke, are not such a big burden on healthcare providers. There are no good drugs for Alzheimer's disease. Those that we have can only relieve symptoms for less than a year. As both the number and proportion of elderly people grows, we desperately need new drugs that can prevent, cure or even just delay the onset of Alzheimer's. We therefore seem to be heading for a world of elderly people with functioning bodies, but demented minds.

Once we understand the science behind a disease, we can devise solutions. These do not always need to be expensive or high-tech. Measures such as vaccines, water filters, soap, and fluids for rehydration cost little, so should be available to all. As always, clean drinking water and sanitation is vital. International borders are products of our imaginations and are not respected by infectious microorganisms. Successes against polio, guinea worm, malaria and many others can only be achieved if every country participates in programmes. For instance, if we had neglected Somalia or Bangladesh in the 1970s, then we would still have smallpox. Failed states or war zones that are inaccessible to healthcare workers are a danger to us all, as they will be reservoirs of disease. Polio lingering on in Nigeria, Pakistan and Afghanistan is a miserable example of this. Similarly, groups of people who refuse to participate in vaccination, or other measures aimed at disease elimination, ensure that the diseases stay with us. We were fortunate that there was no substantial anti-vaccination campaign against the smallpox vaccine in the 1970s. If you really think that children should not be vaccinated by the measles, mumps and rubella jab, then paradoxically you should campaign hard for worldwide immunisation. Then, when the three diseases are eradicated, there will be no need to use the MMR vaccine ever again. Polio, guinea worm, elephantiasis, yaws, lymphatic filariasis, measles, mumps, rubella, river blindness, syphilis and hookworm are all current targets for total eradication.[4] More challenging, but more important, would be to eradicate malaria, HIV/AIDS and tuberculosis.

Dealing with epidemics, famines and other catastrophes not only requires international cooperation, but also blowing the whistle as soon as possible when a potential disaster arises. The world must be alerted when harvests fail or new diseases appear, so that the problems can be dealt with rapidly before they blow up into major disasters. Governments will always be tempted to deny that a problem exists, rather than alerting their neighbours, as they don't want to appear to be failing. The media has responsibility here too. They must report issues fairly, rather than choosing to defend one set of politicians, whatever they do. Nevertheless, taking the long view, and despite continuing tuberculosis, HIV/AIDS, malaria and flare-ups like Covid-19, infectious disease has been in retreat since the nineteenth century. If we continue with this progress, we can get more countries through the demographic transition, working together to reach a place where we all live long and healthy lives.

Humans are the great destroyers. We use most of the land on Earth for our purposes, leaving precious little room for other species. We spread a small number of species (such as rice and chickens), while driving many others towards extinction. The ultimate reason for the environmental damage that we cause is too many people. If we are to reduce human population and the damage that we do, then this can be done in two ways: the first is catastrophe, where our civilisation collapses due to nuclear war, unstoppable climate change, a devastating epidemic (most likely a new strain of influenza, far more deadly than Covid-19), super-volcanoes (Yellowstone is a prime candidate), an asteroid strike or some other disaster. There is not a lot that we can do if a ten-mile-wide rock is heading in our direction at high speed. If so, the list of top ten causes of death will need a swift rewrite.

The alternative is to reduce the stress we place on the planet by having fewer children, ultimately moving to a stable state in harmony with our world. Counter-intuitively, birth rates drop and populations start to fall if we extend life, particularly if we reduce the death of children to negligible levels, educate girls and make contraception accessible.[5] A steady population decrease is our best hope to avoid ruin. Falling birth rates worldwide give hope that this is achievable.

How might our causes of death change in the next few decades? Hopefully, the Covid-19 epidemic will soon be gone. Extrapolating other current trends seems reasonable, for a few years at least, so we can expect heart disease, lung conditions and stroke to continue to decline, while type 2 diabetes and dementia will rise. Cancer is a more complicated story, as trends vary depending on the affected organ. More people are getting cancer as other diseases are overcome, but we are finding better chemotherapies, diagnostics and treatment methods. Drug discovery, medical advances and science in general will continue to motor on. Even with dementia, there are glimmers that we may finally be able to develop drugs that can halt its progression or prevent its onset.[6]

A more interesting question is whether any novel medical breakthroughs might happen, transforming the ways we die. Will any of our present-day causes of death be largely overcome, gone the ways of the complications of childbirth, measles and plague? If so, how could this be done?

Genetic disease has always been around, since DNA replication is never perfect, and mutations are inevitable. All we have ever been able to do with genetic problems so far is to screen for them and treat their symptoms. Now, however, we are on the verge of the next healthcare revolution, where we can defeat genetic disease absolutely at its source, by taking out disease-causing mutations, as we saw in Chapter 16. Severe conditions that result from a single unwanted mutation like haemophilia, cystic fibrosis, early-onset Alzheimer's disease and fumarase deficiency are prime candidates. More complex polygenic conditions may follow, and even ageing itself.

Many hundreds of SNPs have been reported to affect ageing and life expectancy. For example, one study looked at genetic variation in 801 centenarians (median age 104 years) from New England and compared them to 914 controls of the same ethnicity.[7] They found 281 SNPs, within 130 genes, that appeared to influence lifespan. Many of these genes were already known to be involved with ageing processes like Alzheimer's, diabetes, heart disease, cancer and hypertension. Two in particular stood out, namely *APOE* and *FOXO3*. Variations in *APOE* were already known to strongly influence the likelihood of getting Alzheimer's disease.[8] The *FOXO3* gene encodes a protein that switches genes on and off in many cellular activities, such as cell death, the immune system, cardiovascular disease, stem-cell generation and cancer.[9] It seems that the centenarians have SNPs that can delay many of the usual problems arising from ageing, opening the possibility of extending lifespan by introducing these changes into our DNA.

Knowing the sequence of the DNA that we are born with has the potential to predict the likelihood of disease throughout our lives.

Furthermore, we could track how our bodies are behaving from day to day, keeping a close eye on our health. The concentrations of biological molecules could be regularly measured in small samples of blood, saliva, stool, urine or breath. Stool is particularly useful, as it shows which bacteria are living in our guts. To catch an accurate snapshot of how an organ is working, we could find out what is going on inside, specifically by measuring the concentrations, sequences and structures of the DNA, RNA, proteins and other chemicals within a tissue or even individual cells.[10] Malfunctioning cells will deviate from the normal levels of their biomolecules or acquire mutations, particularly if we have a new infection or they are cancerous, when expression of the genes regulating cell growth goes haywire. We could wear sensors to track the state of our bodies, measuring brain activity, the way we talk, walk and move, and whether we are active or sleeping. Smartwatches are small steps in this direction.

Keeping track of all these data gives millions of numbers to describe the condition of a body. They would be interpreted by computers running sophisticated machine-learning algorithms, trained to perform pattern recognition, using the data in an optimal way to make predictions. The computers would be able to detect the onset of a health condition by noticing warning signs, well before any symptoms are apparent. The potential power of monitoring the states of our bodies, coupled with artificial intelligence systems trained on data from billions of people, will allow us to step in at the earliest stages of disease. Cancer, neurological problems and metabolic disorders will be detected years earlier than they are now. Treatments will be personalised, targeting the precise nature of our condition, such as exactly which mutations we have in our tumours, rather than grouping all people with the same diagnosis together.

The current supply of organs for transplants is already much smaller than the demand. Kidney-transplant patients can have to endure years of being regularly hooked up to a dialysis machine, waiting for an organ that might never arrive. With an increasing lifespan, the situation is getting worse.

Rather than wait for a donor, soon we may be able to meet the demand for new organs by growing them from our own cells. Stem cells have the ability to grow and differentiate into new cell types. We already know how to take skin cells, change them into stem cells, grow them in culture, and then transform them into the cell type of our choice. Since we start with our own cells, the resulting organ will be genetically identical to ourselves, so will not be rejected by our immune system. We could make new pancreas islets cells that secrete insulin to help diabetics, for instance. Alternatively, we can collect cells from our bodies when we are in peak shape, say age twenty, and deep-freeze them, ready to be used decades later. Persuading cells to form a structure large enough and functional enough to replace an entire organ isn't easy,[11] though a mould or framework made by a 3D printer to match the exact shape of the organ we want to replace might help. Perhaps we will 3D-print cells, arranging them layer by layer to sculpt a new organ. Deaths from organ failure could then become largely a thing of the past. Even more radically, if an organ is steadily losing function due to age, we could replace it with a new one, even if it isn't yet diseased. Perhaps it would become routine to go into hospital at the age of sixty to freshen up with new sets of lungs, kidneys, liver, pancreas and heart.[12]

In addition, before growing a new organ from stem cells, we could change its DNA. If we are going to grow a new liver, we could put in DNA sequences that we know will optimise liver function and eliminate any genetic problems. Stem cells have already been edited to try to make them resistant to HIV or treat sickle-cell disease before being put into bone marrow, for example,[13] and genes have been edited in the livers of living monkeys to lower their cholesterol levels.[14] At present, our DNA is the same in every cell and thus is a compromise, as a gene sequence that is good for the heart might be not so good for the pancreas. By DNA editing as part of stem-cell-based organ-replacement therapy, we can give every organ the optimal DNA for its function. We could then have hearts like Usain Bolt and lungs like Serena Williams. Many more of us would only die when our brains can no longer function, as everything else would have been upgraded. Years of living with chronic disability would end.

All the scientific advances described here, among many others,[15,16] are under development now. There seem to be no insurmountable obstacles to stop their use in humans, so soon we will have to address the ethical issues and choose whether or not to implement them.

Appendix

Life Table Data

Table A1 shows life table data for the UK, showing how many people died at ages from 0 to 100 from 2014 to 2016. Life tables are the standard way in which ages of death are presented and are an essential tool in all kinds of fields, such as public health, insurance and government. In the top left of the table we start with 100,000 newborns. The 'survivors' columns show how many will live to the age (x) in the left column. 'Deaths at age x' shows how many will die at that age. For example, from 100,000 newborns, 423 males and 352 females will die before their first birthdays, taking the numbers of survivors down to 99,578 and 99,649, respectively rounded to the nearest whole number. The 'Life expectancy from Age x' columns show the mean number of years that someone can be expected to live from the age x in the left column. Working out life expectancies is a complex calculation using all the data in the table, as we need to know how many people there are of each age and how likely they are likely to die at that age.

The big assumption here is that nothing will change in the next hundred years. If, for example, a cure for cancer is discovered, then the number of deaths for each age in the table will reduce, with ages most affected by cancer showing the largest changes.

Table A1. *Life table from UK averaged over years 2014–16. Data is from the UK Office for National Statistics.*[24]

Age	Males			Females		
x	Survivors	Deaths at age x	Life expectancy from age x	Survivors	Deaths at age x	Life expectancy from age x
0	100,000	423	79.2	100,000	352	82.9
1	99,578	31	78.5	99,649	25	82.2
2	99,547	16	77.5	99,624	14	81.2
3	99,531	13	76.5	99,610	10	80.2
4	99,518	9	75.6	99,600	8	79.2
5	99,509	9	74.6	99,592	7	78.2
6	99,500	9	73.6	99,585	7	77.2
7	99,491	9	72.6	99,578	7	76.2
8	99,483	7	71.6	99,570	6	75.2
9	99,476	9	70.6	99,564	7	74.2
10	99,468	9	69.6	99,558	6	73.2
11	99458	10	68.6	99,552	6	72.2
12	99,448	10	67.6	99,546	6	71.2
13	99,439	10	66.6	99,540	11	70.2
14	99,429	12	65.6	99,529	11	69.2
15	99,416	16	64.6	99,518	14	68.3
16	99,401	21	63.6	99,504	16	67.3
17	99,380	29	62.7	99,488	15	66.3
18	99,350	41	61.7	99,473	21	65.3
19	99,309	45	60.7	99,452	21	64.3
20	99,264	47	59.7	99,431	20	63.3

Age	Males			Females		
x	Survivors	Deaths at age x	Life expectancy from age x	Survivors	Deaths at age x	Life expectancy from age x
21	99,217	50	58.8	99,411	22	62.3
22	99,167	50	57.8	99,389	22	61.3
23	99,117	55	56.8	99,367	23	60.4
24	99,062	54	55.8	99,344	23	59.4
25	99,008	58	54.9	99,321	25	58.4
26	98,950	62	53.9	99,297	27	57.4
27	98,888	62	52.9	99,269	27	56.4
28	98,825	66	52.0	99,243	33	55.4
29	98,760	69	51.0	99,210	35	54.4
30	98,691	73	50.0	99,175	38	53.5
31	98,617	75	49.1	99,137	41	52.5
32	98,542	89	48.1	99,096	46	51.5
33	98,453	87	47.2	99,050	49	50.5
34	98,366	95	46.2	99,001	53	49.6
35	98,271	101	45.2	98,949	58	48.6
36	98,170	108	44.3	98,890	65	47.6
37	98,063	112	43.3	98,826	67	46.6
38	97,950	130	42.4	98,759	75	45.7
39	97,821	134	41.4	98,684	80	44.7
40	97,687	153	40.5	98,604	93	43.7
41	97,534	165	39.6	98,511	96	42.8

Age	Males			Females		
x	Survivors	Deaths at age x	Life expectancy from age x	Survivors	Deaths at age x	Life expectancy from age x
42	97,369	170	38.6	98,415	107	41.8
43	97,199	186	37.7	98,308	114	40.9
44	97,013	207	36.8	98,194	126	39.9
45	96,806	215	35.8	98,068	144	39.0
46	96,591	231	34.9	97,924	150	38.0
47	96,361	256	34.0	97,774	160	37.1
48	96,105	263	33.1	97,614	173	36.1
49	95,842	289	32.2	97,441	183	35.2
50	95,553	320	31.3	97,259	208	34.3
51	95,233	331	30.4	97,051	228	33.3
52	94,902	354	29.5	96,823	246	32.4
53	94,548	378	28.6	96,577	269	31.5
54	94,170	415	27.7	96,308	289	30.6
55	93,755	467	26.8	96,020	322	29.7
56	93,288	501	26.0	95,698	347	28.8
57	92,787	542	25.1	95,351	380	27.9
58	92,245	597	24.2	94,971	403	27.0
59	91,649	654	23.4	94,568	454	26.1
60	90,995	726	22.6	94,115	495	25.2
61	90,269	786	21.7	93,620	529	24.4
62	89,483	844	20.9	93,090	586	23.5

Age	Males			Females		
x	Survivors	Deaths at age x	Life expectancy from age x	Survivors	Deaths at age x	Life expectancy from age x
63	88,639	931	20.1	92,504	629	22.6
64	87,708	1005	19.3	91,876	676	21.8
65	86,703	1070	18.5	91,200	721	20.9
66	85,633	1137	17.8	90,479	790	20.1
67	84,496	1208	17.0	89,689	840	19.3
68	83,288	1310	16.2	88,849	935	18.5
69	81,978	1433	15.5	87,915	1,012	17.6
70	80,545	1558	14.8	86,903	1,131	16.8
71	78,987	1702	14.0	85,772	1,236	16.1
72	77,284	1844	13.3	84,536	1,356	15.3
73	75,441	1986	12.7	83,180	1,502	14.5
74	73,455	2202	12.0	81,677	1,628	13.8
75	71,253	2350	11.3	80,049	1,780	13.1
76	68,903	2478	10.7	78,269	1,968	12.3
77	66,425	2651	10.1	76,301	2,104	11.6
78	63,774	2822	9.5	74,197	2,291	11.0
79	60,953	2994	8.9	71,906	2,496	10.3
80	57,959	3220	8.3	69,409	2,775	9.7
81	54,739	3365	7.8	66,634	2,988	9.0
82	51,374	3577	7.3	63,646	3,256	8.4
83	47,797	3759	6.8	60,389	3,530	7.9

Age	Males			Females		
x	Survivors	Deaths at age x	Life expectancy from age x	Survivors	Deaths at age x	Life expectancy from age x
84	44,038	3859	6.3	56,860	3,775	7.3
85	40,179	3966	5.9	53,085	3,963	6.8
86	36,213	3961	5.5	49,121	4,176	6.3
87	32,252	3943	5.1	44,946	4,330	5.8
88	28,310	3890	4.7	40,616	4,396	5.4
89	24,420	3684	4.4	36,219	4,435	5.0
90	20,737	3482	4.0	31,785	4,398	4.6
91	17,255	3143	3.8	27,387	4,144	4.3
92	14,112	2829	3.5	23,243	3,915	4.0
93	11,283	2502	3.2	19,329	3,580	3.7
94	8,782	2146	3.0	15,749	3,296	3.4
95	6,636	1742	2.8	12,453	2,822	3.2
96	4,894	1384	2.6	9,631	2,361	3.0
97	3,510	1030	2.5	7,270	1,898	2.8
98	2,480	807	2.3	5,372	1,538	2.6
99	1,673	574	2.2	3,834	1,198	2.4
100	1,099	410	2.1	2,636	871	2.2

We can work out all sorts of statistics on a population using this data: For example, the age at which you are least likely to die is eight – only seven boys and six girls out of 100,000 die at this age. From this age, death rates steadily climb, peaking at the ages of eighty-five for males and eighty-nine for females. These are the modal ages of death

– the ages at which you are most likely to die. The first year after birth is by far the most dangerous period of childhood. Once you reach the age of one, death rates plummet and do not reach the same levels until you are fifty-five for a man or fifty-seven for a woman. Babies are at especial risk from genetic problems, may be born prematurely, have other problems associated with childbirth, or can die from the still mysterious sudden infant death syndrome.

For a 54-year-old male, the life expectancy from Table A1 is 27.7 years. The probability that a 54-year-old male will die within the next year is:

$$probability\ male\ dying\ at\ 55 =$$
$$1 - \frac{number\ of\ male\ 55\ year\ olds}{nunber\ of\ male\ 54\ year\ olds} = 1 - \frac{93755}{94170} = 0.4\%$$

A 0.4 per cent chance of dying per year is still highly unlikely. If the man is ninety, though, the chance of dying that year jumps up to 16.8 per cent and the life expectancy is only four years. What are the chances of a 54-year-old making it to ninety anyway?

$$probability\ male\ age\ 54\ living\ to\ 90$$
$$= \frac{number\ of\ male\ 90\ year\ olds}{number\ of\ male\ 54\ year\ olds} = \frac{20737}{94170} = 22\%$$

Living to ninety would be a lot more likely for a female:

$$probability\ female\ age\ 54\ living\ to\ 90$$
$$= \frac{number\ of\ female\ 90\ year\ olds}{number\ of\ female\ 54\ year\ olds} = \frac{31785}{96308} = 33\%$$

33/22 = 1.5, so you are 50 per cent more likely to live to be ninety if you are female and this discrepancy grows with age. The oldest people are therefore mostly women. The chances of dying before fifty-four for a man are:

$$probability\ male\ dying\ before\ 54 = 1 - \frac{94170}{100000} = 6\%$$

So about 6 per cent of men die before the age of fifty-four; for women it is 4 per cent. It is relatively easy, then, to work out life expectancy probabilities for yourself. Of course, these are average values for the whole UK population. It is possible to change your own odds by good behaviour (running, maintaining a healthy weight, good diet…) or bad (smoking, eating too much junk food, using crack cocaine…).

Acknowledgements

In 1981, at the age of fourteen, I watched the *Cosmos* TV series, written and presented by the astronomer Carl Sagan – a masterpiece in science and history. Within the accompanying book, in a section that discussed astrology, I read:

> *John Graunt compiled the mortality statistics in the City of London in 1632. Among the terrible losses from infant and childhood diseases and such exotic illnesses as 'the rising of the lights' and 'the King's evil,' we find that, of 9,535 deaths, 13 people succumbed to 'planet,' more than died of cancer. I wonder what the symptoms were.*[1]

I wondered too. These few sentences thus planted a seed in my head that eventually germinated and grew into this book.

When I first conceived of the idea of writing a book on how causes of death have changed, I thought it would be about medicine. To my surprise, however, I kept finding that the ways we solved many of our greatest problems had little to do with healthcare. Instead, progress was frequently a result of better law, politics, engineering, statistics, economics, or simply came from driven and talented people having some really good ideas and pushing hard to get them accepted in the face of much resistance. This meant that when trying to cover the history of causes of death, I needed to get to grips with many more fields than I first anticipated. No matter – I have never liked artificial divisions into distinct fields of knowledge. The world is a product of the interaction of disparate forces, only some of which come from decisions made by humans.

This Mortal Coil is a result of four decades reading, pondering and chatting with very many friends, colleagues and students. I have benefitted from encouragement and criticism (both are tremendously valuable) from a huge number of people. In particular, I must thank my agent, Caroline Hardman, for giving a new author a chance, and her support, expertise, advice and time. My excellent editors at Bloomsbury, Jasmine Horsey, Bill Swainson, Alexis Kirschbaum, Lauren Whybrow and Kate Quarry helped enormously to improve the text, from getting me to write entirely new chapters to the correct use of capital letters. Catherine Best, Stephanie Rathbone, Amy Wong, Akua Boateng and Anna Massardi were also part of the great Bloomsbury team who helped with proofreading, artwork, production, marketing and publicity. Matthew Cobb and Dan Davis patiently talked me through how to get published. (You don't just write a book and then send it to a publisher, as I had naively originally thought.) Emyr Benbow kindly explained the procedure that the medical and legal systems use for assigning a cause of death. Susan Barker, Alistair MacDonald, Paul Redman, Lucy Doig, Penny Doig, Sarah Doig, Peter Tallack, Andrew Lownie, Dan Davis, Helen Stuart, Emyr Benbow, Mohammad Husain, John Caddis, Sasha Golovanov, Marina Golovanova, Geoff Hooper, Shivani Kaura, Amanda Dalton, Jeremy Derrick, Jen McBride, Simon Pearce, Ali Ashkanani, Anna Mayall and Steve Deane all gave invaluable feedback on the text. In particular, Sarah Dowd very kindly read and checked the whole thing. Antony Adamson told me about advances in CRISPR. Lorna Fraser, Samaritans Media Officer, Monica Hawley, Samaritans Media Adviser, and all at Huddersfield Samaritans taught me about suicide and helped me compose this section in a responsible manner.

I am grateful to my employer, the University of Manchester, for allowing me to spend an inordinate amount of time on this project, when I should have been writing grant proposals. To accusations of over-simplification and omission, I plead guilty with the excuse that I only had 100,000 words to play with. All mistakes are my responsibility.

Notes

INTRODUCTION: THE FOUR HORSEMEN OF SIENA

1 W.M. Bowsky, 'The Plague in Siena: An Italian Chronicle, Agnolo di Tura del Grasso, Cronica Maggiore', in *The Black Death: A Turning Point in History?*, Holt, Rinehart & Winston: 1971, pp. 13–14.
2 A. White, 'The Four Horsemen', in *Plague and Pleasure. The Renaissance World of Pius II*, Catholic University of America Press: Washington DC, 2014, pp. 21–47.

PART I

1 J. Graunt, 'Natural and Political Observations Mentioned in a Following Index, and Made Upon the Bills of Mortality', in *Mathematical Demography*, Vol. 6, *Biomathematics*, Springer: Berlin, Heidelberg, 1977.

1 WHAT IS DEATH?

1 N. Browne-Wilkinson, 'Airedale National Health Service Trust v Bland [1993] AC 789', 1993, https://lucidlaw.co.uk/criminal-law/hom icidemurder/unlawful-killing/airedale-nhs-trust-v-bland/ (accessed 11 May 2021).
2 M. Cascella, 'Taphophobia and "life preserving coffins" in the nineteenth century', *History of Psychiatry*, 27, 2016, 345–9.
3 L. Davies, ' "Dead" man turns up at own funeral in Brazil', *Guardian*, 24 October 2012.

4 A.K. Goila and M. Pawar, 'The diagnosis of brain death', *Indian Journal of Critical Care Medicine* 13, 2009, 7–11.

5 J. Clark, 'Do You Really Stay Conscious After Being Decapitated?', 2011, https://science.howstuffworks.com/science-vs-myth/extrasen soryperceptions/lucid-decapitation.htm (accessed 25 June 2021).

6 L. Volicer et al., 'Persistent vegetative state in Alzheimer disease – Does it exist?', *Archives of Neurology* 54, 1997, 1382–4.

7 H. Arnts et al., 'Awakening after a sleeping pill: Restoring functional brain networks after severe brain injury', *Cortex* 132, 2020, 135–46.

2 OBSERVATIONS MADE UPON THE BILLS OF MORTALITY

1 N. Boyce, 'Bills of Mortality: tracking disease in early modern London', *The Lancet* 395, 2020, 1186–7.

2 R. Munkhoff, 'Searchers of the Dead: Authority, Marginality, and the Interpretation of Plague in England, 1574–1665', *Gender & History* 11, 1999, 1–29.

3 L. Barroll, *Politics, Plague, and Shakespeare's Theater: The Stuart Years*, Cornell University Press: Ithaca, New York, 1991.

4 N. Cummins et al., 'Living standards and plague in London, 1560–1665', *Economic History Review* 69, 2016, 3–34.

5 J. Graunt, 'Natural and Political Observations Mentioned in a Following Index, and Made Upon the Bills of Mortality', *Mathematical Demography*, Vol. 6, *Biomathematics*, Springer: Berlin, Heidelberg, 1977.

6 J. Aubrey, 'John Graunt: A Brief Life', in *Brief Lives and Other Selected Writings*, ed. A. Powell, Charles Scribner's Sons: New York, 1949.

7 W. Farr, in 'Annual Report of the Registrar-General for England and Wales', HMSO: 1842, p. 92.

8 World Health Organization, 'History of the development of the ICD', http://www.who.int/classifi cations/icd/en/HistoryOfICD.pdf

9 World Health Organization, 'ICD-11 for Mortality and Morbidity Statistics (Version: 05/2021)', 2021, https://icd.who.int/browse11/l-m/en (accessed 6 July 2021).

10 World Health Organization, 'International Statistical Classification of Diseases and Related Health Problems (ICD)', 2021, https://www.who.int/standards/classifications/classification-of-diseases (accessed 6 July 2021).

11 World Health Organization, 'The top 10 causes of death', 2020, https://www.who.int/news-room/fact-sheets/detail/the-top-10-causes-ofdeath (accessed 6 July 2021).

12 R. Rajasingham and D.R. Boulware, 'Cryptococcosis', 2019, https://bestpractice.bmj.com/topics/en-gb/917 (accessed 6 July 2021).

3 LIVE LONG AND PROSPER

1 World Health Organization, 'World health statistics 2016: monitoring health for the SDGs, sustainable development goals, Annex B: tables of health statistics by country, WHO region and globally', 2016.

2 Office for National Statistics, 'National life tables, UK: 2014 to 2016', 2017, https://www.ons.gov.uk/releases/nationallifetablesuk2014to2016 (accessed 6 July 2021).

3 J.L. Angel, 'The Bases of Paleodemography', *American Journal of Physical Anthropology*, 30, 1969, 427–38.

4 J. Whitley, 'Gender and hierarchy in early Athens: The strange case of the disappearance of the rich female grave', *Mètis. Anthropologie des mondes grecs anciens*, 1996, 209–32.

5 B.W. Frier, 'Demography', in *The Cambridge Ancient History XI: The High Empire, A.D. 70–192*, ed. Peter Garnsey, Alan K. Bowman and Dominic Rathbone, Cambridge University Press: Cambridge, 2000, pp. 787–816.

6 R.S. Bagnall and B.W. Frier, *The Demography of Roman Egypt*, Cambridge University Press: Cambridge, 2006.

7 B.W. Frier, 'Roman Life Expectancy: Ulpian's Evidence', *Harvard Studies in Classical Philology*, 86, 1982, 213–51.

8 P. Pflaumer, 'A Demometric Analysis of Ulpian's Table', *JSM Proceedings*, 2014, 405–19.

9 R. Duncan-Jones, *Structure and Scale in the Roman Economy*, Cambridge University Press: Cambridge, 1990, pp. 100–1.

10 M. Morris, *A Great and Terrible King: Edward I and the Forging of Britain*, Windmill Books: London, 2008.

11 S.N. DeWitte, 'Setting the Stage for Medieval Plague: Pre-Black DeathTrends in Survival and Mortality', *American Journal of Physical Anthropology* 158, 2015, 441–51.

12 The Human Mortality Database, 2018,https://www.mortality.org/hmd/FRATNP/STATS/Eoper.txt

13 L. Alkema et al., 'Probabilistic projections of the total fertility rate for all countries', *Demography*, 48, 2011, 815–39.

14 S. Harper, *How Population Change Will Transform Our World*, Oxford University Press: Oxford, 2016.

15 The World Bank, 'DataBank', 2019, https://databank.worldbank.org/home.aspx

16 UNICEF, 'Child Mortality Estimates', 2019, https://childmortality.org/data

17 J.S.N. Anderson and S. Schneider, 'Brazilian Demographic Transition and the Strategic Role of Youth', *Espace Populations Sociétés* [Online], 2015, http://eps.revues.org/

18 Causes_of_Death, 'Leading Causes of death in Ethiopia', 2017, http://causesofdeathin.com/causes-of-death-in-ethiopia/2 (accessed 6 July 2021).

19 S.E. Vollset et al., 'Fertility, mortality, migration, and population scenarios for 195 countries and territories from 2017 to 2100: a forecasting analysis for the Global Burden of Disease Study', *The Lancet* 2020, 396, 1285–1306

20 TES_Educational_Resources, 'World Statistics: GDP and Life Expectancy', 2013, https://www.tes.com/teaching-resource/worldstatistics-gdp-and-life-expectancy-6143776# (accessed 6 July 2021).

21 OECD, 'Life expectancy at birth', OECD Publishing: Paris, 2015.

22 E.C. Schneider, 'Health Care as an Ongoing Policy Project', *New England Journal of Medicine*, 383, 2020, 405–8.

23 J.A. Schoenman, 'The Concentration of Health Care Spending', *NIHCM Foundation Brief* [Online], 2012.

24 S.H. Preston, 'The changing relation between mortality and level of economic development (Reprinted from Population Studies, Vol. 29, July 1975)', *International Journal of Epidemiology*, 36, 2007, 484–90.

25 D.E. Bloom and D. Canning, 'Commentary: The Preston Curve 30 years on: still sparking fires', *International Journal of Epidemiology*, 36, 2007, 498–9.

26 M.J. Husain, 'Revisiting the Preston Curve: An Analysis of the Joint Evolution of Income and Life Expectancy in the 20th Century', 2011, https://www.keele.ac.uk/media/keeleuniversity/ri/risocsci/docs/economics/workingpapers/LeY_KeeleEconWP_JamiHusain.pdf

27 J.W. Lynch et al., 'Income inequality and mortality: importance to health of individual income, psychosocial environment, or material conditions', *British Medical Journal*, 320, 2000, 1, 200–4.

28 P. Martikainen et al., 'Psychosocial determinants of health in social epidemiology', *International Journal of Epidemiology*, 31, 2002, 1,091–3.

29 R. Wilkinson and K. Pickett, *The Spirit Level: Why Equality is Better for Everyone*, Penguin, 2010.

PART II

1 J. Snow, 'On the Mode of Communication of Cholera', *J. Churchill* 1849.

4 THE BLACK DEATH

1 World Health Organization, 'Global Health Observatory (GHO) data', 2019, https://www.who.int/gho/mortality_burden_disease/life_tables/situation_trends/en/ (accessed 6 July 2021).

2 A.M.T. Moore et al., *Village on the Euphrates: From Foraging to Farming at Abu Hureyra*, Oxford University Press: Oxford, 2000.

3 A. Mummert et al., 'Stature and robusticity during the agricultural transition: Evidence from the bioarchaeological record', *Economics & Human Biology*, 9, 2011, 284–301.

4 J.C. Scott, *Against the Grain*, Yale University Press: Yale, CT, 2017.

5 L.H. Taylor et al., 'Risk factors for human disease emergence', *Philosophical Transactions of the Royal Society B: Biological Sciences*, 356, 2001, 983–9.

6 W. Farber, 'Health Care and Epidemics in Antiquity: The Example of Ancient Mesopotamia', in *Health Care and Epidemics in Antiquity: The Example of Ancient Mesopotamia*, Oriental Institute, 2006.

7 W.R. Thompson, 'Complexity, Diminishing Marginal Returns, and Serial Mesopotamian Fragmentation', *Journal of World-Systems Research*, 3, 2004, 613–52.

8 K.R. Nemet-Nejat, *Daily Life in Ancient Mesopotamia*, Hendrickson: Peabody, MA, 1998.

9 D.C. Stathakopoulos, *Famine and Pestilence in the late Roman and early Byzantine Empire*, Routledge: Abingdon, 2004.

10 E. Burke and K. Pomeranz, *The Environment and World History*, University of California Press: Oakland, CA, 2009.

11 G.J. Armelagos et al., 'The Origins of Agriculture – Population-Growth During a Period of Declining Health', *Population and Environment*, 13, 1991, 9–22.

12 J.M. Diamond, 'The Worst Mistake in the History of the Human Race', 1999, https://www.discovermagazine.com/planet-earth/the-worstmistake-in-the-history-of-the-human-race (accessed 6 July 2021).

13 N.P. Evans et al., 'Quantification of drought during the collapse of the classic Maya civilization', *Science*, 361, 2018, 498–501.

14 W.T. Treadgold, *A Concise History of Byzantium*, Palgrave: Basingstoke, 2001.

15 A. Hashemi Shahraki et al., 'Plague in Iran: its history and current status', *Journal of Epidemiology and Community Health*, 38, 2016, e2016033-e2016033.

16 W. Naphy and A. Spicer, *The Black Death. A History of Plagues 1345–1730*, Tempus Publishing: Stroud, UK, 2000.

17 G.D. Sussman, 'Was the black death in India and China?', *Bulletin of the History of Medicine*, 85, 2011, 319–55.

18 L. Wade, 'Did Black Death strike sub-Saharan Africa?', *Science*, 363, 2019, 1022.

19 M. Wheelis, 'Biological warfare at the 1346 Siege of Caffa', *Emerging Infectious Diseases*, 8, 2002, 971–5.

20 R. Horrox, *The Black Death*, Manchester University Press, 1994, pp. 14–26.

21 L.H. Nelson, 'The Great Famine (1315–1317) and the Black Death (1346–1351)', 2017, http://www.vlib.us/medieval/lectures/black_death.html (accessed 6 July 2021).

22 O.J. Benedictow, 'The Black Death: The Greatest Catastrophe Ever', *History Today*, 55, 2005.

23 P. Daileader, *The Late Middle Ages*, The Teaching Company, 2007.

24 S. Cohn, 'Patterns of Plague in Late Medieval and Early-Modern Europe', in *The Routledge History of Disease*, Routledge: Abingdon, UK and New York, 2017, pp. 165–82.

25 W. Jewell, *Historical Sketches of Quarantine*, T.K. and P.G. Collins: Philadelphia, 1857.

26 S.M. Stuard, *A State of Deference: Ragusa/Dubrovnik in the Medieval Centuries*, Philadelphia: University of Pennsylvania Press, 1992.

27 P.A. Mackowiak and P.S. Sehdev, 'The Origin of Quarantine', *Clinical Infectious Diseases*, 35, 2002, 1071–2.

28 K.I. Bos et al., 'Eighteenth century Yersinia pestis genomes reveal the long-term persistence of an historical plague focus', *Elife*, 5, 2016.

29 C.A. Devaux, 'Small oversights that led to the Great Plague of Marseille (1720–1723): Lessons from the past', *Infection Genetics and Evolution*, 14, 2013, 169–85.

30 D.J. Grimes, 'Koch's Postulates – Then and Now', *Microbe*, 1, 2006, 223–8.

31 E. Marriott, *Plague*, Metropolitan Books/Henry Holt & Co: New York, 2003.

32 M. Simond et al., 'Paul-Louis Simond and his discovery of plague transmission by rat fleas: a centenary', *Journal of the Royal Society of Medicine*, 91, 1998, 101–4.

33 D. Wootton, *Bad Medicine: Doctors Doing Harm Since Hippocrates*, Oxford University Press, 2007, p. 127.

34 C. Demeure et al., 'Yersinia pestis and plague: an updated view on evolution, virulence determinants, immune subversion, vaccination and diagnostics', *Microbes and Infection*, 21, 2019, 202–12.

35 G. Alfani and C. Ó Gráda, 'The timing and causes of famines in Europe', *Nature Sustainability* 1, 2018, 283–8.

36 D.M. Wagner et al., 'Yersinia pestis and the Plague of Justinian 541–543 AD: a genomic analysis', *Lancet Infectious Diseases*, 14, 2014, 319–26.

37 G.A. Eroshenko et al., 'Yersinia pestis strains of ancient phylogenetic branch 0.ANT are widely spread in the high-mountain plague foci of Kyrgyzstan', *PLoS One*, 12, 2017, e0187230-e0187230.

38 P.D. Damgaard et al., '137 ancient human genomes from across the Eurasian steppes', *Nature*, 557, 2018, 369–74.

39 D.W. Anthony, *The horse, the wheel, and language: How Bronze-Age riders from the Eurasian steppes shaped the modern world*, Princeton University Press, 2007.

40 N. Rascovan et al., 'Emergence and Spread of Basal Lineages of Yersinia pestis during the Neolithic Decline', *Cell*, 176, 2019, 1–11.

41 S. Rasmussen et al., 'Early Divergent Strains of Yersinia pestis in Eurasia 5,000 Years Ago', *Cell*, 163, 2015, 571–82.

42 J. Manco, *Ancestral Journeys: The Peopling of Europe from the First Venturers to the Vikings*, Thames and Hudson: London, 2015.

43 S.K. Verma and U. Tuteja, 'Plague Vaccine Development: Current Research and Future Trends', *Frontiers in Immunology*, 7, 2016.

44 A. Guiyoule et al., 'Transferable plasmid-mediated resistance to streptomycin in a clinical isolate of Yersinia pestis', *Emerging Infectious Diseases*, 7, 2001, 43–8.

45 T.J. Welch et al., 'Multiple Antimicrobial Resistance in Plague: An Emerging Public Health Risk', *PLoS One*, 2, 2007, e309.

5 THE MILKMAID'S HAND

1 N. Barquet and P. Domingo, 'Smallpox: The triumph over the most terrible of the ministers of death', *Annals of Internal Medicine*, 127, 1997, 635–42.

2 S. Riedel, 'Edward Jenner and the history of smallpox and vaccination', *Proceedings (Baylor University Medical Center)*, 18, 2005, 21–5.

3 A.S. Lyons and R.J. Petrucelli, *Medicine – An Illustrated History*, Abradale Press, Harry N. Abrams Inc: New York, 1987.

4 A.G. Carmichael and A.G. Silverstein, 'Smallpox in Europe before the Seventeenth Century: Virulent Killer or Benign Disease?', *Journal of the History of Medicine and Allied Sciences*, 42, 1987, 147–68.

5 R. Ganev, 'Milkmaids, ploughmen, and sex in eighteenth-century Britain', *Journal of the History of Sexuality*, 16, 2007, 40–67.

6 E. Jenner, *An Inquiry into the Causes and Effects of Variolæ Vaccinæ*, Samuel Cooley, 1798.

7 J.F. Hammarsten et al., 'Who discovered smallpox vaccination? Edward Jenner or Benjamin Jesty?', *Transactions of the American Climatological Association*, 90, 1979, 44–55.

8 P.J. Pead, 'Benjamin Jesty: new light in the dawn of vaccination', *The Lancet*, 362, 2003, 2,104–9.

9 The_Jenner_Trust, 'Dr Jenner's House Museum and Gardens', 2020, https://jennermuseum.com/ (accessed 22 June 2020).

10 J. Romeo, 'How Children Took the Smallpox Vaccine around the World', 2020, https://daily.jstor.org/how-children-took-the-smallpox vaccine-around-the-world/ (accessed 22 June 2020).

11 C. Mark and J.G. Rigau-Pérez, 'The World's First Immunization Campaign: The Spanish Smallpox Vaccine Expedition, 1803–1813', *Bulletin of the History of Medicine*, 83, 2009, 63–94.

12 Editorial, 'The spectre of smallpox lingers', *Nature*, 560, 2018, 281.

13 World Health Organization, 'Global polio eradication initiative applauds WHO African region for wild polio-free certification', 2020, https://www.who.int/news/item/25-08-2020-global-polio-eradicatio ninitiative-applauds-who-african-region-for-wild-polio-freecertificat ion (accessed 6 July 2021).

14 F. Godlee et al., 'Wakefield's article linking MMR vaccine and autism was fraudulent', *British Medical Journal (BMJ)*, 342, 2011.

15 R. Dobson, 'Media misled the public over the MMR vaccine, study says', *BMJ*, 326, 2003, 1,107.

16 Centers for Disease Control and Prevention, 'Historical Comparisons of Vaccine-Preventable Disease Morbidity in the U.S. – Comparison of 20th Century Annual Morbidity and Current Morbidity: Vaccine-Preventable Diseases', 2018, https://stacks.cdc.gov/view/cdc/58586 (accessed 4 August 2021).

17 US Food and Drug Administration, 'First FDA-approved vaccine for the prevention of Ebola virus disease, marking a critical milestone in public health preparedness and response', 2019, https://www.fda.gov/ news-events/press-announcements/first-fda-approved-vaccinepre vention-ebola-virus-disease-marking-critical-milestone-publichealth (accessed 6 July 2021).

18 A. Gagnon et al., 'Age-Specific Mortality During the 1918 Influenza Pandemic: Unravelling the Mystery of High Young Adult Mortality', *PLoS One*, 8, 2013, e69586.

19 M. Worobey et al., 'Genesis and pathogenesis of the 1918 pandemic H1N1 influenza A virus', *Proceedings of the National Academy of Sciences of the USA*, 111, 2014, 8,107–12.

20 C.H. Ross, 'Maurice Ralph Hilleman (1919–2005)', *The Embryo Project Encyclopedia* [Online], 2017.

21 A.E. Jerse et al., 'Vaccines against gonorrhea: Current status and future challenges', *Vaccine*, 32, 2014, 1,579–87.

6 TYPHUS AND TYPHOID IN THE SLUMS OF LIVERPOOL

1 H. Southall, 'A Vision of Britain Through Time: 1801 Census', 2017, http://www.visionofbritain.org.uk/census/GB1801ABS_1/1 (accessed 6 July 2021).

2 Anon., *The Economist*, 1848.

3 S. Halliday, 'Duncan of Liverpool: Britain's first Medical Officer', *Journal of Medical Biography*, 11, 2003, 142–9.

4 W. Gratzer, *Terrors of the Table: The Curious History of Nutrition*, Oxford University Press: Oxford, 2005.

5 E. Chadwick, *Report on the Sanitary Conditions of the Labouring Poor of Great Britain*, W. Clowes & Son: London, 1843, p. 661.

6 S. Halliday, *The Great Filth: The War Against Disease in Victorian England*, Sutton Publishing: Stroud, Gloucestershire, UK, 2007.

7 ONS, 'How has life expectancy changed over time?', 2015, https://www.ons.gov.uk/peoplepopulationandcommunity/birthsdeathsandmarriages/lifeexpectancies/articles/howhaslifeexpectancychangedovertime/2015-09-09 (accessed 6 July 2021).

8 S. Bance, 'The "hospital and cemetery of Ireland": The Irish and Disease in Nineteenth-Century Liverpool', 2014, https://warwick.ac.uk/fac/arts/history/chm/outreach/migration/backgroundreading/disease (accessed 6 July 2021).

9 A. Karlins, 'Kitty Wilkinson – "Saint of the Slums"', 2015, http://www.theheroinecollective.com/kitty-wilkinson-saint-of-the-slums/ (accessed 6 July 2021).

10 K. Youngdahl, 'Typhus, War, and Vaccines', 2016, https://www.historyofvaccines.org/content/blog/typhus-war-and-vaccines (accessed 6 July 2021).

11 A. Allen, *The Fantastic Laboratory of Dr. Weigl: How Two Brave Scientists Battled Typhus and Sabotaged the Nazis*, W.W. Norton: London, 2015.

12 H.R. Cox and E.J. Bell, 'Epidemic and Endemic Typhus: Protective Value for Guinea Pigs of Vaccines Prepared from Infected Tissues of the Developing Chick Embryo', *Public Health Reports (1896–1970)*, 55, 1940, 110–15.

13 B.E. Mahon et al., 'Effectiveness of typhoid vaccination in US travelers', *Vaccine*, 32, 2014, 3,577–9.

7 THE BLUE DEATH

1   Centers for Disease Control and Prevention, 'Cholera in Haiti', 2021, https://www.cdc.gov/cholera/haiti/ (accessed 6 July 2021).

2   S.J. Snow, 'Commentary: Sutherland, Snow and water: the transmission of cholera in the nineteenth century', *International Journal of Epidemiology*, 31, 2002, 908–11.

3   S. Almagro-Moreno et al., 'Intestinal Colonization Dynamics of Vibrio cholerae', *PLoS Pathogens*, 11, 2015.

4   S.N. De et al., 'An experimental study of the action of cholera toxin', *Journal of Pathology and Bacteriology*, 63, 1951, 707–17.

5   S.N. De and D.N. Chatterje, 'An experimental study of the mechanism of action of Vibriod cholerae on the intestinal mucous membrane', *Journal of Pathology and Bacteriology*, 66, 1953, 559–62.

6   K. Bharati and N.K. Ganguly, 'Cholera toxin: A paradigm of a multifunctional protein', *Indian Journal of Medical Research*, 133, 2011, 179–87.

7   P.K. Gilbert, 'On Cholera in Nineteenth-Century England', *BRANCH:Britain, Representation and Nineteenth-Century History* [Online], 2012, http://www.branchcollective.org/?ps_articles=pamela-k-gilberton-cholera-in-nineteenth-century-england (accessed 24 November 2020).

8   M. Pelling, *Cholera, Fever and English Medicine, 1825–1865*, Clarendon Press: Wotton-under-Edge, 1978, pp. 4–5.

9   Royal College of Physicians of London, 'Report of the General Board of Health on the Epidemic Cholera of 1848 and 1849', *British and Foreign Medico-Chirurgical Review*, 1851, 1–40.

10 J. Snow, *On the Mode of Communication of Cholera*, John Churchill: London, 1849.

11 S. Garfield, *On the Map*, Profile Books: London, 2012.

12 R.R. Frerichs, 'Reverend Henry Whitehead', 2019, https://www.ph.ucla.
    edu/epi/snow/whitehead.html (accessed 6 July 2021).

13 H. Whitehead, *Special investigation of Broad Street*, 1854.

14 R.R. Frerichs, 'Birth and Death Cerificates of Index Case', 2019, https://
    www.ph.ucla.edu/epi/snow/indexcase2.html (accessed 6 July 2021).

15 F. Pacini, 'Osservazioni microscopiche e deduzioni patologiche sul
    cholera asiatico', *Gazzetta Medica Italiana: Toscana*, 4, 1854, 397–401,
    405–12.

16 M. Bentivoglio and P. Pacini, 'Filippo Pacini: A Determined Observer',
    Brain Research Bulletin, 38, 1995, 161–5.

17 N. Howard-Jones, 'Robert Koch and the cholera vibrio: a centenary',
    BMJ, 288, 1984, 379–81.

18 Centers for Disease Control and Prevention, 'Cholera – Vibrio cholerae
    infection. Treatment', 2018.

8 CHILDBIRTH

1   C. Niemitz, 'The evolution of the upright posture and gait– a review and
    a new synthesis', *Naturwissenschaften*, 97, 2010, 241–63.

2   L. Brock, 'Newborn horse stands up for the first time', 2011, https://
    www.youtube.com/watch?v=g1Qc28PfKpU (accessed 6 July 2021).

3   P.M. Dunn, 'The Chamberlen family (1560–1728) and obstetric forceps',
    Archives of Disease in Childhood – Fetal and Neonatal Edition, 81, 1999,
    F232–F234.

4   D. Pearce, 'Charles Delucena Meigs (1792–1869)', 2018, https://www.
    general-anaesthesia.com/people/charlesdelucenameigs.html (accessed 6
    July 2021).

5   I. Loudon, *The Tragedy of Childbed Fever*, Oxford University Press:
    Oxford, 2000.

6   P.M. Dunn, 'Dr Alexander Gordon (1752–99) and contagious puerperal
    fever', *Archives of Disease in Childhood*, 78, 1998, F232–F233.

7   O. Holmes, 'On the contagiousness of puerperal fever', *New England
    Quarterly Journal of Medicine and Surgery*, 1, 1842, 503–30.

8   E.P. Hoyt, *Improper Bostonian: Dr. Oliver Wendell Holmes*, William
    Morrow & Co: New York, 1979.

9   I. Semmelweis, *The Etiology, Concept, and Prophylaxis of Childbed
    Fever*, 1861.

10 S. Halliday, *The Great Filth: The War Against Disease in Victorian
    England*, Sutton Publishing: Stroud, Gloucestershire, 2007.

9 DEADLY ANIMALS

1 CBS News, 'The 20 Deadliest Animals on Earth', 2020, https://www.cbsnews.com/pictures/the-20-deadliest-animals-on-earth-ranked/ (accessed 15 June 2020).

2 H. Ritchie and M. Roser, 'Our World in Data: Deaths by Animal', 2018, https://ourworldindata.org/causes-of-death#deaths-by-animal (accessed 15 June 2020).

3 J. Flegr et al., 'Toxoplasmosis – a global threat: Correlation of latent toxoplasmosis with specific disease burden in a set of 88 countries', *PLoS One*, 9, 2014, e90203.

4 G. Desmonts and J. Couvreur, 'Congenital toxoplasmosis: A prospective study of 378 pregnancies', *New England Journal of Medicine*, 290, 1974, 1,110–16.

5 Centers for Disease Control and Prevention, 'Parasites – Guinea Worm: Biology', 2015, https://www.cdc.gov/parasites/guineaworm/biology.html (accessed 6 July 2021).

6 The Carter Center, 'Guinea Worm Eradication Program', 2021, https://www.cartercenter.org/health/guinea_worm/index.html (accessed 6 July 2021).

7 World Health Organization, 'Dracunculiasis eradication: global surveillance summary, 2020', 2021, https://www.who.int/dracunculiasis/eradication/en (accessed 6 July 2021).

8 World Health Organization, 'Dengue and severe dengue', 2021, https://www.who.int/news-room/fact-sheets/detail/dengue-and-severedengue (accessed 6 July 2021).

9 Centers for Disease Control and Prevention, 'Yellow Fever', 2018, https://www.cdc.gov/globalhealth/newsroom/topics/yellowfever/index.html (accessed 16 June 2020).

10 World Health Organization, 'Yellow Fever', 2019, https://www.who.int/news-room/fact-sheets/detail/yellow-fever (accessed 6 July 2021).

11 P.H. Futcher, 'Notes on Insect Contagion', *Bulletin of the Institute of the History of Medicine*, 4, 1936, 536–58.

12 B.S. Kakkilaya, 'Malaria Site. Journey of Scientific Discoveries', 2015, https://www.malariasite.com/history-science/ (accessed 26 June 2020).

13 E. Pongponratn et al., 'An ultrastructural study of the brain in fatal Plasmodium falciparum malaria', *American Journal of Tropical Medicine and Hygiene*, 69, 2003, 345–59.

14 Institute of Medicine (US) Committee on the Economics of Antimalarial Drugs, 'The Parasite, the Mosquito, and the Disease', in *Saving Lives,*

Buying Time: Economics of Malaria Drugs in an Age of Resistance, ed. K.J. Arrow, C. Panosian and H. Gelband, National Academies Press: Washington, DC, 2004, pp. 136 –67.

15 Centers for Disease Control and Prevention, 'Malaria Disease', 2019, https://www.cdc.gov/malaria/about/disease.html (accessed 18 June 2020).

16 F.E.G. Cox, 'History of the discovery of the malaria parasites and their vectors', *Parasites & Vectors*, 3, 2010, 5.

17 Institute of Medicine (US) Committee on the Economics of Antimalarial Drugs, 'A Brief History of Malaria', in *Saving Lives, Buying Time*, pp. 136–67.

18 E. Faerstein and W. Winkelstein, Jr., 'Carlos Juan Finlay: Rejected, Respected, and Right', *Epidemiology*, 21, 2010.

19 UNESCO, 'Biography of Carlos J. Finlay', 2017, http://www.unesco.org/new/en/natural-sciences/science-technology/basic-sciences/lifesciences/carlos-j-finlay-unesco-prize-for-microbiology/biography/ (accessed 24 June 2020).

20 A.N. Clements and R.E. Harbach, 'History of the discovery of the mode of transmission of yellow fever virus', *Journal of Vector Ecology*, 2017, 42, 208–22.

21 W. Reed et al., 'Experimental yellow fever', *Transactions of the Association of American Physicians*, 1901, 16, 45–71.

22 W.L. Craddock, 'The Achievements of William Crawford Gorgas', *Military Medicine*, 1997, 162, 325–7.

23 D. McCullough, *The Path Between the Seas: The Creation of the Panama Canal, 1870–1914*, Simon & Schuster: New York, 1977.

24 P.D. Curtin, *Death by Migration: Europe's Encounter with the Tropical World in the Nineteenth Century*, Cambridge University Press: Cambridge, 2008.

25 R. Carter and K.N. Mendis, 'Evolutionary and historical aspects of the burden of malaria', *Clinical Microbiology Reviews*, 2002, 15, 564–94.

26 J. Whitfield, 'Portrait of a serial killer', *Nature* [Online], 2002. https://doi.org/10.1038/news021001-6 (accessed 3 October 2002).

27 C. Shiff, 'Integrated approach to malaria control', *Clinical Microbiology Reviews*, 2002, 15, 278–93.

28 B. Greenwood and T. Mutabingwa, 'Malaria in 2002', *Nature*, 2002, 415, 670–2.

29 R.L. Miller et al., 'Diagnosis of Plasmodium Falciparum Infections in Mummies Using the Rapid Manual Parasight (TM)-F Test', *Transactions of the Royal Society of Tropical Medicine and Hygiene*, 1994, 88, 31–2.

30 W. Liu et al., 'Origin of the human malaria parasite Plasmodium falciparum in gorillas', *Nature*, 2010, 467, 420–5.

31 D.E. Loy et al., 'Out of Africa: origins and evolution of the human malaria parasites Plasmodium falciparum and Plasmodium vivax', *International Journal for Parasitology*, 2017, 47, 87–97.

32 G. Höher et al., 'Molecular basis of the Duffy blood group system', *Blood Transfusion*, 2018, 16, 93–100.

33 G.B. de Carvalho and G.B. de Carvalho, 'Duffy Blood Group System and the malaria adaptation process in humans', *Revista Brasileira de Hematologia e Hemoterapia*, 2011, 33, 55–64.

34 R.E. Howes et al., 'The global distribution of the Duffy blood group', *Nature Communications*, 2011, 2, 266.

35 M.T. Hamblin and A. Di Rienzo, 'Detection of the signature of natural selection in humans: evidence from the Duffy blood group locus', *American Journal of Human Genetics*, 2000, 66, 1,669–79.

36 W. Liu et al., 'African origin of the malaria parasite Plasmodium vivax', *Nature Communications*, 2014, 5, 3,346.

37 F. Prugnolle et al., 'Diversity, host switching and evolution of *Plasmodium vivax* infecting African great apes', *Proceedings of the National Academy of Sciences of the USA*, 2013, 110, 8,123–8.

38 A. Demogines et al., 'Species-specific features of DARC, the primate receptor for Plasmodium vivax and Plasmodium knowlesi', *Molecular Biology and Evolution*, 2012, 29, 445–9.

39 A. Zijlstra and J.P. Quigley, 'The DARC side of metastasis: Shining a light on KAI1-mediated metastasis suppression in the vascular tunnel', *Cancer Cell*, 2006, 10, 177–8.

40 X.-F. Liu et al., 'Correlation between Duffy blood group phenotype and breast cancer incidence', *BMC Cancer*, 2012, 12, 374–9.

41 K. Horne and I.J. Woolley, 'Shedding light on DARC: the role of the Duffy antigen/receptor for chemokines in inflammation, infection and malignancy', *Inflammation Research*, 2009, 58, 431–5.

42 G.J. Kato et al., 'Sickle cell disease', *Nature Reviews Disease Primers*, 2018, 4, 18,010.

43 Centers for Disease Control and Prevention, 'Elimination of Malaria in the United States (1947–1951)', 2018, https://www.cdc.gov/malaria/about/history/elimination_us.html (accessed 6 July 2021).

44 Centers for Disease Control and Prevention, 'Malaria's Impact Worldwide', 2021, https://www.cdc.gov/malaria/malaria_worldwide/impact.html (accessed 6 July 2021).

45 M. Wadman, 'Malaria vaccine achieves striking early success', *Science*, 2021, 372, 448.

46 M. Scudellari, 'Self-destructing mosquitoes and sterilized rodents: the promise of gene drives', *Nature*, 2019, 571, 160–2.

47 S. James et al., 'Pathway to Deployment of Gene Drive Mosquitoes as a Potential Biocontrol Tool for Elimination of Malaria in Sub-Saharan Africa: Recommendations of a Scientific Working Group', *American Journal of Tropical Medicine and Hygiene* 2018, 98, 1–49.

48 E. Waltz, 'First genetically modified mosquitoes released in the United States', *Nature*, 2021, 593, 175–6.

49 R.G.A. Feachem et al., 'Malaria eradication within a generation: ambitious, achievable, and necessary', *The Lancet*, 2019, 394, 1,056–112.

10 THE MAGIC BULLET

1 R. Woods and P.R.A. Hinde, 'Mortality in Victorian England: Models and Patterns', *Journal of Interdisciplinary History*, 1987, 18, 27–54.

2 R.W. Fogel, *The Escape from Hunger and Premature Death, 1700–2100: Europe, America, and the Third World*, Cambridge University Press: Cambridge, 2004.

3 F. Bosch and L. Rosich, 'The contributions of Paul Ehrlich to pharmacology: A tribute on the occasion of the centenary of his Nobel Prize', *Pharmacology*, 2008, 82, 171–9.

4 S. Riethmiller, 'From Atoxyl to Salvarsan: Searching for the magic bullet', *Chemotherapy*, 2005, 51, 234–42.

5 F.R. Schaudinn and E. Hoffmann, 'Vorläufiger Bericht über das Vorkommen von Spirochaeten in syphilitischen Krankheitsprodukten und bei Papillomen' [Preliminary report on the occurrence of Spirochaetes in syphilitic chancres and papillomas], *Arbeiten aus dem Kaiserlichen Gesundheitsamte*, 1905, 22, 527–34.

6 J. Mann, *The Elusive Magic Bullet: The Search for the Perfect Drug*, Oxford University Press: New York, 1999.

PART III

1 E. Jenner, 'An Inquiry into the Causes and Effects of Variolæ Vaccinæ', Samuel Cooley, 1798.

11 HANSEL AND GRETEL

1 T.R. Malthus, 'An Essay on the Principle of Population As It Affects the Future Improvement of Society, with Remarks on the Speculations of Mr. Goodwin, M. Condorcet and Other Writers', 1st edn, J. Johnson in St. Paul's Churchyard: London, 1798.

2 G. Alfani and C. Ó Gráda, 'The timing and causes of famines in Europe', *Nature Sustainability*, 2018, 1, 283–8.

3 W. Rosen, *The Third Horseman: A Story of Weather, War, and the Famine History Forgot*, Penguin, 2015.

4 C.S. Witham and C. Oppenheimer, 'Mortality in England during the 1783–4 Laki Craters eruption', *Bulletin of Volcanology*, 2004, 67, 15–26.

5 T. Thordarson and S. Self, 'The Laki (Skaftar-Fires) and Grimsvotn Eruptions in 1783–1785', *Bulletin of Volcanology*, 1993, 55, 233–63.

6 T. Thordarson and S. Self, 'Atmospheric and environmental effects of the 1783–1784 Laki eruption: A review and reassessment', *Journal of Geophysical Research: Atmospheres*, 2003, 108.

7 L. Oman et al., 'High-latitude eruptions cast shadow over the African monsoon and the flow of the Nile', *Geophysical Research Letters*, 2006, 33, L18711.

8 C. Ó Gráda, *Famine: A Short History*, Princeton University Press: Princeton, USA, 2009.

9 T. Vorstenbosch et al., 'Famine food of vegetal origin consumed in the Netherlands during World War II', *Journal of Ethnobiology and Ethnomedicine*, 2017, 13.

10 W.W. Farris, *Japan to 1600: A Social and Economic History*, University of Hawaii Press, 2009.

11 J. Aberth, *From the Brink of the Apocalypse: Confronting Famine, War, Plague, and Death in the Later Middle Ages*, Routledge, 2000.

12 A. Keys et al., *The Biology of Human Starvation*, University of Minnesota Press, 1950.

13 L.M. Kalm and R.D. Semba, 'They Starved So That Others Be Better Fed: Remembering Ancel Keys and the Minnesota Experiment', *The Journal of Nutrition*, 2005, 135, 1,347–52.

14 D.R. Curtis and J. Dijkman, 'The escape from famine in the Northern Netherlands: a reconsideration using the 1690s harvest failures and a broader Northwest European perspective', *The Seventeenth Century*, 2017, 1–30.

15 J. Hearfield, 'Roads in the 18th Century', 2012, http://www.johnhearfield.com/History/Roads.htm .

16 Anon, 'Friendly advice to the industrious poor: Receipts for making soups', s.n.: England, 1790.

17 A. Smith, 'An Inquiry into the Nature and Causes of the Wealth of Nations', Strahan & Cadell: London, 1776.

18 A. Sen, *Poverty and Famines: An Essay on Entitlement and Depravation*, Oxford University Press: USA, 1990.

19 A. Sen, *Development as Freedom*, Alfred Knopf: New York, 1999.

20 F. Burchi, 'Democracy, institutions and famines in developing and emerging countries', *Canadian Journal of Development Studies / Revue canadienne d'études du développement*, 2011, 32, 17–31.

21 W.L.S. Churchill, in *The World Crisis*, New York Free Press, 1931, p. 686.

22 G. Kennedy, 'Intelligence and the Blockade, 1914–17: A Study in Administration, Friction and Command', *Intelligence and National Security*, 2007, 22, 699–721.

23 D.A. Janicki, 'The British Blockade During World War I: The Weapon of Deprivation', *Inquiries Journal/Student Pulse* [Online], 2014. http://www.inquiriesjournal.com/a?id=899 (accessed 11 May 2018).

24 I. Zweiniger-Bargielowska et al., *Food and War in Twentieth Century Europe*, Burlington: Ashgate Publishing Limited, 2001, p. 15.

25 I. Materna and W. Gottschalk, *Geschichte Berlins von den Anfängen bis 1945*, Dietz Verlag Berlin, 1987, p. 540.

26 W. Philpott, *War of Attrition: Fighting the First World War*, Overlook Press, 2014.

27 W. Van Der Kloot, 'Ernst Starling's Analysis of the Energy Balance of the German People During the Blockade 1914–1919', *Notes and Records of the Royal Society of London*, 2003, 57, 189–90.

28 H. Strachan, 'The First World War', in *The First World War*, Penguin: New York, 2005, p. 215.

29 C.P. Vincent, *The Politics of Hunger: The Allied Blockade of Germany, 1915–1919*, Ohio University Press, 1986.

30 L. Grebler, 'The Cost of the World War to Germany and Austria-Hungary', in *The Cost of the World War to Germany and Austria-Hungary*, Yale University Press, 1940, p. 78.

31 M.E. Cox, 'Hunger games: or how the Allied blockade in the First World War deprived German children of nutrition, and Allied food aid subsequently saved them', *Economic History Review*, 2015, 68, 600–31.

32 C.E. Strickland, 'American aid to Germany, 1919 to 1921', *Wisconsin Magazine of History*, 1962, 45, 256–70.

33 V.J.B. Martins et al., 'Long-Lasting Effects of Undernutrition', *International Journal of Environmental Research and Public Health*, 2011, 8, 1,817–46.

34 D.J.P. Barker, 'Maternal nutrition, fetal nutrition, and disease in later life', *Nutrition*, 1997, 13, 807–13.

35 C. Li and L.H. Lumey, 'Exposure to the Chinese famine of 1959–61 in early life and long-term health conditions: a systematic review and metaanalysis', *International Journal of Epidemiology*, 2017, 46, 1,157–70.

36 L.H. Lumey et al., 'Association between type 2 diabetes and prenatal exposure to the Ukraine famine of 1932–33: a retrospective cohort study', *Lancet Diabetes & Endocrinology*, 2015, 3, 787–94.

37 L.H. Lumey et al., 'Prenatal Famine and Adult Health', in *Annual Review of Public Health*, Vol. 32, ed. J.E. Fielding, R.C. Brownson and L.W. Green, Annual Reviews: Palo Alto, 2011, pp. 237–62.

38 D. Wiesmann, 'A global hunger index: measurement concept, ranking of countries, and trends', *FCND discussion papers*, International Food Policy Research Institute (IFPRI), 2006, 212.

39 P. French, *North Korea: State of Paranoia*, Zed Books, 2014.

40 BBC News, 'North Korea hunger: Two in five undernourished, says UN', 2017, https://www.bbc.co.uk/news/world-asia-39349726 (accessed 6 July 2021).

41 NationMaster, 'Current military expenditures as an estimated percent of gross domestic product', 2007. https://www.nationmaster.com/country-info/stats/Military/Expenditures/Percent-of-GDP

42 A. Rice, 'The Peanut Solution', *New York Times Magazine*, 2010.

12 A TREATISE ON THE SCURVY

1 R.W. Fogel, *The Escape from Hunger and Premature Death, 1700–2100: Europe, America, and the Third World*, Cambridge University Press: Cambridge, 2004.

2 G.J.Mulder,'UeberdieZusammensetzungeinigerthierischenSubstanzen', *Journal für praktische Chemie*, 1839, 16, 129.

3 J.F. von Liebig and W. Gregory, *Researches on the chemistry of food, and the motion of the juices in the animal body*, Taylor & Wharton: London, 1848.

4 J. Sire de Joinville, *Histoire de Saint-Louis écrite par son compagnon d'armes le Sire de Joinville*, Paris, 2006.

5 W. Gratzer, *Terrors of the Table: The Curious History of Nutrition*, Oxford University Press: Oxford, 2005.

6 J. Lind, *A Treatise on the Scurvy in Three Parts*, Sands, Murray and Cochran for A. Kincaid and A. Donaldson: Edinburgh, 1753.

7 M. Bartholomew, 'James Lind's Treatise of the Scurvy (1753)', *Postgraduate Medical Journal*, 2002, 78, 695–6.

8 D.I. Harvie, *Limey: The Conquest of Scurvy*, Sutton Publishing: Stroud, 2002.

9 K.J. Carpenter, 'The Discovery of Vitamin C', *Annals of Nutrition & Metabolism*, 2012, 61, 259–64.

10 A.Cherry-Garrard,*The World Journey in the World*,Vintage:London,2010.

11 K.J. Carpenter et al., 'Experiments That Changed Nutritional Thinking', *Nutrition*, 1997, 127, 1017S–1053S.

12 L.R. McDowell, *Vitamin History, the Early Years*, First Edition Design Publishing: Sarasota, FL, 2013.

13 Y. Sugiyama and A. Seita, 'Kanehiro Takaki and the control of beriberi in the Japanese Navy', *Journal of the Royal Society of Medicine*, 2013, 106, 332–4.

14 A. Holst and T. Frolich, 'Experimental studies relating to ship-beri-beri and scurvy', *Journal of Hygiene*, 1907, 7, 634–71.

15 G. Drouin et al., 'The Genetics of Vitamin C Loss in Vertebrates', *Current Genomics*, 2011, 12, 371–8.

16 World Health Organization, 'Investing in the future: A united call to action on vitamin and mineral deficiencies', 2009. https://www. who.int/vmnis/publications/investing_in_the_future.pdf (accessed 17 Sept 2021).

17 H. Ritchie and M. Roser, 'Micronutrient Deficiency', 2019. https:// ourworldindata.org

18 Centers for Disease Control and Prevention, 'Micronutrients', 2021, https://www.cdc.gov/nutrition/micronutrient-malnutrition/index.html (accessed 6 July 2021).

13 THE BODY OF VENUS

1 World Health Organization, 'Overweight and Obesity', 2019. https:// www.who.int/gho/ncd/risk_factors/overweight/en/

2 M. Di Cesare et al., 'Trends in adult body-mass index in 200 countries from 1975 to 2014: a pooled analysis of 1698 population-based measurement studies with 19.2 million participants', *The Lancet*, 2016, 387, 1,377–96.

3 R.W. Fogel, *The Escape from Hunger and Premature Death, 1700–2100: Europe, America, and the Third World*, Cambridge University Press: Cambridge, 2004.

4　G. Eknoyan, 'A history of obesity, or how what was good became ugly and then bad', *Advances in Chronic Kidney Disease*, 2006, 13, 421–7.

5　C.Y. Ye et al., 'Decreased Bone Mineral Density Is an Independent Predictor for the Development of Atherosclerosis: A Systematic Review and Meta-Analysis', *PLoS One*, 2016, 11.

6　World Population Review, 'Kuwait Population 2019', 2019. http://worldpopulationreview.com/countries/kuwait-population (accessed 6 July 2021).

7　S. Al Sabah et al., 'Results from the first Kuwait National Bariatric Surgery Report', *BMC Surgery*, 2020, 20, 292.

8　H. Leow, 'Kuwait', 2019. https://www.everyculture.com/Ja-Ma/Kuwait.html.

9　World Health Organization, 'Obesity', 2021. https://www.who.int/topics/obesity/en/ (accessed 6 July 2021).

10　A.J. Zemski et al., 'Body composition characteristics of elite Australian rugby union athletes according to playing position and ethnicity', *Journal of Sports Sciences*, 2015, 33, 970–8.

11　A.J. Zemski et al., 'Differences in visceral adipose tissue and biochemical cardiometabolic risk markers in elite rugby union athletes of Caucasian and Polynesian descent', *European Journal of Sport Science*, 2020, 20, 691–702.

12　J.S. Friedlaender et al., 'The genetic structure of Pacific islanders', *PLoS Genetics*, 2008, 4.

13　J.M. Diamond, 'The double puzzle of diabetes', *Nature*, 2003, 423, 599–602.

14　J.V. Neel, 'Diabetes Mellitus – A Thrifty Genotype Rendered Detrimental by Progress', *American Journal of Human Genetics*, 1962, 14, 353–362.

15　J.R. Speakman, 'Thrifty genes for obesity, an attractive but flawed idea, and an alternative perspective: the "drifty gene" hypothesis', *International Journal of Obesity*, 2008, 32, 1,611–17.

16　A. Qasim et al., 'On the origin of obesity: identifying the biological, environmental and cultural drivers of genetic risk among human populations', *Obesity Reviews*, 2018, 19, 121–49.

17　R.L. Minster et al., 'A thrifty variant in CREBRF strongly influences body mass index in Samoans', *Nature Genetics*, 2016, 48, 1,049–54.

18　D. Hart and R.W. Sussman, 'Man the Hunted: Primates, Predators, and Human Evolution', Westview Press: Boulder, CO, 2002.

19　Minstero Della Cultura, 'Neanderthal, dalla Grotta Guattari al Circeo nuove incredibili scoperte', 2021. https://cultura.gov.it/neanderthal (accessed 17 May 2021).

20 M. Pigeyre et al., 'Recent progress in genetics, epigenetics and metagenomics unveils the pathophysiology of human obesity', *Clinical Science*, 2016, 130, 943–86.

21 C.W. Kuzawa, 'Adipose tissue in human infancy and childhood: An evolutionary perspective', in *Yearbook of Physical Anthropology*, Vol. 41, ed. C. Ruff, 1998, Wiley-Liss, Inc: New York, 1998, pp. 177–209.

22 C.M. Kitahara et al., 'Association between Class III Obesity (BMI of 40–59 kg/m(2)) and Mortality: A Pooled Analysis of 20 Prospective Studies', *Plos Medicine*, 2014, 11.

23 B. Lauby-Secretan et al., 'Body Fatness and Cancer – Viewpoint of the IARC Working Group', *New England Journal of Medicine*, 2016, 375, 794–8.

24 C.P. Kovesdy et al., 'Obesity and Kidney Disease: Hidden Consequences of the Epidemic', *Canadian Journal of Kidney Health and Disease*, 2017, 4, 2054358117698669-2054358117698669.

25 W.L. Xu et al., 'Midlife overweight and obesity increase late-life dementia risk: A population-based twin study', *Neurology*, 2011, 76, 1,568–74.

26 N.H. Lents, 'Maladaptive By-Product Hypothesis', in *Encyclopedia of Evolutionary Psychological Science*, ed. T.K. Shackelford and V.A. Weekes-Shackelford, Springer International Publishing: Cham, Switzerland, 2019, pp. 1–6.

27 P.A.S. Breslin, 'An Evolutionary Perspective on Food and Human Taste', *Current Biology*, 2013, 23, R409–R418.

28 P.L. Balaresque et al., 'Challenges in human genetic diversity: demographic history and adaptation', *Human Molecular Genetics*, 2007, 16, R134–R139.

29 E. McFadden et al., 'The Relationship Between Obesity and Exposure to Light at Night: Cross-Sectional Analyses of Over 100,000 Women in the Breakthrough Generations Study', *American Journal of Epidemiology*, 2014, 180, 245–50.

30 J. Theorell-Haglow et al., 'Both habitual short sleepers and long sleepers are at greater risk of obesity: a population-based 10-year follow-up in women', *Sleep Medicine*, 2014, 15, 1204–11.

31 J. Wheelwright, 'From Diabetes to Athlete's Foot, Our Bodies Are Maladapted for Modern Life', 2015. https://www.discovermagazine.com/the-sciences/from-diabetes-to-athletes-foot-our-bodies-aremal adapted-for-modern-life (accessed 6 July 2021).

32 New England Centenarian Study, 'Why Study Centenarians? An Overview', 2019. https://www.bumc.bu.edu/centenarian/overview/ (accessed 6 July 2021).

33 B.J. Willcox et al., 'Demographic, phenotypic, and genetic characteristics of centenarians in Okinawa and Japan: Part 1 – centenarians in Okinawa', *Mechanisms of Ageing and Development*, 2017, 165, 75–9.

34 Okinawa Research Center for Longevity Science, 'The Okinawa Centenarian Study', 2019. https://www.orcls.net/ocs

35 B. Schumacher et al., 'The central role of DNA damage in the ageing process', *Nature*, 2021, 592, 695–703.

36 B.J. Willcox et al., 'Caloric restriction, the traditional Okinawan diet, and healthy aging – The diet of the world's longest-lived people and its potential impact on morbidity and life span', in *Healthy Aging and Longevity*, Vol. 1,114, ed. N.J. Weller and S.I.S. Rattan, Wiley-Blackwell: Malden, 2007, pp. 434–55.

37 L. Fontana et al., 'Extending Healthy Life Span – From Yeast to Humans', *Science*, 2010, 328, 321–6.

38 S.Z. Yanovski and J.A. Yanovski, 'Long-term Drug Treatment for Obesity: A Systematic and Clinical Review', *Journal of the American Medical Association*, 2014, 311, 74–86.

39 National Institute of Diabetes and Digestive and Kidney Diseases, 'Prescription Medications to Treat Overweight and Obesity', 2021. https://www.niddk.nih.gov/healthinformation/weight-management/prescription-medications-treatoverweight-obesity (accessed 17 February 2021).

40 J.P.H. Wilding et al., 'Once-Weekly Semaglutide in Adults with Overweight or Obesity', *New England Journal of Medicine*, 2021.

PART IV

1 L. Pasteur, 'Germ Theory and Its Applications to Medicine and Surgery', *Comptes Rendus de l' Academie des Sciences* 1878, 86, 1037–1043.

14 WOODY GUTHRIE AND THE BLONDE ANGEL OF VENEZUELA

1 A. Lange and G.B. Müller, 'Polydactyly in Development, Inheritance, and Evolution', *Quarterly Review of Biology*, 2017, 92, 1–38.

2 J. Klein, *Woody Guthrie: A Life*, Dell Publishing/Random House, Inc.: New York, 1980.

3 Woody Guthrie, 'This Land is Your Land', 1944, https://www.youtube.com/watch?v=wxiMrvDbq3s (accessed 6 July 2021).

4   K.B. Bhattacharyya, 'The story of George Huntington and his disease', *Annals of Indian Academy of Neurology*, 2016, 19, 25–8.

5   G. Huntington 'On Chorea', *Medical and Surgical Reporter of Philadelphia*, 1872, 26, 317–21.

6   J. Huddleston and E.E. Eichler, 'An Incomplete Understanding of Human Genetic Variation', *Genetics*, 2016, 202, 1,251–4.

7   Genomes Project Consortium, 'A global reference for human genetic variation', *Nature*, 2015, 526, 68–74.

8   G. Mendel, 'Versuche über Pflanzenhybriden', *Verhandlungen des naturforschenden Vereines in Brünn*, 1866, IV, 3–47.

9   R. Marantz Henig, *The Monk in the Garden: The Lost and Found Genius of Gregor Mendel, the Father of Genetics*, Houghton Mifflin: Boston, 2001.

10   E.W. Crow and J.F. Crow, '100 Years Ago: Walter Sutton and the Chromosome Theory of Heredity', *Genetics*, 2002, 160, 1–4.

11   C.D. Darlington, 'Meiosis in perspective', *Philosophical Transactions of the Royal Society of London*, 1977, B277, 185–9.

12   N.S. Wexler, 'Huntington's Disease: Advocacy Driving Science', in *Annual Review of Medicine*, Vol. 63, ed. C.T. Caskey, C.P. Austin and J.A. Hoxie, 2012, pp. 1–22.

13   J.F. Gusella et al., 'A Polymorphic DNA Marker Genetically Linked to Huntington's Disease', *Nature*, 1983, 306, 234–8.

14   F. Saudou and S. Humbert, 'The Biology of Huntingtin', *Neuron*, 2016, 89, 910–26.

15   H. Paulson, 'Repeat expansion diseases', *Handbook of clinical neurology*, 2018, 147, 105–23.

16   M. Jimenez-Sanchez et al., 'Huntington's Disease: Mechanisms of Pathogenesis and Therapeutic Strategies', *Cold Spring Harbor Perspectives in Medicine*, 2017, 7.

17   I. Ionis Pharmaceuticals, 'Ionis Pharmaceuticals Licenses IONIS-HTT Rx to Partner Following Successful Phase 1/2a Study in Patients with Huntington's Disease', 2017. http://ir.ionispharma.com/news-releases/news-release-details/ionis-pharmaceuticals-licenses-ionis-htt-rxpartner-following (accessed 6 July 2021).

18   D. Kwon, 'Failure of genetic therapies for Huntington's devastates community', *Nature*, 2021, 180, 593.

19   Z. Li et al., 'Allele-selective lowering of mutant HTT protein by HTT–LC3 linker compounds', *Nature*, 2019, 575, 203–9.

20   D. Grady, 'Haunted by a Gene', *New York Times* [Online], 2020. https://www.nytimes.com/2020/03/10/health/huntingtons-disease-wexler.html

15 DAUGHTERS OF THE KING

1 Genetics Home Reference, 'Fumarase deficiency', 2020. https://ghr.nlm. nih.gov/condition/fumarase-deficiency (accessed 6 July 2021).

2 J. Dougherty, 'Forbidden Fruit', *Phoenix New Times* [Online], 2005. https://www.phoenixnewtimes.com/news/forbidden-fruit-6438448

3 M. Oswaks, 'Tiny Tombstones: Inside the FLDS Graveyard for Babies Born from Incest', *Vice.com* [Online], 2016. https://www.vice.com/ en_us/article/qkgymp/tiny-tombstones-inside-the-flds-graveyard-forbabies-born-from-incest (accessed 17 Sept 2021).

4 R. Sanchez, 'Fort Knox has nothing on polygamist compound', *Anderson Cooper Blog 360°* [Online], 2006. http://edition.cnn.com/CNN/Progr ams/anderson.cooper.360/blog/2006/05/fort-knox-has-nothingon-pol ygamist.html (accessed 17 Sept 2021).

5 J. Hollenhorst, 'Sex banned until Warren Jeffs' prison walls crumble, FLDS relatives say', 2011. https://www.deseret.com/2011/12/30/20391 030/sex-banned-until-warren-jeffs-prison-walls-crumble-fl ds-relatives-say (accessed 5 July 2021).

6 T.K. Danovich, 'The Forest Hidden Behind the Canyons', 2019. https://www.theringer.com/2019/6/24/18692816/fl ds-short-creek-polygamyfeature (accessed 5 July 2021).

7 L. Yengo et al., 'Extreme inbreeding in a European ancestry sample from the contemporary UK population', *Nature Communications*, 2019, 10.

8 H. Hamamy, 'Consanguineous marriages: Preconception consultation in primary health care settings', *Journal of Community Genetics*, 2012, 3, 185–92.

9 N. Al-Dewik et al., 'Clinical genetics and genomic medicine in Qatar', *Molecular Genetics and Genomic Medicine*, 2018, 6, 702–12.

10 P.K. Joshi et al., 'Directional dominance on stature and cognition in diverse human populations', *Nature*, 2015, 523, 459–462.

11 C.R. Scriver, 'Human genetics: Lessons from Quebec populations', *Annual Review of Genomics and Human Genetics*, 2001, 2, 69–101.

12 A.M. Laberge et al., 'A "Fille du Roy" introduced the T14484C Leber hereditary optic neuropathy mutation in French Canadians', *American Journal of Human Genetics*, 2005, 77, 313–17.

13 N.J.R. Fagundes et al., 'How strong was the bottleneck associated to the peopling of the Americas? New insights from multilocus sequence data', *Genetics and Molecular Biology*, 2018, 41, 206–14.

14 M.N. Leathlobhair et al., 'The evolutionary history of dogs in the Americas', *Science*, 2018, 361, 81–5.

15 Z.Y. Gao et al., 'An Estimate of the Average Number of Recessive Lethal Mutations Carried by Humans', *Genetics*, 2015, 199, 1,243–54.
16 V. Grech et al., 'Unexplained differences in sex ratios at birth in Europe and North America', *British Medical Journal*, 2002, 324, 1,010–11.
17 E.I. Rogaev et al., 'Genotype Analysis Identifies the Cause of the "Royal Disease"', *Science*, 2009, 326, 817.
18 S.M. Carr, 'Hemophilia in Victoria pedigree', 2012. https://www.mun. ca/biology/scarr/Hemophilia_in_Victoria_pedigree.jpg (accessed 27 May 2020).
19 E.I. Rogaev et al., 'Genomic identification in the historical case of the Nicholas II royal family', *Proceedings of the National Academy of Sciences of the USA*, 2009, 106, 5,258–63.

16 THE BRAIN OF AUGUSTE D

1 K. Maurer et al., 'Auguste D and Alzheimer's disease', *The Lancet*, 1997, 349, 1,546–9.
2 T.G. Beach, 'The History of Alzheimer's Disease – 3 Debates', *Journal of the History of Medicine and Allied Sciences*, 1987, 42, 327–49.
3 R. Katzman, 'Prevalence and Malignancy of Alzheimer Disease – A Major Killer', *Archives of Neurology*, 1976, 33, 217–18.
4 R.H. Swerdlow, 'Pathogenesis of Alzheimer's disease', *Clinical Interventions in Aging*, 2007, 2, 347–59.
5 G.G. Glenner and C.W. Wong, 'Alzheimer's disease: Initial report of the purification and characterization of a novel cerebrovascular amyloid protein', *Biochemical and Biophysical Research Communications*, 1984, 120, 885–90.
6 S.N. Chen and G. Parmigiani, 'Meta-analysis of BRCA1 and BRCA2 penetrance', *Journal of Clinical Oncology*, 2007, 25, 1,329–33.
7 M.N. Braskie et al., 'Common Alzheimer's Disease Risk Variant within the CLU Gene Affects White Matter Microstructure in Young Adults', *Journal of Neuroscience*, 2011, 31, 6,764–70.
8 C.C. Liu et al., 'Apolipoprotein E and Alzheimer disease: risk, mechanisms and therapy', *Nature Reviews Neurology*, 2013, 9, 106–18.
9 C.J. Smith et al., 'Putative Survival Advantages in Young Apolipoprotein ε4 Carriers are Associated with Increased Neural Stress', *Journal of Alzheimer's Disease*, 2019, 68, 885–923.
10 M. Wadman, 'James Watson's genome sequenced at high speed', *Nature*, 2008, 452, 788.

11 K.A. Wetterstrand, 'The Cost of Sequencing a Human Genome', 2020. https://www.genome.gov/about-genomics/fact-sheets/Sequencing-Human-Genome-cost (accessed 6 July 2021).

12 M.J. Owen et al., 'Rapid Sequencing-Based Diagnosis of Thiamine Metabolism Dysfunction Syndrome', *New England Journal of Medicine*, 2021, 384, 2,159–61.

13 D. Dimmock et al., 'Project Baby Bear: Rapid precision care incorporating rWGS in 5 California children's hospitals demonstrates improved clinical outcomes and reduced costs of care', *American Journal of Human Genetics*, 2021, 108, 1231–1238.

14 Human Fertilisation and Embryology Authority, 'Pre-implantation genetic diagnosis (PGD)', 2019. https://www.hfea.gov.uk/treatments/embryo-testing-and-treatments-for-disease/pre-implantation-genetic-testing-for-monogenic-disorders-pgt-m/ (accessed 6 July 2021).

15 T. Jonsson et al., 'A mutation in APP protects against Alzheimer's disease and age-related cognitive decline', *Nature*, 2012, 488, 96–9.

16 L.S. Wang et al., 'Rarity of the Alzheimer Disease-Protective APP A673T Variant in the United States', *JAMA Neurology*, 2015, 72, 209–16.

17 S.J. van der Lee et al., 'A nonsynonymous mutation in PLCG2 reduces the risk of Alzheimer's disease, dementia with Lewy bodies and frontotemporal dementia, and increases the likelihood of longevity', *Acta Neuropathologica*, 2019, 138, 237–50.

18 E. Evangelou et al., 'Genetic analysis of over 1 million people identifies 535 new loci associated with blood pressure traits', *Nature Genetics*, 2018, 50, 1,412–25.

19 R. Ray et al., 'Nicotine Dependence Pharmacogenetics: Role of Genetic Variation in Nicotine-Metabolizing Enzymes', *Journal of Neurogenetics*, 2009, 23, 252–61.

20 G. Alanis-Lobato et al., 'Frequent loss-of-heterozygosity in CRISPRCas9-edited early human embryos', *Proceedings of the National Academy of Sciences*, 2021, 202004832.

21 D. Cyranoski, 'Russian "CRISPR-baby" scientist has started editing genes in human eggs with goal of altering deaf gene', *Nature*, 2019, 574, 465–6.

22 R. Stein, 'Gene-Edited "Supercells" Make Progress In Fight Against Sickle Cell Disease', *Shots: Health News from NPR* [Online], 2019. https://www.npr.org/sections/health-shots/2019/11/19/780510277/geneedited-supercells-make-progress-in-fight-against-sickle-cell-disease

23 McKusick-Nathans Institute of Genetic Medicine, 'Online Mendelian Inheritance in Man, OMIM®', 2021. https://www.omim.org (accessed 6 July 2021).

24 L. Yengo et al., 'Meta-analysis of genome-wide association studies for height and body mass index in ~700,000 individuals of European ancestry', *Human Molecular Genetics* 2018, 27, 3,641–9.
25 J.E. Savage et al., 'Genome-wide association meta-analysis in 269,867 individuals identifies new genetic and functional links to intelligence', *Nature Genetics*, 2018, 50, 912–19.

17 DEATH BEFORE BIRTH

1 J.L.H. Down, 'Observations on an ethnic classification of idiots', *Clinical Lecture Reports, London Hospital*, 1866, 3, 259–62.
2 N. Howard-Jones, 'On the diagnostic term "Down's disease"', *Medical History*, 1979, 23, 102–4.
3 G. Allen et al., '"MONGOLISM"', *The Lancet*, 1961, 277, 775.
4 T. Cavazza et al., 'Parental genome unification is highly error-prone in mammalian embryos', *Cell*, 2021, 2,860–77.
5 P. Cerruti Mainardi, 'Cri du Chat syndrome', *Orphanet Journal of Rare Diseases*, 2006, 1, 33.
6 Five P-Society, 'Five P-Society Home Page', 2020. https://fivepminus.org (accessed 6 July 2021).
7 M. Medina et al., 'Hemizygosity of delta-catenin (CTNND2) is associated with severe mental retardation in cri-du-chat syndrome', *Genomics*, 2000, 63, 157–64.
8 K. Bender, 'Cri du Chat Syndrome (Cry of the Cat)', 2009. http://ji-criduchat.blogspot.com/ (accessed 5 July 2021).
9 K. Oktay et al., 'Fertility Preservation in Women with Turner Syndrome: A Comprehensive Review and Practical Guidelines', *Journal of Pediatric and Adolescent Gynecology*, 2016, 29, 409–16.

PART V

1 Martin Luther King, *Stride Toward Freedom: The Montgomery Story*, Harper & Brothers: New York, 1958.

18 THOU SHALT NOT KILL

1 'In Africa: The role of East Africa in the evolution of human diversity', 2021. http://in-africa.org/in-africa-project/ (accessed 6 July 2021).

2 M.M. Lahr et al., 'Inter-group violence among early Holocene hunter-gatherers of West Turkana, Kenya', *Nature*, 2016, 529, 394.

3 M.M. Lahr, 'Finding a hunter-gatherer massacre scene that may change history of human warfare', 2016. https://theconversation.com/finding-a-hunter-gatherer-massacre-scene-that-may-change-history-of-human-warfare-53397 (accessed 6 July 2021).

4 C. Boehm, *Moral Origins: The Evolution of Virtue, Altruism, and Shame*, Basic Books: New York, 2012.

5 L.H. Keeley, *War Before Civilization: The Myth of the Peaceful Savage*, Oxford University Press: Oxford, 1997.

6 M. Roser, 'Ethnographic and Archaeological Evidence on Violent Deaths', 2013. https://ourworldindata.org/ethnographic-and-archaeologicalevidence-on-violent-deaths (accessed 6 July 2021).

7 D.P. Fry and P. Soderberg, 'Lethal Aggression in Mobile Forager Bands and Implications for the Origins of War', *Science*, 2013, 341, 270–3.

8 J.M. Diamond, 'A Longer Chapter, About Many Wars', in *The World Until Yesterday*, Penguin: London, 2012, pp. 129–70.

9 L.W. King, 'The Code of Hammurabi', 2008. http://avalon.law.yale.edu/ancient/hamframe.asp (accessed 6 July 2021).

10 T. Delany, *Social Deviance*, Rowman & Littlefield: Lanham, Maryland, 2017.

11 T. Hobbes, *Leviathan*, 1651.

12 M.K.E. Weber, 'Politik als Beruf', in *Gesammelte Politische Schriften*, Duncker & Humblot: München, 1921, pp. 396–450.

13 J.-J. Rousseau, *The Social Contract*, Penguin: London, 1968.

14 C. Tilly, *Coercion, Capital, and European States, AD 990–1992*, Basil Blackwell: Cambridge, MA, 1992.

15 L. Wade, 'Feeding the gods: Hundreds of skulls reveal massive scale of human sacrifice in Aztec capital', *Science*, 2018, 360, 1,288–92.

16 The World Bank, 'Intentional homicides (per 100,000 people)', 2016. https://data.worldbank.org/indicator/vc.ihr.psrc.p5

17 M. Kaldor, *New and Old Wars: Organized Violence in a Global Era*, Polity Press: Cambridge, 2012.

18 World Health Organization, 'Suicide rate estimates, age-standardized Estimates by country', 2021. https://apps.who.int/gho/data/node.main.MHSUICIDEASDR?lang=en (accessed 6 July 2021).

19 World Health Organization, 'Suicide', 2021, https://www.who.int/news-room/fact-sheets/detail/suicide, (accessed 6 July 2021).

20 R.H. Seiden, 'Where are they now? A follow-up study of suicide attempters from the Golden Gate Bridge', *Suicide and Life-Threatening Behavior*, 1978, 8, 203–16.

21 Samaritans, 'Our History', 2019. https://www.samaritans.org/aboutsam aritans/our-history/ (accessed 6 July 2021).

22 'Rev. Dr Chad Varah Obituary', *Guardian*, 8 November 2007.

23 Science Museum, 'Telephones Save Lives: The History of the Samaritans', 2018. https://www.sciencemuseum.org.uk/objects-and-stories/ telephonessave-lives-history-samaritans

19 ALCOHOL AND ADDICTION

1 M. Moreton, 'The Death of the Russian Village', 2012. https://www. opendemocracy.net/en/odr/death-of-russian-village/ (accessed 7 July 2012).

2 D. Zaridze et al., 'Alcohol and mortality in Russia: prospective observational study of 151,000 adults', *Lancet*, 2014, 383, 1,465–73.

3 L. Harding, 'No country for old men', *Guardian*, 11 February 2008.

4 P. McGovern et al., 'Early Neolithic wine of Georgia in the South Caucasus', *Proceedings of the National Academy of Sciences*, 2017, 114, E10309–E10318.

5 A.G. Reynolds, 'The Grapevine, Viticulture, and Winemaking: A Brief Introduction', in *Grapevine Viruses: Molecular Biology, Diagnostics and Management*, ed. B. Meng, G. Martelli, D. Golino and M. Fuchs, Springer: Cham, Switzerland, 2017.

6 D. Tanasia et al., '1H-1H NMR 2D-TOCSY, ATR FT-IR and SEM-EDX for the identification of organic residues on Sicilian prehistoric pottery', *Microchemical Journal* 2017, 135, 140–7.

7 H. Barnard et al., 'Chemical evidence for wine production around 4000 BCE in the Late Chalcolithic Near Eastern highlands', *Journal of Archaeological Science*, 2011, 38, 977–84.

8 M. Cartwright, 'Wine in the Ancient Mediterranean', *Ancient History Encyclopedia* [Online], 2016. https://www.ancient.eu/article/944/

9 H. Li et al., 'The worlds of wine: Old, new and ancient', *Wine Economics and Policy*, 2018, 7, 178–82.

10 L. Liu et al., 'Fermented beverage and food storage in 13,000 y-old stone mortars at Raqefet Cave, Israel: Investigating Natufian ritual feasting', *Journal of Archaeological Science: Reports*, 2018, 21, 783–93.

11 J.J. Mark, 'Beer', *Ancient History Encyclopedia* [Online], 2018. https:// www.ancient.eu/Beer/

12 M. Denny, *Froth! The Science of Beer*, Johns Hopkins University Press: 2009.

13 Tacitus, *Annals*, New English Library, 1966, p. 19.

14 Velleius Paterculus, *Compendium of Roman History: Res Gestae Divi Augusti*, Vol. II, Loeb, 1924, p. 118.

15 World Population Review, 'Beer Consumption by Country 2020', 2020. https://worldpopulationreview.com/countries/beer-consumption-bycountry/ (accessed April 2020).

16 N. McCarthy, 'Which Countries Drink the Most Wine?', 2020. https://www.statista.com/chart/6402/which-countries-drink-the-most-wine/ (accessed April 2020).

17 J. Conway, 'Global consumption of distilled spirits worldwide by country 2015', 2018, (accessed April 2020).

18 A. Nemtsov, *A Contemporary History of Alcohol in Russia*, Södertörn University: Sweden, 2011.

19 S. Sebag Montefiore, *Stalin: The Court of the Red Tsar*, Orion Publishing Co.: London, 2003.

20 Z. Medvedev, 'Russians dying for a drink', *Times Higher Education*, 1996. https://www.timeshighereducation.com/news/russians-dying-for-a-drink/99996.article (accessed 17 Sept 2019).

21 World Health Organization, 'Alcohol Consumption 2014'. https://www.who.int/substance_abuse/publications/global_alcohol_report/msb_gsr_2014_3.pdf

22 M.A. Carrigan et al., 'Hominids adapted to metabolize ethanol long before human-directed fermentation', *Proceedings of the National Academy of Sciences of the USA*, 2015, 112, 458–63.

23 H.J. Edenberg, 'The genetics of alcohol metabolism – Role of alcohol dehydrogenase and aldehyde dehydrogenase variants', *Alcohol Research & Health*, 2007, 30, 5–13.

24 T.V. Morozova et al., 'Genetics and genomics of alcohol sensitivity', *Molecular Genetics and Genomics*, 2014, 289, 253–69.

25 Mayo Clinic Staff, 'Alcohol: Weighing risks and potential benefits', 2018. https://www.mayoclinic.org/healthy-lifestyle/nutrition-and-healthyeating/in-depth/alcohol/art-20044551 (accessed 7 July 2021).

26 T. Marugame et al., 'Patterns of alcohol drinking and all-cause mortality: Results from a large-scale population-based cohort study in Japan', *American Journal of Epidemiology*, 2007, 165, 1,039–46.

27 Alzforum, 'AlzRisk Risk Factor Overview. Alcohol', 2013. http://www.alzrisk.org/riskfactorview.aspx?rfi d=12 (accessed 7 July 2021).

28 J. Case, 'Hubris and the Serpent: The Truth About Rattlesnake Bite Victims', 2019. https://www.territorysupply.com/hubris-truth-about-rattlesnake-bite-victims (accessed 7 July 2021).

29 J.P. Bohnsack et al., 'The lncRNA BDNF-AS is an epigenetic regulator in the human amygdala in early onset alcohol use disorders', *Alcoholism: Clinical and Experimental Research*, 2018, 42, 86A.

30 National Cancer Institute, 'Alcohol and Cancer Risk', 2018. https://www.cancer.gov/about-cancer/causes-prevention/risk/alcohol/alcoholfact-sheet (accessed 7 July 2021).

31 World Health Organization, 'Global action plan on alcohol: 1st draft', 2021. https://www.who.int/substance_abuse/facts/alcohol/en (accessed 7 July 2021).

32 M.G. Griswold et al., 'Alcohol use and burden for 195 countries and territories, 1990–2016: a systematic analysis for the Global Burden of Disease Study 2016', *Lancet*, 2018, 392, 1,015–35.

33 G. Maté, *In the Realm of Hungry Ghosts*, Vermilion: London, 2010.

34 HelpGuide, 'Understanding Addiction', 2021. https://www.helpguide.org/harvard/how-addiction-hijacks-the-brain.htm (accessed 7 July 2021).

35 R.A. Wise and M.A. Robble, 'Dopamine and Addiction', *Annual Review of Psychology*, 2020, 71, 79–106.

36 D.J. Nutt et al., 'The dopamine theory of addiction: 40 years of highs and lows', *Nature Reviews Neuroscience*, 2015, 16, 305–12.

37 J.M. Mitchell et al., 'Alcohol consumption induces endogenous opioid release in the human orbitofrontal cortex and nucleus accumbens', *Science Translational Medicine*, 2012, 4, 116ra6.

38 C.M. Anderson et al., 'Abnormal T2 relaxation time in the cerebellar vermis of adults sexually abused in childhood: potential role of the vermis in stress-enhanced risk for drug abuse', *Psychoneuroendocrinology*, 2002, 27, 231–44.

39 S. Levine and H. Ursin, 'What is Stress?', in *Stress, Neurobiology and Neuroendocrinology*, ed. M.R. Brown, C. Rivier and G. Koob, Marcel Decker: New York, 1991, pp. 3–21.

40 H. Ritchie and M. Roser, 'Drug Use', 2019. https://ourworldindata.org/drug-use (accessed 15 May 2021).

41 D.J. Nutt et al., 'Drug harms in the UK: a multicriteria decision analysis', *Lancet*, 2010, 376, 1,558–65.

42 K. Kupferschmidt, 'The Dangerous Professor', *Science*, 2014, 343, 478–81.

43 A. Travis, 'Alcohol worse than ecstasy – drugs chief', *Guardian*, 29 October 2009.

44 M. Tran, 'Government drug adviser David Nutt sacked', *Guardian*, 30 October 2009.

20 THE BLACK, STINKING FUME

1 C.C. Mann, *1493: Uncovering the New World Columbus Created*, Knopf: New York, 2011.

2 L. Newman et al., 'Global Estimates of the Prevalence and Incidence of Four Curable Sexually Transmitted Infections in 2012 Based on Systematic Review and Global Reporting', *PLoS One*, 2015, 10.

3 R. Lozano et al., 'Global and regional mortality from 235 causes of death for 20 age groups in 1990 and 2010: a systematic analysis for the Global Burden of Disease Study 2010', *Lancet*, 2012, 380, 2,095–128.

4 R.S. Lewis and J.S. Nicholson, 'Aspects of the evolution of Nicotiana tabacum L. and the status of the United States Nicotiana Germplasm Collection', *Genetic Resources and Crop Evolution*, 2007, 54, 727–40.

5 S.J. Henley et al., 'Association between exclusive pipe smoking and mortality from cancer and other diseases', *JNCI: Journal of the National Cancer Institute*, 2004, 96, 853–61.

6 M.C. Stöppler and C.P. Davis, 'Chewing Tobacco (Smokeless Tobacco, Snuff) Center', *MedicineNet* [Online], 2019. https://www.medicinenet.com/smokeless_tobacco/article.htm

7 CompaniesHistory.com, 'British American Tobacco', 2021. https://www.companieshistory.com/british-american-tobacco/ (accessed 7 July 2021).

8 M. Hilton, *Smoking in British Popular Culture 1800–2000*, Manchester University Press: Manchester, UK, 2000, pp. 1–2.

9 P.M. Fischer et al., 'Brand Logo Recognition by Children Aged 3 to 6 Years – Mickey Mouse and Old Joe the Camel', *JAMA: Journal of the American Medical Association*, 1991, 266, 3,145–8.

10 Associated Press, 'Reynolds will pay $10 million in Joe Camel lawsuit', 1997. https://usatoday30.usatoday.com/news/smoke/smoke50.htm (accessed 7 July 2021).

11 S. Elliott, 'Joe Camel, a Giant in Tobacco Marketing, Is Dead at 23', *New York Times*, 11 July 1997.

12 I. Gately, *Tobacco: A Cultural History of How an Exotic Plant Seduced Civilization*, Grove Press: New York, 2001.

13 J.A. Dani and D.J.K. Balfour, 'Historical and current perspective on tobacco use and nicotine addiction', *Trends in Neurosciences*, 2011, 34, 383–92.

14 N.L. Benowitz, 'Nicotine Addiction', *New England Journal of Medicine*, 2010, 362, 2,295–303.

15 R. Ray et al., 'Nicotine Dependence Pharmacogenetics: Role of Genetic Variation in Nicotine-Metabolizing Enzymes', *Journal of Neurogenetics*, 2009, 23, 252–61.

16 N. Monardes, *Medicinall historie of things brought from the West Indies*, London, 1580.

17 G. Everard, *Panacea; or the universal medicine, being a discovery of the wonderfull vertues of tobacco*, London, 1659.

18 E. Duncon, *Rules for the preservation of health*, London, 1606.

19 T. Venner, *A briefe and accurate treatise concerning the taking of tobacco*, London, 1637.

20 J. Lizars, *Practical observations on the use and abuse of tobacco*, Edinburgh, 1868.

21 M. Jackson, '"Divine stramonium": the rise and fall of smoking for asthma', *Medical History*, 2010, 54, 171–94.

22 R. Doll and A. Bradford Hill, 'The Mortality of Doctors in Relation to their Smoking Habits: A Preliminary Report', *British Medical Journal*, 1952, 1, 1,451–5.

23 G.P. Pfeifer et al., 'Tobacco smoke carcinogens, DNA damage and p53 mutations in smoking-associated cancers', *Oncogene* 2002, 21, 7,435–51.

24 R. Doll and A. Bradford Hill, 'Smoking and Carcinoma of the Lung – Preliminary Report', *British Medical Journal* 1950, 2, 739–48.

25 D. Wootton, *Bad Medicine: Doctors Doing Harm Since Hippocrates*, Oxford University Press: 2007, p. 127.

26 A.J. Alberg et al., 'The 2014 Surgeon General's Report: Commemorating the 50th Anniversary of the 1964 Report of the Advisory Committee to the US Surgeon General and Updating the Evidence on the Health Consequences of Cigarette Smoking', *American Journal of Epidemiology*, 2014, 179, 403–12.

27 C. Bates and A. Rowell, 'Tobacco Explained: The truth about the tobacco industry… in its own words', Center for Tobacco Control Research and Education, UC San Francisco: 2004.

28 World Health Organization, 'Prevalence of Tobacco Smoking', 2016. http://gamapserver.who.int/gho/interactive_charts/tobacco/use/atlas.html (accessed 7 July 2021).

29 World Health Organization, 'Tobacco', 2021. https://www.who.int/health-topics/tobacco#tab=tab_1 (accessed 7 July 2021).

30 G. Iacobucci, 'BMA annual meeting: doctors vote to ban sale of tobacco to anyone born after 2000', *British Medical Journal*, 2014, 348.

21 UNSAFE AT ANY SPEED

1 Ford Motor Company, 'Highland Park', 2020. https://corporate.ford.com/articles/history/highland-park.html (accessed 7 July 2021).

2 'Motor Vehicle Traffic Fatalities and Fatality Rates, 1899–2015', *Traffic Safety Facts Annual Report* [Online], 2017. https://cdan. nhtsa.gov/TSFTables/Fatalities%20and%20Fatality%20Rates%20 (1899–2015).pdf.

3 National Highway Traffic Safety Administration, 'National Statistics', 2019, https://www-fars.nhtsa.dot.gov/Main/index.aspx (accessed 7 July 2021).

4 J. Doyle, 'GM and Ralph Nader, 1965–1971', 2013. https://www.pophis torydig.com/topics/g-m-ralph-nader1965-1971/ (accessed 7 July 2021).

5 D.P. Moynihan, 'Epidemic on the Highways', *The Reporter*, 1959, 16–22.

6 R. Nader, *Unsafe at Any Speed: The Designed-In Dangers of the American Automobile*, Grossman: New York, 1965.

7 C. Jensen, '50 Years Ago, "Unsafe at Any Speed" Shook the Auto World', *New York Times*, 2015.

8 M. Green, 'How Ralph Nader Changed America', 2015. https://www. thenation.com/article/how-ralph-nader-changed-america/ (accessed 7 July 2021).

9 A.D. Branch, 'National Traffic and Motor Vehicle Safety Act', 2019. https://www.britannica.com/topic/National-Traffic-and-Motor-Vehi cle-Safety-Act (accessed 7 July 2021).

10 'Congress Acts on Traffic and Auto Safety', in *CQ Almanac 1966*, Congressional Quarterly: Washington, DC, 1967, pp. 266–8.

11 Automobile Association, 'The Evolution of Car Safety Features: From windscreen wipers to crash tests and pedestrian protection', 2019. https://www.theaa.com/breakdown-cover/advice/evolution-of-carsaf ety-features (accessed 7 July 2021).

12 E. Dyer, 'Why Cars Are Safer Than They've Ever Been', 2014. https:// www.popularmechanics.com/cars/a11201/why-cars-are-safer-thanthe yve-ever-been-17194116/ (accessed 7 July 2021).

13 Press Room, 'On 50th Anniversary of Ralph Nader's "Unsafe at Any Speed", Safety Group Reports Auto Safety Regulation Has Saved 3.5 Million Lives', 2015. https://www.thenation.com/article/on-50th anniversary-of-ralph-naders-unsafe-at-any-speed-safety-group-repo rtsauto-safety-regulation-has-saved-3-5-million-lives/ (accessed 7 July 2021).

14 I.M. Cheong, 'Ten Most Harmful Books of the 19th and 20th Centuries', 2005. https://humanevents.com/2005/05/31/ten-most-harmful-booksof-the-19th-and-20th-centuries/ (accessed July 7 2021).

15 M. Novak, 'Drunk Driving and The Pre-History of Breathalyzers', 2013, https://paleofuture.gizmodo.com/drunk-driving-and-the-pre-historyof-breathalyzers-1474504117 (accessed 7 July 2021).

16 C. Lightner, 'Cari's Story', 2017. https://wesavelives.org/caris-story/ (accessed 7 July 2021).

17 Biography.com Editors, 'Candy Lightner Biography', 2019. https://www.biography.com/activist/candy-lightner (accessed 7 July 2021).

18 National Highway Traffic Safety Administration, 'Drunk Driving', 2018. https://www.nhtsa.gov/risky-driving/drunk-driving (accessed 7 July 2021).

19 World Health Organization, 'Road Safety', 2016. http://gamapserver.who.int/gho/interactive_charts/road_safety/road_traffic_deaths2/atlas.html (accessed 7 July 2021).

CONCLUSION: A BRIGHT FUTURE?

1 M.A. Benarde, *Our Precarious Habitat*, Norton, 1973.

2 A.S. Hammond et al., 'The Omo-Kibish I pelvis', *Journal of Human Evolution*, 2017, 108, 199–219.

3 World Health Organization, 'Global health estimates: Leading causes of death', 2021, https://www.who.int/data/gho/data/themes/mortality-and-global-health-estimates/ghe-leading-causes-of-death (accessed 16 Aug 2021).

4 D.R. Hopkins, 'Disease Eradication', *New England Journal of Medicine*, 2013, 368, 54–63.

5 S.E. Vollset et al., 'Fertility, mortality, migration, and population scenarios for 195 countries and territories from 2017 to 2100: a forecasting analysis for the Global Burden of Disease Study', *The Lancet*, 2020, 396, 1285–1306.

6 J. Cummings et al., 'Alzheimer's disease drug development pipeline: 2020', *Alzheimer's and Dementia: Translational Research and Clinical Interventions*, 2020, 6, e12050.

7 P. Sebastiani et al., 'Genetic Signatures of Exceptional Longevity in Humans', *PLoS One*, 2012, 7.

8 A.D. Roses, 'Apolipoprotein E affects the rate of Alzheimer's disease expression: β-amyloid burden is a secondary consequence dependent on APOE genotype and duration of disease', *Journal of Neuropathology and Experimental Neurology*, 1994, 53, 429–37.

9 B.J. Morris et al., 'FOXO3: A Major Gene for Human Longevity – A Mini-Review', *Gerontology*, 2015, 61, 515–25.

10 E. Pennisi, 'Biologists revel in pinpointing active genes in tissue samples', *Science*, 2021, 371, 1,192–3.

11 J.L. Platt and M. Cascalho, 'New and old technologies for organ replacement', *Current Opinion in Organ Transplantation*, 2013, 18, 179–85.

12 M. Cascalho and J.L. Platt, 'The future of organ replacement: needs, potential applications, and obstacles to application', *Transplantation Proceedings*, 2006, 38, 362–4.

13 L. Xu et al., 'CRISPR-Edited Stem Cells in a Patient with HIV and Acute Lymphocytic Leukemia', *New England Journal of Medicine*, 2019, 381, 1,240–7.

14 K. Musunuru et al., 'In vivo CRISPR base editing of PCSK9 durably lowers cholesterol in primates', *Nature*, 2021, 593, 429–34.

15 M.H. Porteus, 'A New Class of Medicines through DNA Editing', *New England Journal of Medicine*, 2019, 380, 947–59.

16 H. Li et al., 'Applications of genome editing technology in the targeted therapy of human diseases: mechanisms, advances and prospects', *Signal Transduction and Targeted Therapy*, 2020, 5, 1.

ACKNOWLEDGEMENTS

1 C. Sagan, *Cosmos*, Random House, 1980.

Image credits

Pages 17 and 22, Bills of Mortality, Wellcome Collection, Public Domain Mark.

Page 64, The Black Death in Europe, information from historyguide. org, designed by Philip Beresford.

Page 74, Ancient *Y.pestis* strain, reprinted from *Cell* 2019, 176, Rascovan, N., et al., 'Emergence and Spread of Basal Lineages of Yersinia pestis during the Neolithic Decline', 1–11, with permission from Elsevier.

Page 124, Global Distribution of Duffy negativity, Howes, R.E., et al., 'The global distribution of the Duffy blood group', *Nature Communications* 2011, 2, 266.

Page 157, Global Health Index Data, von Grebmer, K., J. Bernstein, C. Delgado, D. Smith, M. Wiemers, T. Schiffer, A. Hanano, O. Towey, R. Ni Chéilleachair, C. Foley, S. Gitter, K. Ekstrom, and H. Fritschel. 2021. "Figure 1: Global and Regional 2000, 2006, 2012, and 2021 Global Hunger Index scores, and their components." In 2021 Global Hunger Index Synopsis: Hunger and Food Systems in Conflict Settings. Bonn: Welthungerhilfe; Dublin: Concern Worldwide.

Page 174, Di Cesare, M., et al., 'Trends in adult body-mass index in 200 countries from 1975 to 2014: a pooled analysis of 1698 population-based measurement studies with 19.2 million participants'. Lancet 2016, 387, 1377–1396.

Page 192, KATERYNA KON/SCIENCE PHOTO LIBRARY, © Getty Images

Page 210, Haemophilia in the descendants of Queen Victoria, material © Steven Carr.

Page 262, Drugs ordered by their overall harm scores, © David Nutt.

Graphs by Philip Beresford, data by Andrew Doig.

Index

A Note on the Type

The text of this book is set in Linotype Stempel Garamond, a version of Garamond adapted and first used by the Stempel foundry in 1924. It is one of several versions of Garamond based on the designs of Claude Garamond. It is thought that Garamond based his font on Bembo, cut in 1495 by Francesco Griffo in collaboration with the Italian printer Aldus Manutius. Garamond types were first used in books printed in Paris around 1532. Many of the present-day versions of this type are based on the *Typi Academiae* of Jean Jannon cut in Sedan in 1615.

Claude Garamond was born in Paris in 1480. He learned how to cut type from his father and by the age of fifteen he was able to fashion steel punches the size of a pica with great precision. At the age of sixty he was commissioned by King Francis I to design a Greek alphabet, and for this he was given the honourable title of royal type founder. He died in 1561.